DATE DUE

Group Psychotherapy for Eating Disorders

Group Psychotherapy for Eating Disorders

Edited by

Heather Harper-Giuffre, B.N., B.Sc., M.Sc.
Former Coordinator of Group Therapy
Eating Disorders Outpatient Clinic
Toronto, Ontario

K. Roy MacKenzie, M.D., F.R.C.P.(C)
Professor of Psychiatry
University of British Columbia
Vancouver, British Columbia

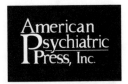

Washington, DC
London, England

Note: The authors have worked to ensure that all information in this book concerning drug dosages, schedules, and routes of administration is accurate as of the time of publication and consistent with standards set by the U.S. Food and Drug Administration and the general medical community. As medical research and practice advance, however, therapeutic standards may change. For this reason and because human and mechanical errors sometimes occur, we recommend that readers follow the advice of a physician who is directly involved in their care or the care of a member of their family.

Copyright © 1992 American Psychiatric Press, Inc.
ALL RIGHTS RESERVED
Manufactured in the United States of America on acid-free paper.
First Edition 95 94 93 92 4 3 2 1

American Psychiatric Press, Inc.
1400 K Street, N.W., Washington, DC 20005

Library of Congress Cataloging-in-Publication Data

   Group psychotherapy for eating disorders / Heather Harper-Giuffre,
     K. Roy MacKenzie, editors.
       p. cm.
     Includes bibliographical references and index.
     ISBN 0-88048-419-5
     1. Eating disorders—Treatment. 2. Group psychotherapy.
   I. Harper-Giuffre, Heather, 1954–   . II. MacKenzie, K. Roy, 1937–   .
     [DNLM: 1. Eating Disorders—therapy. 2. Psychotherapy, Group.
     WM 175 G882]
     RC552.E18G76 1992
     616.85′260651—dc20
     DNLM/DLC
     for Library of Congress   91-25958
                                                                         CIP

British Library Cataloguing in Publication Data

A CIP record is available from the British Library.

Table of Contents

◆ **SECTION ONE** ◆
Eating Disorder Groups in Perspective

◆ **SECTION TWO** ◆
Specialized Group Treatment

Contributors

Fern Cramer-Azima, Ph.D.
Associate Professor, Department of Psychiatry, McGill University; Director, Adolescent Group Psychotherapy Program, Child & Adolescent Service, Allan Memorial Institute, Montreal, Quebec

Ron Davis, Ph.D., C.Psych.
Director, Eating Disorder Outpatient Clinic, The Toronto Hospital; Assistant Professor of Psychiatry, University of Toronto, Ontario

Sarah Dearing, B.A.A.
Former Programme Assistant, National Eating Disorder Information Centre, The Toronto Hospital, Toronto, Ontario

Jacqueline Duncan, M.B., M.R.C.Psych.
Formerly Fellow in Psychiatry, University of Toronto, Ontario

Joan Faulkner, M.S.W.
Executive Director, Federation of Foster Family Associations of Nova Scotia, Halifax, Nova Scotia; Former Coordinator, National Eating Disorder Information Center, The Toronto Hospital, Toronto, Ontario

Paul Garfinkel, M.D., F.R.C.P.(C)
Professor and Chairman of Psychiatry, University of Toronto; Director and Psychiatrist-in-Chief, Clarke Institute of Psychiatry, Toronto, Ontario

Heather Harper-Giuffre, B.N., B.Sc., M.Sc.
Former Coordinator of Group Therapy, Eating Disorders Outpatient Clinic, Toronto, Ontario

Karin Jasper, Ph.D., M.Ed.
Psychotherapist, College Street Women's Centre for Health, Education, and Counselling, Toronto, Ontario

Allan S. Kaplan, M.D., F.R.C.P.(C)
Director, Eating Disorder Day Centre, The Toronto Hospital; Assistant Professor of Psychiatry, University of Toronto, Ontario

Sidney H. Kennedy, M.B., F.R.C.P.(C)
Head, Program for Eating Disorders, The Toronto Hospital; Associate Professor of Psychiatry, University of Toronto, Ontario

Ann Kerr, B.Sc., O.T.
Coordinator of Group Therapy, Eating Disorder Clinic, The Toronto Hospital; Clinical Lecturer in Psychiatry, University of Toronto, Ontario

Jan Lackstrom, M.S.W., R.S.W.
Coordinator of Family Services, Eating Disorder Center, The Toronto Hospital; Adjunct Professor, Faculty of Social Work, University of Toronto; Sessional Lecturer, School of Social Work, York University, Toronto, Ontario

Molyn Leszcz, M.D., F.R.C.P.(C)
Head, Group Therapy Programme, Mount Sinai Hospital and Baycrest Centre for Geriatric Care; Senior Group Psychotherapy Consultant, The Toronto Hospital; Assistant Professor of Psychiatry, University of Toronto, Ontario

K. Roy MacKenzie, M.D., F.R.C.P.(C)
Professor of Psychiatry, University of British Columbia, Vancouver, British Columbia

Sarah E. Maddocks, Ph.D., C.Psych.
Psychologist, Department of Psychology, Women's College Hospital, Toronto, Ontario

Marion P. Olmsted, Ph.D.
Psychologist, Eating Disorder Day Centre, The Toronto Hospital; Research Fellow, Department of Psychology, The Toronto Hospital; Assistant Professor of Psychiatry, University of Toronto, Ontario

Patricia J. Perry, R.N., M.Sc.N.
Director, Eating Disorder Clinic, Toronto, Ontario

Carla Rice, B.A.
Coordinator, National Eating Disorder Information Center, The Toronto Hospital, Toronto, Ontario

Wendi Rockert, B.A.
Research Consultant, The Toronto Hospital, Toronto, Ontario

Lorie F. Shekter-Wolfson, M.S.W., C.S.W.
Director, Department of Social Work, The Toronto Hospital; Field Practice Professor, Faculty of Social Work, University of Toronto; Lecturer, Department of Psychiatry, University of Toronto, Ontario

Denise Sivitilli, M.A.
Program Director, Touchstone Youth Centre, Toronto, Ontario

D. Blake Woodside, M.D., F.R.C.P.(C)
Psychiatrist, Eating Disorder Center, The Toronto Hospital;
Assistant Professor, Department of Psychiatry, University of
Toronto, Ontario

**Correspondence regarding the Eating Disorder Program can be
addressed to:**
Eating Disorder Program
The Toronto Hospital
8 Eaton North, Room 235
200 Elizabeth Street
Toronto, Ontario M5G 2C4 CANADA

Foreword

It is a pleasure to have been asked to provide introductory remarks to this volume on group psychotherapy for eating disorders. This book is the first to relate the subject of the treatment of the eating disorders to the role of group therapies within it; in both areas, there have been exciting developments that can now be transmitted directly to the benefit of our patients.

It is hard to imagine the rate of change in our knowledge and experience of the eating disorders in the past two decades. Until the 1970s, anorexia nervosa was thought to be a rare disorder, and its treatment varied greatly from physician to physician. Prior to the 1950s, the symptoms of bulimia were reported as part of another illness, usually anorexia nervosa. It was only after reports began appearing in the late 1970s, identifying binge eating and purging in nonemaciated individuals, that bulimia nervosa emerged as a syndrome. The volume of research on these disorders and its effects on our patients through the 1980s has been exciting.

One area of significant advance has been in epidemiology. Early reports suffered from major methodological concerns, but in recent years more reliable estimates have noted that 0.5–1% of young women develop anorexia nervosa and another 2–3% develop bulimia nervosa. The typical age distribution of onset—between ages 10 and 25—remains, but with some blurring at both extremes. Similarly, the social class distribution, described more than 100 years ago, seems to have been eroded. Most important has been the recognition of groups of people at high risk for an eating disorder—especially women, and those with particular characteristics. These include women who by occupation have a strong need to be thin (ballet and other dance students, fashion models); those with a family history of depression, alcoholism, or an eating disorder; those who have been premorbidly obese; and those with certain illnesses—insulin dependent diabetes mellitus, depression, or alcoholism. In addition, certain personality characteristics lend a tendency to bulimia nervosa—especially poor impulse control and affective instability. And in both anorexia nervosa and bulimia nervosa, significant defects in self-esteem render a patient vulnerable.

Another area of significant advancement in recent years has been in diagnosis. Some confusion and criticism about earlier criteria have led to diagnostic refinements. Clear recognition of factors that differentiate the eating disorders from other causes of weight loss and vomiting have been described (Garfinkel et al. 1983) and the areas of overlap and differentiation between anorexia nervosa and "normal" excessive dieting have been clarified (Garner et al. 1984). There has also been progress in recognizing that bulimia nervosa and anorexia nervosa share many common features, yet there are differences between bulimic and restricting types of anorexic patients (Garfinkel et al. 1980) and many similarities between bulimic patients with anorexia nervosa and those who never meet criteria for the anorexic syndrome (Garner et al. 1985a, 1985b). Finally, areas of overlap and clear differentiation between the eating disorders and affective disorders have been described, although the reasons behind the shared vulnerabilities to these illnesses require further study.

Great strides have been made in understanding the types of psychopathologies that occur. The fundamental psychopathology in both anorexia nervosa and bulimia nervosa relates to the individual's intense need to maintain her sense of self-worth through undue self-control in the area of weight control. This fear of loss of personal control has been linked to underlying feelings of helplessness (Bruch 1973) and to a sense of personal mistrust (Selvini-Palazzoli 1974); rather than experiencing pleasure from their bodies, anorexic women fear the body as if it were something that must be artificially, rather than naturally, controlled. Because of these feelings about themselves, these patients often fear the demands of maturity and the increased independence that this requires. Not surprisingly, given these other features, people with eating disorders have very low levels of self-worth, and their self-esteem is highly bound to external standards. How parents, teachers, peers, and significant others feel about them is an undue determinant of how they feel about themselves. They are extremely eager to conform to external standards, and for this reason, fueled by the characteristic "all or nothing" thinking style, a particular cultural look or an image can be carried to a pathological extreme.

Both anorexia nervosa and bulimia nervosa are frequently chronic disorders, and there has been increasing awareness of their sequelae. It is not my intent to review these in detail here. However, with the increased frequency of these disorders and their common chronicity, investigators must more clearly delineate the broad range of difficulties that may develop over time, and clinicians must use this information in planning treatment strategies. This is an area that often leads to collaborative efforts among health care professionals.

A few examples of recently derived information can serve as examples. In the last few years, alarming reports have documented the presence of osteoporosis and pathological fractures in these patients (Rigotti et al. 1984), especially those with the bulimic form of anorexia nervosa. About 10 years ago we suggested that estrogen replacement therapy has no role in the management of chronic anorexia nervosa (Garfinkel and Garner

1982). This issue must now be reconsidered. However, there may be multiple contributors to the development of osteoporosis: low levels of calcium in the diet, low body weight itself (as evidenced by the effects on mineral density in the astronauts), purging, high levels of cortisol, and low levels of somatomedin and gonadotropins. At present the best advice for these patients is to maintain: 1) an adequate calcium intake of 1–1.5 g/day (for example, 3 dairy food servings per day); 2) for female patients, a body weight that can sustain menses; 3) adequate Vitamin D intake; and 4) moderate regular activity. Clearly, however, this area requires more careful research.

Another subgroup of patients that requires further study is the group that subsequently goes through pregnancy and childbirth. Some patients have expressed the belief that if they diet during pregnancy the baby will "live off [their] fat and be all right." However, the early literature on this subject does not support this view, and patients must know this. Brinch and colleagues (1985) found a very high rate of prematurity and perinatal deaths in this group. Stewart and colleagues (1987) have found striking differences in those actively ill at the time of conception: this group gains far less weight and has much smaller babies with low Apgar scores.

There are many more examples of complications among people with eating disorders that could be cited, including delayed gastric emptying, dental erosion, cortical pseudoatrophy, impaired cognitive processing, and the high frequency of affective and anxiety disorders that develop over time. These must be studied and addressed if this large group of people are to lead their lives with dignity and as modest an impairment from the illness as possible.

Treatment

To be aware of how great the changes in treatment of patients have been, we need only remind ourselves that in 1970 most patients with anorexia nervosa received either psychoanalytic psychotherapy or a combination of bed rest, chlorpromazine, and insulin. There was little attempt to combine psychosocial treatments with nutritional rehabilitation, outside of one or two treatment programs in Great Britain, and treatments for bulimia were not even being considered.

Treatments for people with eating disorders have been significantly altered by newly acquired knowledge; frequently, these treatments now incorporate components from different theoretical models, as the patient's needs dictate. However, these therapeutic strategies have only infrequently been subject to careful controlled study, and currently there is little factual information to help determine which treatment method is best suited to specific patients.

What will be especially important for the future, as large numbers of patients continue to require treatment, is a sequencing of treatments from the least intrusive and costly to those that are more intensive. Such a tailored approach is currently gaining in acceptance but is based on clinical experience, rather than on the results of controlled empirical studies.

Today, a variety of treatment options are available. For the relatively mild case of bulimia nervosa without personality disorder, an educationally oriented group and support from a family doctor may suffice. Anorexia nervosa patients require more than this because of their intense desire to maintain their thin size and because of their deteriorated physical state.

In Toronto, psychoeducational group therapies are provided to patients with bulimia nervosa over a period of 5 or 6 weeks, often while patients await placement in an ongoing psychotherapy. These groups cover the following subjects: physiologic controls over body weight ("set point"); cognitive, affective, and behavioral effects of starvation; the importance of normal eating patterns; the adverse effects of dieting, bingeing, and purging; sociocultural pressures on women to be thin, to perform, and to please others; food myths and good nutrition; and coping strategies to deal with urges to binge. About 25% of our bulimic patients respond to such group treatment, but unfortunately the relapse rate over the subsequent 2 years is high.

For most patients, individual psychotherapy is the cornerstone of treatment. Both cognitive and psychodynamic approaches have been advocated, and early results indicate that both are effective in bulimia nervosa. Moreover, there has been a trend toward the integration of different therapeutic modalities, with the recognition that no single therapy will suit the needs of every patient. Regardless of theoretical orientation, clinicians have recognized the importance of self-monitoring, along with attention to food, weight, and behavioral control of the cycle of bingeing and vomiting. Correcting faulty misconceptions and "all or nothing" thinking is important. Most therapists also recognize the need to address developmental themes related to separation, identity formation, and self-concept.

Family therapy is often necessary, either as the primary clinical intervention or as an adjunct to other treatments. Specific familial issues vary from family to family, and it is often not known whether these familial problems are involved in the pathogenesis or are due to the eating disorder; however, their successful resolution is important. Issues in the family may often deal with effective parenting, emotional boundaries between individuals, communication, conflict resolution, and affective expression. Early controlled studies from The Maudsley Hospital suggest that for the young patient (i.e., someone less than 18 years of age) with a relatively acute form of anorexia nervosa who is living at home, family therapy should be considered as the primary treatment method (Russell et al. 1987).

Inpatient treatment is now reserved for a minority of our patients—as an initial step if the symptoms pose serious medical risks, the eating is completely out of control (daily bingeing and purging), or outpatient treatment has failed. The in-hospital treatment has a number of components. These include controlled weight gain, beginning with complete bed rest, in a setting of emotional support; dietary reeducation and information; a graduated level of activities; occupational and group therapies; family support; and the beginning of an individual relationship type of psychotherapy. This multifaceted treatment cannot in itself be considered sufficient for patients, but it does restore their health to the point where ongoing outpatient treatments are possible.

For many patients previously requiring in-hospital care, we have found that an intensive day hospital group therapy program provides an excellent and cost-effective alternative. Patients are treated in a variety of groups for 7 hours per day, 5 days each week, for about 10 weeks each. This treatment provides both nutritional rehabilitation and promotes personal autonomy and enhances self-esteem. Initial evaluation of this program has documented its effectiveness (Piran et al. 1989).

Medications have a modest role to play. Insulin, thyroxine, diuretics, and laxatives are to be avoided. A small minority of anorexic patients who are terrified of any weight gain benefit from an anxiolytic (e.g., lorazepam 0.5 mg tid) before meals, for a few weeks. Although neuroleptics have often been recommended for this, their use is to be discouraged because of the increased potential for side effects. The antidepressant medications have not been demonstrated to be effective in anorexia nervosa. By contrast, imipramine, desipramine, phenelzine, isocarboxazid, and fluoxetine have all been found to be clinically effective in the short term in placebo-controlled, double-blind studies in bulimia nervosa. Unfortunately, at present, predictors of which bulimic patients will respond to these medications do not yet exist. Nor have studies documented the efficacy of these medications in the long term.

This brief comment describes a variety of treatment options currently available in Toronto. Group therapies play an important role at all levels: in initial psychoeducation, in outpatient treatments, as adjuncts to in-hospital management, or as the focus in the day hospital program. Groups offer many advantages; not the least of these is the sense of support people derive from sharing a common problem, of learning from peers what has been useful to others. Groups provide patients with an opportunity to explore and discuss feelings, often for the first time, in a setting where they can be accepted and understood. A group is an excellent setting for learning about and working through interpersonal difficulties. The group setting also provides an opportunity for the clinician to treat more patients in a limited time. The evolution of specific types of group therapies that have been developed in response to the various needs of patients is described in this volume and should prove of great value to clinicians treating people with eating disorders.

Although the work of the past two decades has resulted in improvements in the treatment of patients with eating disorders, further challenges exist:

1. Can we develop useful preventive approaches? Group interventions for people at high risk—for example, people with diabetes mellitus, ballet dancers, or people with personal vulnerabilities—should be developed and evaluated.

2. Can comparative treatment studies define the optimal sequencing and integration of these various treatment methods for people with vastly different treatment needs?

3. How can we ensure maintenance of improvements? Can the short-term gains of treatment be maintained over the long term with appropriate, timely interventions?

4. Can we improve understanding of chronically ill patients to help this group live with dignity and with minimal impairment, even though their illnesses persist?

I hope that the work of the 1970s and 1980s will have provided sufficient knowledge and education for both clinicians and the public that specialized treatment units and general clinicians are skilled in treating patients with eating disorders, and that attention to these four challenges in the coming decade will result in further improvements for our patients.

Paul Garfinkel, M.D., F.R.C.P.(C)

References

Brinch M, Isager T, Tolstrup K: Anorexia nervosa: granviditeter indtruffet, under og efter sygdommen. Ugeskr Laeger 147:292–296, 1985

Bruch H: Eating Disorders. New York, Basic Books, 1973

Garfinkel PE, Garner DM: Anorexia Nervosa: A Multidimensional Perspective. New York, Brunner/Mazel, 1982

Garfinkel PE, Moldofsky H, Garner DM: The heterogeneity of anorexia nervosa: bulimia as a distinct subgroup. Arch Gen Psychiatry 37:1036–1040, 1980

Garfinkel PE, Garner DM, Kaplan AS, et al: Emotional disorders that cause weight loss. Can Med Assoc J 129:939–945, 1983

Garner DM, Olmsted MP, Polivy J, et al: Comparison between weight preoccupied women and anorexia nervosa. Psychosom Med 46:255–266, 1984

Garner DM, Garfinkel PE, O'Shaughnessy M: Validity of the distinction between bulimia with and without anorexia nervosa. Am J Psychiatry 142:581–587, 1985a

Garner DM, Olmsted MP, Garfinkel PE: Similarities among bulimic groups selected by weight and weight history. J Psychiatr Res 19:129–134, 1985b

Piran NP, Langdon L, Kaplan A, et al: Initial evaluation of a day hospital program for eating disorders. International Journal of Eating Disorders 8:523–532, 1989

Rigotti NA, Nussbaum SR, Herzog DB, et al: Osteoporosis in women with anorexia nervosa. N Engl J Med 311:1601–1606, 1984

Russell GM, Szmukler GI, Dare C, et al: An evaluation of family therapy in anorexia nervosa and bulimia nervosa. Arch Gen Psychiatry 44:1047–1056, 1987

Selvini-Palazzoli MP: Self-Starvation. London, Chaucer, 1974

Stewart DE, Raskin J, Garfinkel PE, et al: Anorexia nervosa, bulimia and pregnancy. Am J Obstet Gynecol 157:1194–1198, 1987

Preface

This book is a result of the joining of two clinical traditions: the treatment of the eating disorders and the use of the group as a treatment modality. The Eating Disorder Program at The Toronto Hospital is one of the oldest established treatment programs devoted to the treatment of anorexia nervosa (AN) and bulimia nervosa (BN). As a tertiary referral center, it has specialized in the assessment and management of the severely affected patient. A series of structured treatment components have been developed to deal with selected aspects of the disorder. These are based on an understanding of the underlying dimensions of eating disorder (ED) psychopathology. Most of these applications are implemented in a group format.

The etiology of AN and BN remains obscure. Most investigators have adopted a multidimensional view that focuses on the interaction of biologic, psychologic, family, and sociocultural factors. Similarly, treatment has tended to be multifaceted and individually tailored to the needs of each patient. Psychotherapy, pharmacotherapy, and nutrition therapy represent the most common treatment approaches that can be incorporated in either an inpatient or outpatient setting. This book provides practical guidelines regarding the strategies and interventions that can be employed with a variety of treatment approaches. An emphasis is placed on integrating theoretical constructs with clinical application. The reader is presented with background information on why a clinician is conducting a particular group approach, followed by the specific tactics and techniques employed. Where possible, the authors have included empirical data to bridge the gaps between theory, research, and practice.

One goal of this book is to demonstrate how the group environment can be used to enhance the delivery of such treatments. A properly managed group can provide the same therapeutic ingredients more effectively than individual treatment because of the reinforcing properties of the group social system. The group approach also uses clinician time considerably more efficiently—an important consideration in terms of cost containment.

Group psychotherapy is commonly equated with a psychodynamic orientation, and most of the authors in this volume come from this background. However, the nature of the eating disorders dictates that this approach be integrated with behavioral and cognitive-behavioral strategies. Failure to do so may delay the correction of metabolic effects and stereo-

typed eating behaviors that will sabotage the effectiveness of psychological learning. This book provides an unusually broad perspective on how
the group format can be adapted to specialized treatment purposes. It is
the first major publication to compile and synthesize this array of information about group approaches for the eating disorders.

The editors see this book falling into the increasingly influential "in-
tegrative psychotherapy" tradition that seeks to pull together concepts
from various theoretical orientations. The challenge is to apply varied approaches in such a manner that the unique effectiveness of each is re-
tained—that is, these approaches must be used in a truly complementary
fashion, so that specific advantages are not lost in confusion.

The group treatment modality by its very nature addresses a number
of the core features of anorexia nervosa and bulimia nervosa. Distorted or
unrealistic cognitive beliefs concerning eating, body image, and self-concept form the core of the psychopathology of AN and BN. The interpersonal framework of a group provides a forum to examine these
assumptions and to deal with the associated affect. Most group therapists
are not theoretic or strategic purists. They lean toward an eclectic and
utilitarian approach. For instance, a therapist conducting an experiential
psychodynamic group may integrate cognitive-behavioral principles into
the group approach. Similarly, a therapist conducting a structured psychoeducational group may focus on the affect being generated in a session as a particular topic is discussed. Among the different group
approaches there is a consensus about essential components of treatment.
This concerns the fundamental importance of the regulation and normalization of eating behavior as well as the need to address self-esteem deficits. Methods for managing these two target areas form a common thread
linking all chapters.

The book is divided into two sections. Section One begins with an
overview chapter that reviews the history of the eating disorders along
with their diagnostic and epidemiological features. This is followed by
practical information on basic group concepts to familiarize or update the
reader to this particular treatment modality. It also serves as a reference
guide for subsequent chapters. The medical assessment of eating disorder
patients is described in detail and the current literature regarding biological and pharmacological considerations is reviewed. Two major approaches to group treatment are presented at greater length. The first of
these deals with cognitive-behavioral methods and the second with psy-
chodynamic-interpersonal techniques. These two theoretical positions
underlie the various groups described in Section Two.

Section Two is organized around a number of specialized group treatment formats for eating disorder patients. Group treatment approaches
are applied in inpatient, day hospital, outpatient clinic, and private prac-

tice offices. The use of groups in these different treatment settings varies. On inpatient units, for example, groups are an adjunctive treatment used in combination with numerous other techniques. In day hospital programs, groups may be the principal treatment used, and in some outpatient settings they may be the only modality. A careful discussion is provided concerning the types of eating disorder patients most suitably treated in each setting.

Other chapters deal with specific content areas. These include chapters on groups to address body image, family relations, and sexual abuse. These three chapters deal with central and interconnected issues. In a less specialized clinical setting, the ideas presented might be flexibly combined into a general group format. One chapter deals with support groups in which the philosophy of the self-help movement is a major component. Specialized groups for adolescents and for the long-term follow-up of chronic AN patients are described.

Group therapy is best conceptualized as one component in an overall treatment approach to the eating disorders. Treatment decisions must be based on the unique formulation of each patient's situation. Decisions surrounding the selection and sequencing of the various treatment modalities reflect the complexities inherent in the treatment of these difficult problems. A basic philosophy is to begin treatment with the least intrusive method and increase the intensity and depth as response indicates. Many patients with eating disorders are greatly helped by relatively simple measures of support and psychoeducational material. Others need more intensive but brief care to break the eating behavior habit. Still others need longer term hospitalization and ongoing intensive interpersonal psychotherapy. The eating behaviors themselves must be under some degree of control before psychological measures are likely to be helpful. In this regard, there are some parallels to the treatment of addictive behaviors. The idea of a stepped approach permits the apportionment of clinical resources in a manner to benefit the greatest number of patients.

Over the past decade, there has been a growing professional interest in patients presenting with eating disorders. There continues to be an increase in the number of such patients presenting for treatment. This has been particularly true of females with bulimia nervosa. Considerable attention has been devoted to the eating disorders by the media, resulting in active public interest. The need for treatment facilities and for the training of specialized professionals offers a major challenge for the mental health professions. This book is designed primarily as a textbook for the practicing clinician in the hope that it will both stimulate interest in treating these patients and also offer ideas about how such treatment may be approached.

Since the great majority of patients experiencing AN and BN are female, the feminine pronoun is used to refer to these patients throughout this book.

Heather Harper-Giuffre, B.N., B.Sc., M.Sc.
K. Roy MacKenzie, M.D., F.R.C.P.(C)

Eating Disorder Groups in Perspective

◆ ◆ ◆ ◆ ◆ ◆ ◆ ◆ ◆

1

Overview of the Eating Disorders

Heather Harper-Giuffre, B.N., B.Sc., M.Sc.

♦ ♦ ♦ ♦ ♦ ♦ ♦ ♦ ♦

This introductory chapter describes the phenomenology of anorexia nervosa and bulimia nervosa and highlights some of the main controversies in the field. In particular, attention is drawn to the complex nature of these disorders, with manifestations at the personal level, such as low self-esteem; at the family level, with over- or underinvolvement; and with extension into general social and vocational adaptation. Frequently, evidence of major affective syndromes is found, as well as personality traits of disorders or, at times, outright disorders. This chapter, together with Chapter 2, is intended as a basic reference guide for the remainder of the book.—The Editors

There has been significant progress during the past decade in the understanding of two complex and serious eating disorders, anorexia nervosa and bulimia nervosa. Diagnosis has been improved by the implementation of empirically based diagnostic criteria. Anorexia nervosa (AN) and bulimia nervosa (BN) have been clearly distinguished as separate syndromes with a number of interrelated features. New understanding of etiological and physiological factors as well as advances in treatment have emerged. More information regarding epidemiology and psychopathology is available. There has also been a better recognition of eating disorders by patients, families, and health care professionals.

This chapter provides a clinical overview of AN and BN and summarizes ongoing controversies surrounding them. The two disorders are dealt with separately, while emphasizing their common features. Detailed

3

diagnostic criteria as well as the physiological, behavioral, and psychological features of each are provided. The predispositions to both of the disorders as well as their treatment are described.

Strong social pressure concerning diet and exercise, plus a cultural obsession with slenderness, has rendered a substantial number of individuals vulnerable to developing an eating disorder. It has been proposed that over the past two decades, the sociocultural milieu for adolescent and young adult women has become progressively more unstable (Bruch 1982; Garfinkel and Garner 1982; Selvini-Palazzoli 1974). This may partially account for the increase in both the recognition and incidence of eating disorders. Women face multiple, ambiguous, high-achievement-oriented, and often contradictory role expectations that have been precipitated by shifting cultural norms (Bruch 1982; Garfinkel and Garner 1982).

Anorexia Nervosa

The hallmark of anorexia nervosa is the relentless pursuit of thinness, coupled with a morbid fear of weight gain or "fatness," in spite of the fact that the person may be severely emaciated. The severe weight loss seen in AN patients cannot be accounted for by other physical disorders and may become life-threatening.

Diagnostic Criteria

Anorexia nervosa, like many other psychiatric disorders, is regarded as a syndrome encompassing an array of symptoms. Since the publication of Gerald Russell's criteria for anorexia nervosa in 1970, there has been general agreement regarding the diagnostic criteria (Fairburn and Garner 1988). The 1987 DSM-III-R criteria (American Psychiatric Association 1987) comprise physical, behavioral, and body image factors:

DSM-III-R Diagnostic Criteria for Anorexia Nervosa

A. Refusal to maintain body weight over a minimal normal weight for age and height, e.g., weight loss leading to maintenance of body weight 15% below that expected; or failure to make expected weight gain during period of growth, leading to body weight 15% below that expected.

B. Intense fear of gaining weight or becoming fat, even though underweight.

C. Disturbance in the way in which one's body weight, size, or shape is experienced, e.g., the person claims to "feel fat" even when emaciated, believes that one area of the body is "too fat" even when obviously underweight.

D. In females, absence of at least three consecutive menstrual cycles

when otherwise expected to occur (primary or secondary amenorrhea). (A woman is considered to have amenorrhea if her periods
occur only following hormone [e.g., estrogen] administration.)

Anorexia nervosa can usually be differentiated from other medical or
psychiatric disorders readily and accurately. However, the diagnosis may
be missed when it exists concurrently with other disorders, such as schizophrenia, manic-depressive illness, obsessive-compulsive disorder, and diabetes mellitus (Beumont and Touyz 1987). Two current areas of debate
surrounding diagnostic criteria are whether the inclusion of amenorrhea is
valid and what criteria should be used regarding the percentage of weight
loss (Fairburn and Garner 1988). In the 1980 DSM-III criteria, weight loss
had been set at 25% lower than normal body weight, not the present 15%.

Demographics and Epidemiology

Although AN has received considerable recent publicity, it is by no means
a new disorder. Medical documentation regarding psychogenic malnutri-
tion dates back as early as 1694 (Morton 1694). Explicit descriptions of AN
as a distinct syndrome appeared in the 1870s when Gull (1874) and
Lasegue (1873) published their classic clinical articles. However, up until
the 1970s, AN was considered a rare disorder, with clinicians typically seeing only a few cases over all the years of their practices.

Anorexia nervosa is primarily a disorder affecting young females, but
it has been reported in prepubertal children and middle-aged females as
well as in males. Various studies report that 90–96% of AN cases are female (Eckert 1985; Halmi 1974; Jones et al. 1980). The age of onset is con-
centrated between 12 and 25 years, with bimodal peaks of onset at ages 14
and 18 (Eckert 1985). AN in females has frequently been associated with
upper-class status in the Western world (Askevold 1983; Garfinkel and
Garner 1982). However, it is by no means limited to this class. Garfinkel
and Garner (1982) found that since 1976 the number of their AN patients
from the upper social classes has declined from 71% to 52%, which suggests that AN is now distributed more equally across all social classes.

Although the true prevalence and incidence of AN are unknown,
there has been a marked increase in the number of anorexic patients over
the last 15 to 20 years (Garfinkel and Darby 1984). It is not known whether
this rise in case registry is reflective of AN becoming more common or
whether increased public and medical awareness has led to better detection, diagnosis, and referral. Nevertheless, clinical teaching programs
have responded accordingly by devoting more curriculum time to the understanding and treatment of eating disorders.

Two studies have estimated the point prevalence of AN in school populations. Nylander (1971) found a prevalence of one severe case of AN in

155 of the females surveyed in a Swedish school. He also found that nearly 1 in 10 of the female students could be considered to have a mild form of AN. Crisp and colleagues (1976) conducted a survey of nine high schools in England and reported that the risk for AN was 1 in every 100 schoolgirls over the age of 16 years attending private school.

Five studies have addressed the incidence of AN. The case registry method has been the most common method used to calculate incidence, because it entails less methodological bias. Theander (1970) estimated the incidence of AN patients referred for psychiatric help in an area of Sweden to be 0.24 per 100,000 population per year. The average new cases per year increased from 1.1 to 5.8 over the 30-year period investigated. Kendell and colleagues (1973) also reported an increased incidence of AN when they analyzed three case registries from Camberwell in London, northeast Scotland, and Monroe County, New York. Estimates of new cases varied from 0.37 per 100,000 population per year in Monroe County to 1.6 per 100,000 in northeast Scotland. In 1980, Jones and colleagues (1980) analyzed the psychiatric case registry in one New York county over two time frames, 1960–1969 and 1970–1976, and estimated the incidence of AN nearly doubled between the two periods, from 0.35 to 0.64 per 100,000. Willi and Grossman (1983) surveyed the frequency of AN in Zurich and found that its incidence had significantly increased over the years from 0.38 per 100,000 for 1956–1958, to 0.55 per 100,000 for 1963–1965, to 1.12 per 100,000 for 1973–1975. In a recent study using the case registry method in northwest Scotland, the incidence of AN increased to 4.06 per 100,000 for the period 1978–1982 (Szmukler et al. 1986).

Eating Patterns

The term anorexia nervosa means a nervous loss of appetite. This is a misnomer, because the loss of appetite typically only occurs in the later stages of the disease. Most individuals with AN experience normal to intense feelings of hunger, but they vigorously deny its existence. Peculiar patterns of handling food develop and patients find themselves constantly preoccupied with food and its preparation. Many of these are features associated with the starvation process (see Table 1–1). Although AN patients may go to great lengths to restrict their food intake, they frequently show considerable interest in reading and talking about cooking and nutrition. It is common for patients with anorexia to prepare elaborate meals for others. The behaviors employed to produce weight loss are multiple. They include restriction or abstinence from food intake; selection of low caloric food items; excessive exercising and restless overactivity; self-induced vomiting; and the overuse of laxatives, diuretics, and appetite suppressants.

Table 1–1. Cardinal features of anorexia nervosa

Physiologic features

1. Significant weight loss and/or low weight according to population norms
2. Deficits in reproductive functioning

Behavioral features

1. Refusal to maintain normal body weight
2. Restrictive eating, excessive activity, and/or purging (i.e., vomiting, laxative abuse, diuretic abuse)
3. Social withdrawal

Psychologic features

1. Relentless pursuit of thinness
2. Intense fear of becoming fat and losing control over eating
3. Extreme concern with body shape and weight
4. Body image distortion
5. Disturbances of interoceptive awareness
6. Perfectionist tendencies
7. Sense of ineffectiveness and powerlessness over own life situation
8. Dichotomous thinking

Features associated with starvation

1. Preoccupation with food and food preparation
2. Peculiar eating habits
3. Social withdrawal
4. Emotional instability
5. Binge eating
6. Sleep disturbances
7. Hypothermia
8. Bradycardia
9. Amenorrhea
10. Gastrointestinal problems
11. Decreased sexual interest
12. Obsessive-compulsive behaviors
13. Impaired concentration

Psychopathology

The person who develops AN often starts on a diet to lose weight or to reduce the shape of certain body parts. Many people who later become anorexic initially pursue a lower weight for the same reasons as non-anorexic dieters. This is often associated with a desire for increased popularity and enhanced self-esteem. However, unlike most dieters, the future anorexic patient obsessively continues to strive for a thinner shape to the point of emaciation. This ever-decreasing weight becomes equated with a sense of mastery and control. Over time, a vicious cycle emerges in which the physical and psychological effects of self-starvation endanger the person's control over eating. This in turn instills an inordinate sense of fear that is counteracted with further vigorous attempts to lose weight.

Virtually all anorexic patients at some time acknowledge body dissatisfaction, and many experience body image distortion. For instance, they may be unaware of their emaciation or deny the extent of weight loss. Alternatively, they may acknowledge weight loss but experience distortion about certain body parts, such as hips, thighs, and abdomen (Garfinkel and Garner 1982).

The distortion of thinking patterns and attitudes in AN extend beyond those related to food and body shape. Cognitive distortions about one's self and one's environment are also salient in AN (Garfinkel and Garner 1982). Dichotomous reasoning, personalization of situations, and a tendency to overgeneralize are all common. An anorexic patient's self-worth becomes inextricably tied to appearance.

Over time the anorexic patient's interests will narrow in scope to the point where activities are focused solely on dieting, preoccupation with food, and exercise. As with other starving people, patients with AN may exhibit depressed mood, anxiety, impaired concentration, sleep disturbance, obsessive-compulsive behavior, and gradual withdrawal from social experiences into an isolated existence. There is a lack of interest in maintaining or developing friendships. Sexual interests and dating activities (if they were present) typically cease.

Bruch (1973) proposed that AN patients fail to establish a sense of control and autonomy over their lives and that they suffer from an overwhelming sense of ineffectiveness. The drive for thinness and perfectionism is viewed as a compensation for an undifferentiated self and intense feelings of helplessness. The rigid discipline over eating is seen as a defense against intolerable feelings of ineffectiveness and powerlessness. The value AN patients place on self-control and self-discipline, coupled with the other central features of their illness, accounts for much of the resistance they show toward interventions by professionals, parents, or significant others.

Restricting Versus Bulimic Anorexia Nervosa

There are significant differences between those AN patients who restrict their food intake in order to lose weight and those who engage in alternating patterns of food restriction and episodes of bulimia. In comparison to restricting anorexics, those patients with the bulimic subtype of AN (AN+BN) report a higher probability of premorbid obesity, a higher likelihood of family history of affective disorder and obesity, greater disturbance in familial interaction patterns, greater depressive symptomatology, more indications of impulsivity, and more social activity (Garner and Fairburn 1988).

Case 1

Sydney, a 20-year-old single female college student with a 3-year history of AN, was referred to an outpatient intensive eating disorder group at the time of her discharge from a 12-week course of treatment in an eating disorder day hospital program. At age 17, Sydney embarked on a rigid, self-imposed diet following her boyfriend's breakup of their 2-year relationship and his subsequent involvement with another woman. Sydney perceived herself as totally mortified by this loss. She recollected experiencing frequent crying spells, having marked difficulty with her academic studies, isolating herself more from her friends, ruminating excessively about the loss, and fantasizing ways in which she could reconcile the relationship. To "save face" and anticipated embarrassment, Sydney chose to withhold the event from her family members. Once the breakup became known to the family through a sibling, Sydney denied that the event or relationship held any significance for her.

Although Sydney had not previously perceived herself as having a weight problem, she was aware that her boyfriend's new girlfriend was smaller. Feeling like a failure for the first time in her life, she blamed herself for the breakup and convinced herself that one of the ways she could "win back" her boyfriend was by losing weight. Sydney succeeded in losing her desired 10 pounds in only 4 weeks yet recalled feeling dissatisfied with this reduction and her weight of 115 pounds. New weight loss goals were set in 5-pound increments, and she was sure that if she reached 100 pounds she would be happier, prettier, and more successful in any endeavor she undertook. Her interest in reconciling the relationship soon dissipated, as did her interest in establishing any new friendships or heterosexual relations. Academically, Sydney's interests became renewed despite her marked difficulty concentrating. Over the next 2 years, her eating pattern became progressively more restrictive and regimented. By the time her weight had declined to 86 pounds, Sydney had become a vegetarian, skipped the majority of family meals, took on the role of the family cook, avoided the consumption of numerous food items deemed "bad and fattening," developed numerous eating rituals, and implemented a vigorous daily 3-hour exercise program. Her sense of identity and self-esteem totally revolved around her weight.

Initially her parents, two older sisters, and younger brother were enamored by both Sydney's weight reduction and stamina. Both her mother and eldest sister viewed themselves as 10 to 15 pounds overweight and had struggled with weight and body image concerns for years with frequent unsuccessful attempts at dieting. The mother readily relinquished her role as the family cook upon Sydney's voiced interest, believing it could help curb her own tendencies to overeat. Sydney enjoyed being perceived as the family nutritional expert, recalling it was the first time family members had ever regarded her as an authority on something. It wasn't until her mother and sister succeeded in losing a few pounds that Sydney began to resent their consultation for dieting tips. Intense feelings of competition arose, and she recalled the tremendous elation she felt when they regained their weight. As Sydney's weight continued to decline and she became socially isolated, the family began to voice concerns about her weight loss. However, they had considerable difficulty accepting the diagnosis of AN, the seriousness of the disorder, the family physician's treatment recommendations, and, generally, the fact that there was a problem in their family.

Sydney achieved normalized eating and weight stabilization through her involvement in the day hospital eating disorder program. Her family benefited from the psychoeducational information received during their brief family therapy. Upon reflection, she felt as if her life had been on hold for the past 3 years and she had been in a trance. She was receptive to a longer term eating disorder outpatient group to work on self-esteem issues and a number of unresolved interpersonal difficulties.

Case 2

Frances, a 41-year-old homemaker and mother of two, was referred for an outpatient eating disorder group following 3 years of individual psychotherapy. Frances related a long-standing history of low self-esteem, intermittent depressive episodes, and a 16-year history of AN. She was raised in an enmeshed, overprotective, rigid, lower working-class immigrant family with three generations residing in the same household. Her grandmother was the primary caregiver during her early childhood while her parents worked very long hours in their family operated business. Shortly after high school Frances married, and she willingly gave up her clerical position and became a homemaker following the birth of her first son.

Throughout her early adult life, Frances's weight "yo-yoed" in response to ongoing attempts to achieve a slimmer appearance. Although she had never had a serious weight problem, she always considered herself on the "chubby side of normal." Her husband, a slim, athletic individual who was also very weight conscious, attempted to help his wife keep her weight in check by drawing attention to her "little tire-tube forming around her waist" or her developing "gopher cheeks." Frances was secretly devastated by these comments. She entered her marriage with very low self-esteem and found herself growing increasingly dependent on her husband over the years, deriving a sense of self-worth largely through his personhood and his accomplishments.

Following the birth of her second child, Frances suffered a severe postpartum depression and lost a significant amount of weight. She received no treatment at this time. Despite her difficulty coping, Frances believed one of the things that helped pull her through this trying time was her delight at losing weight so effortlessly. She vowed to never allow her weight to increase again. However, Frances soon realized that to maintain this low weight and deny her intense hunger took tremendous effort. It was not long before her every waking hour was consumed with thoughts of food and a quest for greater slimness. With time, she began to engage in episodic binges. She found it very difficult to induce vomiting after these binge episodes and instead turned to excessive exercise as a solution to offset weight gain. Shortly thereafter, exercise became a daily, excessive routine. Her propensity for perfectionism escalated, and her behavior became increasingly regimented and obsessive-compulsive. Socially, Frances felt more confident and popular. She took great delight in hearing people refer to her as cute and tiny, most notably her husband. For the first time in her life, she felt as if she had really succeeded at something special. Although she initially claimed that she took great interest in her role as a mother, she later admitted that she had never really derived any sense of gratification from this. As her AN became more chronic, Frances began to spend less time with her children and devoted her energy to restricting food, exercising, and attending to her appearance.

Bulimia Nervosa

Bulimia nervosa is an eating disorder characterized by strong and intractable urges to overeat followed by maneuvers to combat the "fattening" effects of binge eating (Russell 1979). These compensatory maneuvers include self-induced vomiting; misuse of laxatives, diuretics, or diet pills; restrictive dieting or fasting; and excessive exercise. As with AN, the symptoms of BN are diverse and multiple, encompassing behavioral, psychologic, and physiological features (see Table 1–2).

Diagnostic Criteria

In a historical review of the syndrome of BN, Casper (1983) traced clinical descriptions of bulimia back to the late 1900s. However, it was not until the 1940s that detailed accounts of bulimic symptoms began to appear in the literature. Interest in BN developed in the late 1970s when researchers in the area of AN found bulimic symptoms in many of their AN patients (Casper et al. 1980; Russell 1979). At this time controversy existed about nosology, specifically whether bulimia and AN represented separate syndromes, or extreme ends of the same disorder. Researchers recognized that bulimic behavior was not confined solely to individuals with AN. Studies had already demonstrated that bulimia does occur in normal-weight individuals (Boskind-White 1976) and among overweight and obese individuals (Stunkard 1959). Assimilation of this information eventually led to the classification of bulimia nervosa as a disorder distinct from AN.

Gerald Russell (1979) was the first to document specific diagnostic criteria for BN. His criteria focused on three core issues: the urge to overeat, excessive preoccupation about weight and shape, and the purging measures to counteract the effects of overeating. The DSM-III criteria for BN

Table 1–2.   Cardinal features of bulimia nervosa

Physiologic features

1. Weight fluctuation
2. May be experiencing effects of starvation/semistarvation

Behavioral features

1. Recurrent episodes of uncontrollable binge eating
2. Compensatory efforts to counteract the effects of binge eating and to control body weight, including self-induced vomiting, misuse of laxatives, diuretics or diet pills, excessive exercise, severe dieting or fasting
3. Refusal to maintain "natural" weight may be present

Psychologic features

1. Extreme concern with body shape and weight
2. Affective instability
3. Fear of "fatness"
4. Depression, anxiety, guilt, and shame in response to loss of control over eating/purging
5. Propensity for impulsivity and self-destructive behavior, including substance abuse, shoplifting, self-mutilation, sexual acting out, and suicide attempts
6. High need for approval
7. Social adjustment difficulties
8. Low self-esteem and self-deprecation

---

focused predominantly on binge eating. Distinctions between compulsive overeaters, cyclical or "yo-yo" dieters, and bulimic patients could not be made using these criteria. Although the criteria listed by Russell and DSM-III were devised to describe individuals with essentially the same disorder, they encompassed overlapping but different populations (Fairburn and Garner 1986). Inconsistencies in the research literature are linked in part to the use of these differing definitions. Confusion has resulted from the use of the term "bulimia" interchangeably to describe both a symptom (binge eating) and a diagnostic syndrome (bulimia nervosa).

After being subjected to substantial criticism, the original DSM-III criteria were revised in 1985 and again in 1987. The 1987 DSM-III-R criteria for BN rectify most of the former shortcomings. These include the ambiguity surrounding the use of the term "bulimia," the exclusion of the marked overconcern with body shape, the failure to specify a minimum frequency for overeating, the optional rather than mandatory stipulation of behaviors to allay the effects of overeating, and the segregation from AN (Fairburn and Garner 1986; Garner and Garfinkel 1988).

DSM-III-R Diagnostic Criteria for Bulimia Nervosa

A. Recurrent episodes of binge eating (rapid consumption of a large amount of food in a discrete period of time).

B. A feeling of lack of control over eating behavior during the eating binges.

C. Regularly engaging in either self-induced vomiting, use of laxatives or diuretics, strict dieting or fasting, or vigorous exercise in order to prevent weight gain.

D. A minimum average of two binge-eating episodes a week for at least 3 months.

E. Persistent overconcern with body shape and weight.

Demographics and Epidemiology

Bulimia nervosa occurs predominantly in young adult females in their early 20s, though the age may range widely, with cases reported from the early teens to the early 50s. The age of onset is typically in the late teens. From a review of demographic studies, Johnson and Connors (1987) concluded that most bulimic patients are within a normal weight range at the time of assessment, but approximately one-third to one-half of all cases have been overweight at some point. In addition, approximately 30% of the clinical samples and 10% of the community samples give a history suggestive of AN. The bulimic patient tends to be single, college-educated, upwardly mobile, and from an intact family with more than one child.

The prevalence of BN, like that of AN, is unknown, but it is believed to be particularly prevalent among adolescent and adult females living in countries with Westernized cultures (Johnson and Connors 1987). Cases of BN are difficult to detect because of the secretive nature of the syndrome and the few visible physical symptoms. Investigations estimating the average duration of illness prior to seeking treatment have reported averages of approximately 5 years (Johnson and Connors 1987).

The prevalence of the practice of binge eating among the female student population is widespread, with studies yielding a range of 54–86% (Halmi et al. 1981; Hawkins and Clement 1984; Katzman and Wolchik 1984; Hart and Ollendick 1985). In this subpopulation, the occurrence of BN using DSM-III criteria has been estimated to range from 5% of female college students in one clinical sample (Strangler and Printz 1980) to 20% of female college seniors in another (Pope et al. 1984). When more rigid criteria for BN are used (i.e., binge eating followed by vomiting at least weekly), the prevalence drops to reported ranges of less than 3% (Pyle et al. 1983).

Cooper and Fairburn (1983) found that 1.9% of their sample of adult women attending a British family planning clinic fulfilled Russell's (1979) criteria for BN. In a study of 139 working females, Hart and Ollendick (1985) found that 1% fulfilled DSM-III criteria for bulimia. In reviewing the epidemiological findings, Fairburn and Beglin (1990) noted the difference between the prevalence found in self-report questionnaire surveys compared to those using interview techniques. With the more stringent methodology, the rate among adolescent and young adult women was about 1%. They also noted that in longitudinal studies, the eating disorder symptoms tended to wax and wane over time. However, there appeared to be a subgroup with more severely disturbed eating habits that ran a more chronic course.

The prevalence of BN is much lower for males. Surveys among male college students have reported bulimia to range from none (Clarke and Palmer 1983; Pope et al. 1984) to 5% (Halmi et al. 1981), with the average prevalence across studies estimated at less than 1% (Johnson and Connors 1987).

Eating Patterns

Bulimia nervosa patients typically report very disturbed eating patterns. Dieting for weight control and thinness is regularly disrupted by bouts of binge eating. These episodes are experienced as uncontrollable and extremely distressing. Among clinical populations, binge-eating episodes are almost invariably conducted alone and in secrecy and are most prevalent during the evening (Johnson et al. 1982; Pyle et al. 1981). Caloric intake during a single binge has been reported up to 55,000 calories, with an average of 3,400 to 4,800 calories per binge (Johnson et al. 1982; Mitchell et al.

1981). Binges are often planned and consist of "forbidden" food items that are stringently excluded from the patient's usual dietary regimen.

A binge can be precipitated by a number of factors, including the breaking of a self-imposed diet; feelings of anxiety, depression, anger, boredom, or loneliness; or a general feeling of unhappiness. Often they are associated with unsatisfactory interactions with significant others. By external criteria, most of these triggers are, in themselves, not of great significance. Rather, they appear to operate on a reactive predisposition. The patient's definition of a binge episode is often related to the type of food eaten or to the experience of being out of control, irrespective of the amount of food actually ingested.

Typically, binge-eating episodes end as a result of physical exhaustion, abdominal discomfort, intense anxiety, social interruption, lack of food supplies, or self-induced vomiting/purging behavior (Fairburn 1983). The most frequently used compensatory method of purging is self-induced vomiting. During the aftermath of the binge-purge cycle, it is not uncommon for bulimic patients to experience periods of self-deprecation and depression. Most will restrict their food intake and exclude foods that are "fattening" in between binges. Some may totally refrain from eating and engage in fasting. Pyle and colleagues (1981) found that bulimic patients often refrained from eating for more than 24 hours following a binge. This would lead to intense hunger and prompt another binge episode. A minority of bulimic individuals engage in more unusual eating habits such as rumination, in which swallowed food is voluntarily regurgitated back into the mouth where it is rechewed, reswallowed, or spit out (Fairburn 1983).

Psychopathology

A central characteristic of BN is hypersensitivity to weight and body shape. A desire for "thinness" and a fear of "fatness" are foremost in a bulimic patient's thoughts. Research suggests the profile of a BN patient as someone who is prone to depressive moods, anxiety, poor impulse control, low self-esteem, poor body image, and high self-expectations. There is frequently social maladjustment, with concern over sex-role issues, a high need for approval, hypersensitivity to the impressions of others, and difficulty in identifying and expressing internal states (Johnson and Connors 1987; Mizes 1985). It remains unclear whether these personality characteristics serve initially to predispose an individual to develop BN or are, at least in part, a result of the syndrome. Because there are relatively few studies that have investigated personality features using satisfactory methodology, it would be premature to reach any definitive conclusions at this time.

Body Weight

Most bulimic patients appear to be of normal weight and tend to be secretive about their eating behaviors. Therefore, the syndrome can be difficult to recognize. This contrasts with anorexic patients, whose visible emaciation is an evident hallmark of the disorder. Most BN patients present with a body weight within a normal range according to standardized norms. It has been argued that for many of these individuals, their genetic constitution predisposes them to an above-average weight (Garner et al. 1985). Such individuals may be attempting to maintain an unrealistic weight that is well below their "natural" weight and are consequently experiencing the effects of semistarvation. These bulimic individuals have a hunger-driven biological vulnerability to engage in binge-eating episodes while dieting, and marked weight fluctuation is common. Empirical findings suggest that, over time, many BN patients have lost as much body weight as AN patients, despite never having been emaciated (Garner and Fairburn 1988).

Case 3

Jennifer, a 24-year-old single junior marketing executive, was referred for a group placement in a cognitive behavioral psychoeducational group. Her symptoms began 5 years earlier when she was a student at a university and residing on campus. A number of females on her residency floor embarked on a well-known fad diet together and each week would tally up the total pounds lost among them. They planned to reward themselves with a 5-day vacation if they succeeded in losing a group total of 100 pounds in 3 months. Jennifer followed the diet "faithfully" for the first month and lost 6 pounds. She started to find it increasingly difficult to stay with the diet, claiming she "lost her willpower." One of her fellow roommates, who was experiencing the same difficulty, revealed she had tried vomiting after reading about it in a popular women's magazine. Upon Jennifer's request, she was taught how to self-induce vomiting. Shortly thereafter, the two of them were also experimenting with laxatives and over-the-counter diet pills.

Within 2 years, Jennifer was bingeing and purging an average of once a day; however, during times of stress or boredom this would increase to three or four times a day. Her weight oscillated between 5 and 10 pounds heavier than her predieting weight. Academically, Jennifer's grades declined as her study time became replaced with bingeing. Truancy became a problem for her, and she found herself conjuring up all sorts of fabricated stories to family and friends to excuse herself from her unreliable behavior. She managed to graduate, but she then had similar problems of absenteeism and unreliability at work. She described herself as continually walking around with a cloud of guilt surrounding her and ruminating excessively about losing her job. She also had a tendency to date men for only short periods of time, noting that her BN tended to take precedence over relationships.

Jennifer presented as an amiable and well-spoken woman with a tendency to control the content of the conversation. She labelled herself a "phony" and described the "real" her as feeling very overwhelmed, out of control, guilt-ridden, and prone to mood swings. With regard to past history, Jennifer was the second child in a family of eight children. She grew up in a small town, and during her early teens she assumed a "parentified" role in response to her father being absent for long periods of time while working out of town. When Jennifer's father would return home, he would spend most of his evenings out with his "buddies, drinking and partying," and he continually lamented how difficult it was to support a family of their size.

Jennifer held highly ambivalent feelings toward and perceptions of both her parents. She regarded her mother as being "very tough, a survivor" able to cope and "put up" with her life situation. Yet she also perceived her mother as "very weak" for not attempting to change her situation, for being so overaccommodating, and for lacking self-confidence. Jennifer harbored a lot of anger toward her parents and recalled many incidents of feeling humiliated during her childhood. Had it not been for an educational scholarship and a teacher's strong urging, Jennifer believes she may have remained in her hometown. She struggled with feelings of being abandoned by her parents yet also felt guilty for later abandoning them along with her siblings.

Case 4

Russell, a 30-year-old single lab technician, was referred for a group placement with an 8-year history of BN and borderline personality features. Russell had been overweight since his early childhood and became obese in his mid-teens. Dieting had become a way of life for him and his family for as long as he could remember. During his late teens, Russell was placed on some medically supervised diets, but the weight loss was very short-term. He began binge eating during this time. He considered the dieting experiences as highly traumatic. He loathed his appointments with his physician, claiming they were a source of constant humiliation and shame and contributed to his current negative and suspicious view of the medical profession.

In response to a classmate's dieting success with a well-known commercial center for weight loss, Russell joined the program and lost a considerable amount of weight over a 7-month time frame on a very restrictive diet. During the initial 7 months, he refrained from any bingeing activities and recalled eating far less than the recommended plan. Once he was placed on the maintenance program, his weight began to increase. It was at this time that he resumed bingeing and shortly thereafter started to vomit and abuse laxatives. Within a year he was bingeing and vomiting on a daily basis. He began to steal laxatives off the hospital units during his training. This stealing behavior has since expanded to the ongoing theft of other medical supplies and of money from patients and hospital employees, as well as shoplifting from major department stores. He first sought psychiatric help of his own accord for his intermittent periods of depression, and it was during this time that his eating disorder was identified. Prior to his referral to a day hospital eating disorder program, Russell was seen briefly in individual therapy.

Both Russell's father and grandfather were morbidly obese, diabetic, and died of heart disease in their 50s. His father had suffered from chronic depression that necessitated two lengthy hospitalizations, the latter close to the time of his death when Russell was 25. One of Russell's two sisters and his mother were overweight. Russell disclosed leading a very unhappy and lonely childhood. His parents had a very unhappy marriage, and they tended to be despondent with each other and their children. He described his entire family as a group of "timid and fat skeptics." Russell was involved in an incestuous relationship with his mother between the ages of 14 and 16. He initiated an incestuous relationship with his older sister at age 15. Both incestuous relationships ended abruptly at age 16 when his mother discovered his sexual relations with his sister. Russell was still very unresolved about both of these family secrets and held highly ambivalent feelings toward his mother and older sister.

Academically, Russell was an average student, and he described his school years as particularly painful. He was continually teased by his peers, having been nicknamed "Busty Rusty." Russell began engaging in self-mutilating behaviors (cigarette burns to arms) at age 15. He voiced being bothered by chronic feelings of boredom and emptiness, by affective instability, by his longstanding social isolation and feelings of low self-worth, and by his discontentment with his body image.

Relationship Between Anorexia Nervosa and Bulimia Nervosa

Ideas about the relationship between AN and BN have evolved over the last two decades. There is now a growing consensus that the two disorders are closely related (Garner and Fairburn 1988). This conclusion is based on a number of research findings:

1. Many AN patients also report the symptom of bulimia.
2. Many patients shift between AN and BN over the course of their disorder.
3. BN and AN+BN patients exhibit similar psychopathology on most psychometric and clinical variables.
4. Many BN patients with seemingly "normal" body weight have lost as

much weight as AN patients, the difference being that they began with a higher and possibly genetically predisposed absolute weight.

5. There are many similarities in the components of treatment for BN and AN.

There is also disagreement over whether or not weight status should be used to distinguish AN from BN. Some researchers advocate that a more appropriate diagnostic criterion to distinguish AN from BN is the presence or absence of bulimic behavior (Garner and Fairburn 1988; Johnson and Connors 1987). This would leave a category of patients with pure restricting behavior as a distinct subgroup. Patients with BN and AN+BN would be seen to fall into the same category.

Our understanding of the fundamental causes of AN and BN remains incomplete. Numerous etiological theories have been advanced to explain the eating disorders, including biologic, developmental, learning, psychological, family, and social models. However, few theories are supported by sound empirical evidence. There is common ground in considering the eating disorders to be multidetermined. The interplay of a number of predisposing, precipitating, and perpetuating factors may serve a variety of biologic, psychological, familial, and sociocultural needs (Garfinkel and Garner 1982; Johnson and Connors 1987). These are best thought of as risk or vulnerability factors rather than specific causal agents. As the number of risk factors increases and their intensity grows, an individual would have a greater likelihood of developing an eating disorder. The predisposing, precipitating, and perpetuating factors are not identical for all patients: some factors may be more or less relevant, others completely irrelevant. Tables 1–3, 1–4, and 1–5 identify some of the features that comprise each of these risk categories. These should be used for conjecture and not as established fact. There is considerable overlap among the various risk factors for both AN and BN. It is to be anticipated that future studies will modify these lists and identify the more powerful factors.

Association of Eating Disorders and Affective Disorders

There are currently a variety of opinions concerning the nature of the relationship between eating disorders and affective disorders. An association between the two has been identified from the following types of studies: 1) descriptive investigations of symptom frequency and lifetime prevalence of affective disturbance in AN and BN; 2) studies on the history of affective disorders among family members of probands with eating disorders; 3) neurobiological studies; 4) follow-up investigations of course

---

Table 1–3.   Predisposing factors

Sociocultural predispositions

Anorexia nervosa and bulimia nervosa

1. Glorification of thinness and youth
2. Prejudice against obesity
3. Emphasis on high achievement, perfectionism
4. Sex-role change and confusion for women
5. Femininity equated to appearance

Biologic predispositions

Anorexia nervosa

1. Family history of AN in sisters of probands
2. Genetic component: concordance rates of 50% for monozygotic twins versus 10% for dizygotic twins
3. Parental history of affective disorder and alcoholism
4. Family history of obesity among bulimic anorexic patients
5. Pregnancy and delivery complications

Bulimia nervosa

1. Predisposition toward obesity, affective disorder, and alcohol dependence
2. Family history of affective disorder and obesity

Familial predispositions

Anorexia nervosa

1. Higher social class, older parental age
2. Family magnification of sociocultural accentuation of thinness, outward appearance, and perfectionism
3. Distorted or faulty parent-child interactions
4. Dysfunctional family system

Table 1–3. Predisposing factors (continued)

Bulimia nervosa

1. Higher social class
2. Family magnification of sociocultural emphases on outward appearance, high achievement
3. Highly conflictive, disengaged, and chaotic family system
4. Low expressiveness and emotional isolation

Individual predispositions

Anorexia nervosa

1. Difficulties with autonomy, separation, attachment, and identity: maturation fears, early puberty, female gender, difficulty dealing with stress or failure
2. Weight disturbances as child or adolescent
3. Perceptual disturbances
4. Disturbances in cognitive content and process
5. Personality features: perfectionism, dependence on others for approval, shyness, obsessiveness, social anxiety, denial of inner needs, sense of ineffectiveness

Bulimia nervosa

1. Difficulties with autonomy, separation, attachment, and identity
2. Weight disturbances as child or adolescent
3. Affective instability: highly variable moods, impulsiveness, low tolerance for frustration and anxiety, low moods
4. Alexithymia
5. Disturbances in cognitive content and process
6. Personality features: interpersonal sensitivity, high achievement, self-criticalness, competitiveness, body dissatisfaction, dependence, sense of ineffectiveness, low self-esteem, undifferentiated sex role identity

and outcome; and 5) pharmacological investigations with the use of anti-depressant medication (Strober and Katz 1988).

It has been proposed that AN may be an atypical variant of a major affective disorder, taking on a particular form with the onset of adolescence, when preoccupation with body weight and shape is a common developmental feature. In a review of descriptive studies by Strober and Katz (1987), self-reported and clinically diagnosed depression were generally found to be prominent in AN. Preliminary evidence (Piran et al. 1985) has emerged suggesting that in a significant proportion of AN patients who have a history of major depression, the depressive symptoms preceded the onset of AN by at least 1 year. Moreover, depressive symptoms have been reported to persist in a significant proportion of patients after their AN has

---

Table 1–4.   Precipitating factors

Anorexia nervosa

 1. Puberty
 2. Separation, rejection, losses, and conflict
 3. Disruption of family homeostasis
 4. Threats to self-esteem and coping abilities
 5. New environmental demands and expectations
 6. Personal illness
 7. Interest in dance, sports
 8. Exposure to peers who are dieting
 9. Dieting: body dissatisfaction, need for control, success and enhanced self-worth, influence of culture and significant others, dissatisfaction with self and life
10. Effects of weight loss

Bulimia nervosa

 1. Separation, rejection, losses, and conflict
 2. Sexual victimization
 3. Interest in dance, sports
 4. Heterosexual interests
 5. Loneliness, boredom, anger
 6. Failure
 7. Exposure to peers who are dieting
 8. Dieting: body dissatisfaction, need for control, success and enhanced self-worth, influence of culture and significant others, dissatisfaction with self and life
 9. Effects of weight loss

resolved (Hsu 1980). Depressive symptoms are common in AN when star-vation is pronounced, but they frequently remit following nutritional sta-bilization and weight gain. In this instance, the depressive symptoms may be secondary to the metabolic disturbance (Halmi et al. 1986).

The most compelling evidence affiliating AN and biologically medi-ated depression comes from family studies. The prevalence of affective

Table 1–5. Perpetuating factors

Anorexia nervosa

1. Starvation effects
2. Self-induced vomiting
3. Gastrointestinal problems
4. Hypothalamic dysfunction
5. Cognitive disturbances
6. Perceptual disturbances
7. Interpersonal difficulties
8. Unresolved predisposing factors
9. Secondary gain
10. Sociocultural pressures
11. Body image distortion

Bulimia nervosa

1. Emotional instability
2. Interpersonal difficulties
3. Binge eating: tension regulation, expression of aggressive and erotic impulses, cognitive narrowing and diffusion, defiant acting-out, loss of control and panic, fear of being discovered
4. Purging behavior: tension regulation, undoing of the binge, expression of aggressive and erotic impulses, reassertion of control, legitimizing the binge episode, penitence-expiation of guilt, maintaining commitment to weight control
5. Distortion of hunger and satiation
6. Self-deprecation, guilt, shame, anxiety
7. Cognitive disturbances
8. Body image distortion
9. Failure and depression
10. Narrowing of interests
11. Physical illness
12. Unresolved predisposing factors
13. Sociocultural pressures

disorders in the family members of probands with AN has been reported to be significantly higher than control groups (Gershon et al. 1984; Winoker et al. 1980). It reaches levels almost equal to those found in probands with affective disorders (Winoker et al. 1980). Conversely, an increase in the familial aggregation of eating disorders in probands with affective disorders has not been found (Strober and Katz 1987).

Bulimia nervosa has also been proposed as a variant of a biological predisposition to affective disorder. A number of studies have reported that BN patients exhibit a high prevalence of major affective disorder in their personal histories (Hudson et al. 1983; Walsh et al. 1985). As with AN, there is convincing evidence that major affective disorder frequently occurs among the first- and second-degree relatives of BN patients (Hudson et al. 1983; Strober 1981; Strober et al. 1982). There is no evidence that the converse is true. Studies indicate that bulimic patients present with abnormal dexamethasone suppression tests and with polysomnography sleep profiles that are similar to affective disorder patients (Gwirtsman et al. 1983; Hudson et al. 1982; Katz et al. 1984).

The effectiveness of antidepressant pharmacotherapy has strengthened the view that there is a close association between eating disorders and affective disorders. This appears to be helpful in controlling eating symptoms even in the absence of major overt depressive symptoms. Bulimic symptoms seem more responsive than anorexic features.

In summary, evidence suggests that there is comorbidity for depression in AN and BN and that there is a higher lifetime prevalence of major affective disorder in relatives of eating disorder patients. However, it would be premature to reach absolute conclusions about the connections between eating disorders and affective disorders, particularly in regard to causal interpretations (Halmi 1985; Strober and Katz 1988; Swift et al. 1986). Further research is needed to clarify the meaning of the descriptive associations that have been reported.

Summary

This chapter has emphasized the complexity of eating disorders and the numerous risk factors that may play a role in their formation and perpetuation. Treatment must take this diversity into account by tailoring therapeutic efforts to the needs of each patient. These issues fall under two major management areas, both of which are important for effective treatment. The first area, often labelled as "track one" issues, concerns the normalization of eating, the restoration and stabilization of weight, and maintenance of the patient's physical health. The second area, the "track two" issues, concerns underlying psychological issues that precipitated the onset of the eating disorder and that serve to perpetuate it.

Different treatment modalities are needed to address track one and track two issues. Track one requires nutrition therapy, pharmacotherapy, medical stabilization, and psychological support. Track two calls for psychological approaches including individual, group, family, and marital psychotherapy. These commonly involve a combination of psychoanalytic, psychodynamic, cognitive-behavioral, and psychoeducational principles. The suitability and sequencing of the different therapies will vary widely among patients. Regardless of the therapeutic approach, the therapeutic alliance between the patient and the therapist is of paramount importance. Professionals involved in the treatment of eating disorders need to be comfortable in a multidisciplinary environment that includes physicians, psychologists, nurses, dietitians, social workers, and occupational therapists.

References

American Psychiatric Association: Diagnostic and Statistical Manual of Mental Disorders, 3rd Edition. Washington, DC, American Psychiatric Association, 1980

American Psychiatric Association: Diagnostic and Statistical Manual of Mental Disorders, 3rd Edition, Revised. Washington, DC, American Psychiatric Association, 1987

Askevold F: The diagnosis of anorexia nervosa. International Journal of Eating Disorders 2:39–43, 1983

Beumont PJV, Touyz SW: Anorexia and bulimia nervosa: a personal perspective, in Handbook of Eating Disorders, Part 1. Edited by Beumont PJV, Burrows GD, Casper RC. New York, Elsevier, 1987

Boskind-White M: Cinderella's stepsisters: A feminist perspective on anorexia nervosa and bulimia. Journal of Women in Culture and Society 2:342–35, 1976

Bruch H: Eating Disorders: Obesity, Anorexia Nervosa and the Person Within. New York, Basic Books, 1973

Bruch H: Anorexia nervosa: therapy and theory. Am J Psychiatry 139:1531, 1982

Casper RC: On the emergence of bulimia nervosa as a syndrome: a historical review. International Journal of Eating Disorders 2:3–16, 1983

Casper RC, Eckert ED, Halmi KA, et al: Bulimia. Arch Gen Psychiatry 37:1030–1035, 1980

Clarke MG, Palmer RL: Eating attitudes and neurotic symptoms in university students. Br J Psychiatry 142:139–144, 1983

Cooper PJ, Fairburn CG: Binge-eating and self-induced vomiting in the community: A preliminary study. Br J Psychiatry 142:139–144, 1983

Crisp AH, Palmer RL, Kalucy RS: How common is anorexia nervosa? A prevalence study. Br J Psychiatry 218:549–554, 1976

Eckert ED: Characteristics of anorexia nervosa, in Anorexia Nervosa and Bulimia: Diagnosis and Treatment. Edited by Mitchell JE. Minneapolis, MN, University of Minnesota Press, 1985

Fairburn CG: Bulimia nervosa. Br J Hosp Med 29:537–542, 1983

Fairburn CG, Beglin SJ: Studies of the epidemiology of bulimia nervosa. Am J Psychiatry 147(4):401–408, 1990

Fairburn CG, Garner DM: The diagnosis of bulimia nervosa. International Journal of Eating Disorders 5:403–419, 1986

Fairburn CG, Garner DM: Diagnostic criteria for anorexia nervosa and bulimia nervosa: The importance of attitudes to shape and weight, in Diagnostic Issues in Anorexia Nervosa and Bulimia Nervosa. Edited by Garner DM, Garfinkel PE. New York, Brunner/Mazel, 1988

Garfinkel PE, Darby PL: Anorexia nervosa and bulimia. Medicine (North America) 13:1586–1594, 1984

Garfinkel PE, Garner DM: Anorexia Nervosa: A Multidimensional Perspective. New York, Brunner/Mazel, 1982

Garner DM, Fairburn CG: Relationship between anorexia nervosa and bulimia nervosa, in Diagnostic Issues in Anorexia Nervosa and Bulimia Nervosa. Edited by Garner DM, Garfinkel PE. New York, Brunner/Mazel, 1988

Garner DM, Garfinkel PE (eds): Diagnostic Issues in Anorexia Nervosa and Bulimia Nervosa. New York, Brunner/Mazel, 1988

Garner DM, Rockert W, Olmsted MP, et al: Psychoeducational principles in the treatment of bulimia and anorexia nervosa, in Handbook on Psychotherapy for Anorexia Nervosa and Bulimia. Edited by Garner DM, Garfinkel PE. New York, Guilford, 1985

Gershon ES, Schreiber JL, Hamont JR, et al: Clinical findings with patients with anorexia nervosa and affective illness in their relatives. Am J Psychiatry 141:1419–1422, 1984

Gwirtsman HE, Roy-Byrne P, Yager J, et al: Neuroendocrine abnormalities in bulimia. Am J Psychiatry 140:559–563, 1983

Gull WW: Anorexia nervosa. Trans Clin Soc (London) 7:22–28, 1874. Reprinted in Anderson AE, Practical Comprehensive Treatment of Anorexia Nervosa and Bulimia. Baltimore, MD, Johns Hopkins University Press, 1985

Halmi KA: Anorexia nervosa: demographic and clinical features in 94 cases. Psychol Med 36:18–26, 1974

Halmi KA: Relationship of eating disorders to depression: biological similarities and differences. International Journal of Eating Disorders 4:667–680, 1985

Halmi KA, Falk JR, Schwartz E: Binge-eating and vomiting: a survey of a college population. Psychol Med 11:697–700, 1981

Halmi KA, Eckert E, LaDu T, et al: Anorexia nervosa treatment efficacy of cyproheptadine and amitriptyline. Arch Gen Psychiatry 43:177–181, 1986

Hart JK, Ollendick TH: Prevalence of bulimia in working and university women. Am J Psychiatry 142:851–854, 1985

Hawkins RC, Clement PF: Binge eating: measurement problems and a conceptual model, in The Binge-Purge Syndrome. Edited by Hawkins RC, Fremouw WJ, Clement PF. New York, Springer, 1984

Hsu LKG: Outcome in anorexia nervosa: a review of the literature (1954–1978). Arch Gen Psychiatry 37:1041–1046, 1980

Hudson JI, Laffer PS, Pope HG: Bulimia related to affective disorder by family history and response to the dexamethasone suppression test. Am J Psychiatry 137:695–698, 1982

Hudson JI, Pope HG, Jonas JM, et al: Phenomenologic relationship of eating disorders to major affective disorder. Psychiatric Research 9:345–354, 1983

Johnson C, Connors ME: The Etiology and Treatment of Bulimia Nervosa: A Biopsychosocial Perspective. New York, Basic Books, 1987

Johnson C, Stuckey MK, Lewis LD, et al: Bulimia: a descriptive study of 316 cases. International Journal of Eating Disorders 2:3–16, 1982

Jones DJ, Fox MM, Babigan HM, et al: Epidemiology of anorexia nervosa in Monroe County, New York 1960–1976. Psychosom Med 42:551–558, 1980

Katz JL, Kuperberg A, Pollack CP, et al: Is there a relationship between eating disorder and affective disorder? New evidence from sleep recordings. Am J Psychiatry 141:753–759, 1984

Katzman MA, Wolchik SA: Bulimia and binge eating in college women: a comparison of personality and behavioral characteristics. J Consult Clin Psychol 52:423–428, 1984

Kendell RE, Hall DJ, Hailey A, et al: The epidemiology of anorexia nervosa. Psychol Med 3:200–203, 1973

Lasegue C: De l'anorexia hysterique. Arch Gen de Med 385, 1873. Reprinted in Anderson AE (ed): Practical Comprehensive Treatment of Anorexia Nervosa and Bulimia. Baltimore, MD, Johns Hopkins University Press, 1985

Mitchell JE, Pyle RL, Eckert ED: Frequency and duration of binge-eating episodes in patients with bulimia. Am J Psychiatry 138:835–836, 1981

Mizes JS: Bulimia: A review of its symptomatology and treatment. Advances in Behavior, Research, and Therapy 7:91–142, 1985

Morton R: Phthisiologica: or a Treatise of Consumptions. London, S. Smith and B. Walford, 1694. Reprinted in Anderson AE (ed): Practical Comprehensive Treatment of Anorexia Nervosa and Bulimia. Baltimore, MD, Johns Hopkins University Press, 1985

Nylander I: The feeling of being fat and dieting in a school population: Epidemiologic, interview investigation. Acta Sociomedica Scandinavica 3:17–26, 1971

Piran N, Kennedy S, Garfinkel PE, et al: Affective disturbance in eating disorders. J Nerv Ment Dis 173:395–400, 1985

Pope HG Jr, Hudson JI, Yurgelun-Todd D, et al: Prevalence of anorexia nervosa and bulimia in three student populations. International Journal of Eating Disorders 3:45–51, 1984

Pyle RL, Mitchell JE, Eckert ED: Bulimia: A report of 34 cases. J Clin Psychiatry 42:60–64, 1981

Pyle RL, Mitchell JE, Eckert ED, et al: The incidence of bulimia in freshman college students. International Journal of Eating Disorders 2:75–85, 1983

Russell GFM: Anorexia nervosa: its identity as an illness and its treatment, in Modern Trends in Psychosomatic Medicine, Vol 2. Edited by Price JH. London, Butterworths, 1970

Russell GFM: Bulimia nervosa: an ominous variant of anorexia nervosa. Psychol Med 9:429–448, 1979

Selvini-Palazzoli MP: Self-Starvation. New York, Jason Aronson, 1974

Strangler RS, Printz AM: DSM-III: psychiatric diagnosis in a university population. Am J Psychiatry 137:937–940, 1980

Strober M: The significance of bulimia in juvenile anorexia nervosa: an exploration of possible etiological factors. International Journal of Eating Disorders 1:28–43, 1981

Strober M, Katz JL: Do eating disorders share a common etiology? A dissenting opinion. International Journal of Eating Disorders 6:171–180, 1987

Strober M, Katz JL: Depression in the eating disorders: A review and analysis of descriptive, family, and biological findings, in Diagnostic Issues in Anorexia Nervosa and Bulimia Nervosa. Edited by Garner DM, Garfinkel PE. New York, Brunner/Mazel, 1988

Strober M, Salkin B, Burroughs J, et al: Validity of the bulimia-restrictor distinction in anorexia nervosa. Parental personality characteristics and family psychiatric history. J Nerv Ment Dis 170:345–351, 1982

Stunkard AJ: Eating patterns and obesity. Psychiatr Q 33:284–295, 1959

Swift WJ, Andrews D, Barklage NE: The relationship between affective disorder and eating disorders: A review of the literature. Am J Psychiatry 143:290–299, 1986

Szmukler GI, Eisler I, Gillies C, et al: Anorexia nervosa and bulimic disorders: Current perspectives, Proceedings, in Journal of Psychiatric Research. Edited by Smukler GI, Slade PD, Harris P, et al. London, Pergamon, 1986

Theander S: Anorexia nervosa: A psychiatric investigation of 94 female patients. Acta Psychiatr Scand Suppl 214:1–194, 1970

Walsh BT, Roose SP, Glassman AH, et al: Depression and bulimia. Psychosom Med 47:123–131, 1985

Willi J, Grossman S: Epidemiology of anorexia nervosa in a defined region of Switzerland. Am J Psychiatry 140:564–567, 1983

Winoker A, March V, Mendels J: Primary affective disorder in relatives of patients with anorexia nervosa. Am J Psychiatry 137:695–698, 1980

2

Introduction to Group Concepts

K. Roy MacKenzie, M.D., F.R.C.P.(C)
Heather Harper-Giuffre, B.N., B.Sc., M.Sc.

♦ ♦ ♦ ♦ ♦ ♦ ♦ ♦ ♦

This chapter provides an introduction to the central principles and techniques necessary to organize and conduct the types of eating disorder groups described in this book. It should be stressed that specific skill in managing groups can enhance the value to the members by offering helpful conditions not found in individual therapy. At the same time, failure to manage group events competently may lead to harmful experiences of perceived failure or to interpersonal events that are damaging to the already fragile self-esteem of these patients. This chapter is designed to serve as a guide with regard to the specialized types of groups described in other chapters.—The Editors

In this chapter, we provide a survey of current trends in group psychotherapy, emphasizing basic theoretical approaches to conducting effective groups. Many mental health professionals are skilled in individual therapy and in the psychological management of patients with eating disorders. Such skills do not automatically transfer into effective group management. Systematic training in group psychotherapy allows the therapist to capitalize on the use of the group environment. Groups have therapeutic possibilities that are in addition to, and quite distinct from, those found in individual work. The use of these group properties can enhance the management of patients with eating disorders. This applies to brief psychoeducational group formats as well as to more intensive, interpersonally oriented therapy. Numerous studies indicate that the results of group psychotherapy are equivalent to those of individual work (Budman et al. 1988; Garfield and Bergin 1986; Pilkonis et al. 1984; Piper et al. 1984; Toseland and Siporin 1986). For the interested reader, an expansion of the material in this chapter can be found in MacKenzie (1990), Yalom (1985), and Rutan and Stone (1984).

The understanding and management of groups can be approached from three sequential perspectives: 1) the series of tasks involved in assessing the patient, composing the group, and preparing the patient for participation; 2) the various facets of the "nature of groupness" dealing with the predictable group phenomena that must be managed effectively; and 3) specific therapeutic strategies useful in the group. The first two of these perspectives are applicable to all group formats whether they be of a brief or longer term nature. The third perspective moves into material that is more critical for the management of longer term group psychotherapy.

Before the Group Begins

Time spent on the tasks of assessment, composition, and pretherapy preparation will prevent loss of members and will maximize the effectiveness of the early group sessions. In order to capitalize on the therapeutic potential of a group, it is necessary to create a sense of "groupness." This includes the development of group cohesion as well as a sense of the group working together on its tasks. If this does not occur, the likelihood of premature terminations is greatly increased. The great majority of group dropouts occur in the first six to eight sessions. After this point, premature terminations are infrequent and usually the result of quite specific events, either within the group or in outside circumstances.

Assessing the Patient

Patients presenting with eating symptoms frequently meet diagnostic criteria for other psychiatric and medical disorders. It is particularly important to assess the patient for the presence of organic impairment related to starvation or metabolic imbalance and for major depressive symptoms. If severe, these conditions will preclude effective participation in a group setting. The effects of severe starvation usually constitute a contraindication for group psychotherapy; they will hamper the appreciation of psychoeducational material and dilute the usefulness of other group interactions. Effective treatment of organic impairment and depression will improve the clinical status, and at that point group involvement may be reconsidered.

It is also important to assess for the presence of Axis II personality features. If severe, these may also constitute a contraindication for group involvement. A patient with major antisocial characteristics will prove at least disruptive and perhaps actively destructive for the therapy group, particularly in longer term interpersonal groups. Similarly, the patient with major borderline features may respond to the group environment with an exacerbation of histrionic and manipulative behaviors. To manage such patients in groups requires a therapist with particular expertise. Patients who demonstrate severe paranoid or schizoid traits or who use extremely brittle denial will not take to a group environment easily. Such patients are prone to experience this difficulty as vindication of their beliefs or as a further episode of personal failure.

Each of these assessment dimensions can be seen as a continuum. At the severe end, they may constitute an absolute contraindication to group involvement, whereas in the middle range they will serve to alert the therapist regarding questions of group composition. At lower levels of character disturbance, the assessment information can be valuable in preparing the therapist to deal most effectively with predictable issues and thus ensure that these patients will maximize the benefits of the group experience. An additional advantage of a careful diagnostic process is that it serves to sensitize the patient to the interpersonal and psychosocial implications of the primary diagnosis of eating disorder. For groups with limited goals such as a brief psychoeducational experience, the criteria for acceptance can be broad. Only those patients likely to be actively disruptive to the sessions need to be managed elsewhere.

The assessment process provides an opportunity to evaluate the patient's motivation and commitment to a therapeutic undertaking. This may be particularly challenging with the patient with an eating disorder. A common feature of the disorder is a powerful inclination to please or appease significant others. Enthusiasm for therapy may represent such a dynamic. Often, referral information is helpful in this respect. Who made the first contact? How intrusive are the parents, the spouse, or the individual therapist in contributing to the assessment interviews? Are there frequent phone calls from significant others? Is the patient portrayed as a helpless victim of circumstances? One useful function of a preliminary time-limited psychoeducational group is the opportunity to assess behavior over a longer time period. This allows motivation to be observed away from the context of significant others.

Composing the Group

Group composition decisions must be made in relation to the purpose of the group experience. For patients with eating disorders, three major categories can be defined. The first type of group is that with a psychoeducational purpose. The second is for patients whose eating patterns are severely out of control, often requiring inpatient or day hospital settings. The third group format is designed for more intensive interactional work where the relationships within the group will form a focus for much of the therapeutic activity. The implications of these three categories of groups will have a major effect on composition decisions. For psychoeducational groups, only the most disruptive of patients need to be excluded. Intensive treatment settings have the most severely ill patients and rely on milieu factors to reinforce the small group effects. Outpatient interactional groups are generally designed for longer term therapy and require stronger evidence of motivation and ability to use the interactional environment of the group in an effective manner.

Group size.   The question of how many members to have in the group is dependent on the objectives. If the group is designed to provide a relatively brief psychoeducational or supportive function, then the size may be larger than in the other two categories. As the membership increases beyond 10 or 12 members, the interactional characteristics shift. Of necessity, such groups become more leader-oriented. It becomes inappropriate to focus to a major extent on interpersonal events in such settings. Larger groups are most useful for the provision of educational information, for boosting morale and motivation, and for screening patients for additional therapy.

   If the group is designed for the control or containment functions of intensive treatment programs or for psychotherapeutic work focusing on interpersonal learning, then group size needs to be kept to a maximum of about 10 members. Over this limit, the number of possible relationship connections within the group rapidly increases and becomes unmanageable for both the members and the therapist. It is the responsibility of the therapist to clearly define the expectations for the group in advance and make size decisions accordingly.

Homogeneous versus heterogeneous groups.   The next composition decision is whether to treat the patient with an eating disorder in a general psychotherapy group or in one that is homogeneous to the disorder. Here there is greater variability of opinion. In eating disorder clinics, the general preference is for homogeneous groups. In a private office setting, low numbers may make this unrealistic. Because the majority of patients with eating disorder problems are able to present a controlled and effective social front, they often fail to benefit from therapy in heterogeneous groups because the group cannot come to grips with the more subtle nature of their "hidden" psychopathology. This is a strong rationale for homogeneous groups.

   If it is necessary to use heterogeneous groups, the patient with an eating disorder should be carefully prepared for the group experience. This should include an explicit expectation that the patient will review for the group the nature of general adaptational problems at an early point. The specifics of the eating pattern are best dealt with in parallel individual sessions, so that they do not become the focus of group concern and a mechanism by which the patient can control and divert the group interaction. In heterogeneous groups, it is best to consider the group experience as being for the person, not the eating symptoms per se.

A more subtle issue in terms of group composition is whether to mix patients who are primarily suffering from restrictive eating problems with those who have bulimic symptoms. A common problem with mixing the two disorders is that the group members view the restrictive patient as having been more "successful" in her control of body image. This may stimulate reactions of envy and competition. On the other hand, patients with restrictive disorders do not view themselves as having psychological difficulties to the same extent as those with bulimic symptoms. A group setting may prove more effective than an individual therapist at breaking through this denial. Thus, it may benefit a patient with restrictive eating problems to be in a group that is heterogeneous for eating disorders. There are enough overlapping features that mixing the two diagnostic categories can usually be accomplished. These include hypersensitivity to the judgment and criticism of others, low self-esteem, secretiveness, isolation, difficulty identifying and expressing affect, interpersonal difficulties, and family dysfunction (Bruch 1982; Hendren et al. 1987; Rosman et al. 1977; Strober 1980). Homogeneity can also be achieved by composing groups according to age. This is discussed in more detail in Chapter 5.

Overall, groups for patients with eating disorders are more effective when there is a significant degree of homogeneity within the membership. In this group environment, defensive behaviors are more readily identified and less easily denied. In eating disorder clinic settings, there is often an opportunity to begin all patients in a brief information based program and then to select from that experience those who need and can tolerate a more intensive group approach. Homogeneity is particularly important when the group experience is time-limited. A group in which members can quickly identify with each other will move more quickly through preliminary group stages; therefore, such a group will have more time available for intensive work (MacKenzie et al. 1986).

Pretherapy Preparation

There is substantial evidence in the empirical group literature that the systematic preparation of patients for the group experience helps to diminish the number of early dropouts and to promote the development of group cohesion (Piper and Perrault 1989). The effects of such preparation will likely wash out after the first few sessions as the actual group experiences are encountered. Pretherapy preparation, if it results in lower early drop-out rates, ensures that the new members are in the group long enough to have an exposure to group therapeutic factors. The pretherapy material can be presented in a group format, on an individual basis, or through some combination of the two. The advantage of the group format is that it is a more realistic setting and allows a controlled entry into the experience of the group process. Simple structured group exercises can be used to desensitize the members to the anxiety of participating in a small group. Such a pretherapy approach also allows the therapist to make final assessment decisions regarding the suitability of the individual for group work.

The pretherapy material can be effectively presented in individual sessions, but there is a danger that the patient will develop a strong therapeutic alliance with the individual therapist. The transition into a group may be seen as the loss of a privileged status. Therefore, such individual sessions should be limited in number and should be constantly reframed as primarily for the purpose of assessment and preparation for the group experience. There are some advantages to this being done by the future group therapist. Identification with the group therapist may facilitate a patient's entry into the group and deter premature termination during the early stage of engagement, when disillusionment and disappointment are commonly experienced. When cotherapy is used, the preparation tasks should also be done together to lessen the risk of future splitting.

Retention of pretherapy preparation material is enhanced by a handout that is reviewed in detail with the potential group member (MacKenzie 1990). It is useful to give the patient a general orientation to the use of group psychotherapy and the idea that the group situation is one in which there is an opportunity to look at the effects of the eating disorder on close relationships. Some group programs have a former group member meet with a prospective member to discuss their impressions of the group experience. Patients have found these meetings with former group members to be particularly useful in allaying some of their fears about group therapy and instilling hope about the efficacy of the treatment.

Some common misconceptions about groups should be specifically addressed. These include the idea that group psychotherapy is a cheaper, second-rate treatment. Most new group members fear that the group will become a forced confessional and that they may get worse by being with other patients. This idea of "mental contagion" and loss of control is particularly common. Members also commonly fear that they will not be able to fit into the group or that they will be judged harshly by the other members. All of these anticipatory fears should be normalized and explained.

It is then useful to discuss with the patients how to get the most out of the group, a "role induction" for effective group membership. They should be told of the importance of speaking as openly and honestly as possible and of trying to understand and make sense of what others say to them and what they say to others. One way of putting this is to say that the group is a living laboratory in which they can try out new ways of relating. It should be emphasized that the more they put into this interaction, the more they will get out of it. A simple discussion of the mechanisms of self-disclosure, feedback between members, and application to outside circumstances can be stressed.

The importance of confidentiality, attendance, punctuality, and no use of drugs or alcohol in or preceding the sessions should be mentioned. Group observation, the use of two-way mirrors, and video procedures should be reviewed if they are to be part of the group format. It is important that patients understand the time frame for the group experience. A number of issues require particular clarification for patients with eating disorders who are in more intensive groups: the role of the leader; dealing with negativity and feelings of dissatisfaction regarding an individual or group progress; attendance concerns; and extra-group socializing.

The leader should be defined as one who encourages interaction and helps to focus issues but who does not supply specific answers. It is also useful to predict that, with time, the members may find themselves experiencing negative reactions of irritation or disagreement. These should be described as expected and in need of discussion. Many patients with eating disorders have specific difficulty dealing with negative affect. This prediction will probably not be taken seriously initially but can be used as a point of reference later in the group. Similarly, it is useful to speculate that occasions will arise when the members might feel frustrated and disillusioned about their progress in the group or with the group itself. They may find themselves thinking about dropping out. These experiences are also discussed as normal reactions to the difficult tasks of therapy. It is stressed that it is what the member does with these feelings that is important, not the fact that they arise. The member is strongly encouraged to talk about them with the group, preferably at the time they occur.

It is common for patients with eating disorders to be fearful and reluctant to negotiate time off with their employers. To ensure their punctuality at group meetings, it is crucial that this situation be managed prior to the group's beginning. Some members have found it helpful to practice this negotiation process through role-playing. In addition, the therapist may need to provide employers of some group members with a covering letter.

Because members in eating disorder groups usually have a great many concerns in common, there is a particularly strong pull toward extra-group contacts. In all but strictly support and psychoeducational groups, extra-group social contacts are not encouraged. These contacts may take the form of acting out against "parental" figures. The tendency toward enmeshed relationships with ambivalence about independence and control makes such relationships potentially disruptive to the interpersonal work of the intensive group. For instance, a member may become reluctant to give a friend open and honest feedback in the group to avoid hurting or betraying that member. Furthermore, a member may be reluctant to turn full attention to another member in the anticipation that the friend may become jealous. A developing friendship may quickly take precedence over group involvement—something which, in retrospect, members typically voice regretting (MacKenzie et al. 1985). Members who are not included in the extra-group socializing often report feeling left out, rejected, and insignificant (MacKenzie et al. 1985).

The fact that members may want to befriend or socialize with one another is normalized. Verbalizing these extra-group desires as they occur in the group is encouraged, and these revelations can be very important in the patients' understanding of themselves and their relationships. What they are encouraged to refrain from is acting on these wishes outside the group. It is useful to remind the group that its function is to help one another in learning how to form close, meaningful relationships, but not to actually provide the relationships (Yalom 1985). The group members are asked to establish a contract that in the event they do meet outside the group, they will assume responsibility for disclosing the key aspects of that encounter inside the group. An exception to these cautions concerning extra-group socializing is found in the specialized support group format described in Chapter 13.

Pretherapy preparation may be presented in a few minutes to members going into a brief psychoeducational group, or it may occupy several individual sessions for patients going into more intensive psychotherapy groups. Clinic settings may present it in a group context. The important basic idea is that pretherapy preparation is helpful in diminishing the number of early dropouts and fostering group cohesion and should be a systematic part of any group program.

The Group System

In the early stages of any group, the therapist must pay particular attention to the emerging sense of group identity. In technical terms, this refers to the establishment of the group as a separate social system with committed members engaged in important tasks.

Group Cohesion

The most critical task of a new group is the development of a sense of group cohesion. It is relatively easy to tell when there is a high level of group spirit and commitment to the group task. This feeling of groupness evokes a basic sense of belonging to and acceptance from the group that is above and beyond the relationship with any single member, including the leader. Groups that are cohesive are characterized by regular and punctual attendance; few premature terminations; high levels of active participation, risk-taking, and self-disclosure; and low levels of defensiveness and tensions. This idea of group cohesion is analogous to that of the "therapeutic alliance" in individual psychotherapy (Bordin 1979; Docherty 1985). The establishment of a strong positive alliance early in therapy is a good predictor of positive outcome.

In the early group, the role of the leader is particularly prominent, and members will take their cue from the therapist's behavior. The group therapist must conceptualize the leadership role during the early sessions in terms of the primary need to develop cohesion. The leader can facilitate cohesion by prompting, reinforcing, and, if necessary, modeling behaviors drawn from the "supportive" therapeutic factors described in the next section. A manifest display of expectation, enthusiasm, and eagerness to get to work will help. Professionals experienced in individual therapy sometimes find this difficult to contemplate, because it seems to smack of nontherapeutic situations such as sports teams or social situations. However, the group will take its lead from the attitudes of the leader, who must emphasize this sense of a joint undertaking of a common task.

Reinforcing Therapeutic Factors

There is a considerable body of literature concerning the positive contribution of a number of therapeutic factors operating in groups (Bloch and Crouch 1985). Although some of these are found in individual therapy, a number are unique to the group situation or at least are expressed in a markedly different fashion. All of these therapeutic factors are more likely to occur in cohesive groups, and groups that show a lot of these factors will also be described as cohesive. There is thus a natural interaction between the two ways of describing the group. The therapeutic factors can be usefully clustered into four major categories (see Table 2–1).

Supportive factors. The first category may be called the "supportive" factors. Instillation of hope is a common factor to all therapeutic endeavors. It relieves anxiety and enhances motivation. Acceptance by the group is another powerful common factor. It is also important in individual therapy, but in groups it takes on a special significance. Acceptance by peers in the group will be seen to be earned rather than taken as a given of the therapeutic situation. Another therapeutic factor in this cluster is that of universality, the understanding that one's experience is not unique and

Table 2–1.   Therapeutic factors

Supportive factors
  Instillation of hope
  Acceptance
  Universality
  Altruism

Self-revelation factors
  Self-disclosure
  Catharsis

Learning from others factors
  Modeling
  Vicarious learning
  Guidance
  Education

Psychological work factors
  Receiving feedback
  Trying out new behaviors
  Insight
  Corrective emotional experience

that others have had similar experiences or reactions. This sense of commonality is a strong motivator to increase group interaction and serves to address the distress of social isolation. The final supportive factor is that of altruism. In groups, as opposed to individual therapy, it is common for members to experience helpful interactions with others in the group. This idea that one can help someone else strongly reinforces self-esteem. These four therapeutic factors are highly correlated. However, it is useful to identify them specifically so that the therapist can reinforce their emergence. This group of factors is particularly crucial during the early sessions of a group but continues as an important sustaining dimension throughout the group's life.

Self-revelation factors.   There are two "self-revelation" factors, self-disclosure of factual information and catharsis of deeply felt emotion. These are worth considering separately, because they may not necessarily occur simultaneously. Self-disclosure refers to the revelation of factual information about the self. Usually this begins with relatively superficial information, a process facilitated by pretherapy preparation. The therapist must be alert to patients who begin to reveal highly charged personal information too early. Such secret material is often tinged with reactions of guilt or shame. Patients who are ahead of the group in such self-disclosure are at increased risk for premature termination: it is as if they get in over their depth, regret the disclosure, and handle the situation by withdrawing altogether.

Catharsis of deep emotion is a powerful therapeutic factor. The therapist's role is to modulate the expression so that it can be constructively contained. This may be accomplished by asking patients to talk about how the revelation was experienced, if they feel in control again, and if they are able to manage after the session. It is often helpful to encourage patients to link the meaning of the events with the affect produced. This cognitive work helps to bind the affect. Similarly, patients who self-disclose without accompanying affect may need to be encouraged to probe their reactions to the events being described. The therapist must make operational decisions regarding the appropriateness of the self-revelation in the context of the stage of the group and its objectives. If it seems wise to dampen self-revelation, it must be done sensitively so that the patient does not interpret the intervention to mean that the material is objectionable or too powerful ever to be addressed. The therapist might comment that what the patient is discussing is clearly very important and that it will be useful to explore it further when the members have gotten to know each other better, or in the next phase of treatment, or in individual sessions, and so on.

Learning from others factors. A third category of therapeutic factors can be termed "learning from others." These are more cognitive in nature. Learning may occur through modeling new behavior on that of other members or the leader. Group members routinely report the importance of vicarious learning in a group. They observe the interaction between other group members and then privately apply it to their own circumstances. All groups provide a substantial amount of guidance that may be explicit, as in cognitive behavioral therapeutic strategies, or buried in the general group interaction. This may be made more specific in terms of educational information, a common component for patients with eating disorders. The language of education is quite appropriate with such terms as learning, new ways of understanding, and homework. These factors are not emphasized in the psychodynamic group psychotherapy literature, but they occur with great regularity in all groups. The therapist needs to be alert to the presence of these factors in order to reinforce them and to ensure that they are being used in a constructive fashion.

Psychological work factors. The final set of therapeutic factors contains "psychological work" factors. These include interpersonal learning both through trying out new behaviors and receiving feedback concerning one's own behavior. This may be connected with the development of insight into new ways of understanding the self. These processes tend to become mixed together in the interpersonal learning process. One advantage of the group context is the variety of relationships available for such learning and the accelerated tempo of this once the group becomes cohesive. These "psychological work" factors are more characteristic of advanced group work, because they are dependent on a well-established sense of group membership and familiarity with the other members.

A major responsibility of the therapist early in the group's life is to mold the development of a therapeutic group milieu. The factors listed here are important ingredients of such a milieu. The therapeutic task may be conceptualized as one of reinforcing these types of events as they emerge in the natural group interaction. Simple, encouraging "uh-huh"s and identifying comments, such as "it sounds like you two have had pretty similar experiences," allow the therapeutic processes to be more explicitly recognized by the group members. In general, groups undertake their work eagerly, and these factors, particularly the "supportive" group, emerge spontaneously at an early point. When this is the case, the therapist can ease out of the interaction and monitor its ongoing evolution. When the factors are not developing readily, the therapist may need to model them or specifically elicit them from the members.

In the early stages of a group, the therapist must place priority on the evolving group system. Failure to do so will result in a fragmented group in which members become disillusioned or nonproductively anxious. It is important to monitor that all members are participating during the early sessions and that no member is becoming overly self-disclosing or excessively attacked.

Managing Developmental Stages

Another useful way of understanding groups is the idea that social systems progress through a series of stages, each of which can be characterized as having a set of common tasks (MacKenzie and Livesley 1983). This is a parallel conceptualization to that of individual growth and development. A simple model of group development consists of four stages: engagement stage, differentiation stage, interpersonal work stage, and termination stage (see Table 2–2).

Engagement stage.   The first stage, engagement, is critical to the development of a sense of groupness. This process is particularly driven by experiences of universality, when members appreciate that they have had similar experiences and so can understand each other. These experiences provide material around which the group may coalesce. This process usu-

Table 2–2.   Developmental stages in groups

Stage	Group task	Individual task	Therapist task
1. Engagement	Develop group identity and cohesion through preliminary self-disclosure and universality	A willingness to become part of the group social system demonstrated by a commitment to participate and establish regular attendance	Promote group cohesion by actively encouraging self-revelation and providing a safe, noncritical holding environment
2. Differentiation	Develop mechanism of conflict resolution through cooperative exploration, assertion of ideas and beliefs	Learn to tolerate and deal with differences, conflict, and anger	Actively facilitate the expression of differences and anger. Promote the exploration of the members' perceptions and understanding of the conflict
3. Working Phase			
a) Individuation	Develop a deeper understanding of the individual through self-disclosure and reflective introspection	Develop receptivity to psychological exploration and demonstrate increased acceptance of self and others	Facilitate introspective, collaborative exploration and accompanying affective states. Help patient integrate group content with group process to maximize interpersonal awareness
b) Intimacy	Experience, manage, and explore implications of close interpersonal involvement. Allow reciprocal influence	Accept self as capable of closeness and having significance to someone else	Promote intermember interactions. Model and encourage nondefensive openness. Emphasize interpretations that encourage generalizability to patient's current difficulties
c) Mutuality	Develop understanding of mutual responsibility and equality in relationships. Appreciate fundamental uniqueness of each member	Accept implications of one's actions	Facilitate the acceptance of personal responsibility in relationships through direct translation and application of here-and-now to outside relations
4. Termination	Incorporate group experience as beneficial and applicable to external situations. Allow individual autonomy	Acceptance of responsibility for self. Deal with loss and separation	Promote reflection on history of group. Encourage exploration of projected objectives, future plans

ally comprises relatively superficial and often factual self-disclosure. For the participant, this may be quite anxiety producing, but once accomplished, it consolidates each member's sense of participation. The therapeutic factors from the "supportive" cluster are particularly in evidence during this first stage.

Differentiation stage. The second stage, differentiation, moves the group on from the theme of commonality of the engagement stage. The members begin to demonstrate their own personal identity in the group and become differentiated as more complex individuals. This is accompanied by an increase in tension or conflict and may be characterized by a high degree of polarization. The task for the group is to develop a mechanism for the cooperative exploration of differences. When developed, this allows the group to be both supportive and constructively confronting. Individual members may feel quite threatened by this process, as may the leader, particularly when the group as a whole becomes polarized regarding leadership activity. However, this process is a critical one if the group is to advance to a more complex working atmosphere. The differentiation stage has some resemblance to the features of early adolescence.

Interpersonal work stage. Once the tasks of engagement and differentiation have been mastered, the group is ready to move on to more complex interpersonal work. The focus on the individual member increases and is usually accompanied by higher degrees of introspective work. Although the content focus is initially concerned with how each member works internally, the process remains an interactive one. The group now has the capability of being both supportive and confronting. The process of self-exploration is accompanied by deeper levels of self-revelation that may deal with hidden material critical to self-esteem. As the members begin to understand themselves in more complex ways, they are also drawn into closer relationships. These will deal with the experience of intimacy and the implications of being important to another. They will also raise the question of responsibility in relationships, a balance between excessive dependency or exploitation of others. During this stage, interpersonal learning is maximized, and the therapist needs to keep the members focused on the meaning of group events in terms of their relationships with each other.

Termination stage. It is critical that the group address the final stage, termination. The disengagement process is a delicate one and, if avoided, may undo earlier group work. It is useful to review the history of the group and compare and contrast its evolution. Issues of sadness and loss, as well as anger at having to discontinue the group, will commonly need to be addressed. If these themes are adequately worked through, they are accompanied by an increased acceptance of responsibility for self.

Social roles. The work of the engagement stage is facilitated by those members who tend to see relationships in positive terms and can provide support and structure. These members are important throughout the group's life in promoting cohesive events. In the differentiation stage, the activities of members who tend to be more confronting and critical are particularly important. This idea of different social roles can be used by the therapist in making decisions about what sorts of activities from what sorts of members are best elicited and reinforced—or best dampened and discouraged. Often such guidelines can be applied to specific critical incidents that can be evaluated in terms of their appropriateness to a particular stage in the group's life. One might consider effective therapy as a process by which the individual learns a greater degree of role flexibility so that responses can be tailored to the situation rather than made in a stereotyped or automatic fashion.

The idea of group developmental tasks is particularly useful in the context of therapeutic objectives. If a group is designed primarily for psychoeducational activities, or will be meeting for only a brief time, then it is unlikely that the style of group interaction will progress beyond that of the engagement stage. In this situation, the leader may need to be active in dampening more negative dimensions and instead should promote a learning process that centers around the experiences described previously under the therapeutic factors of the "supportive" and "learning from others" categories and the tasks of the engagement stage. This can also be viewed from the opposite direction. If a group is designed to address the more confrontational objectives of interpersonal learning and has the time available to do so, then the therapist must encourage the group through the first two stages so that the group will return to a more positively valenced working atmosphere before it ends. The group experience will be seen by the members through the filter of the final sessions. If these are quite tumultuous in nature, then useful therapeutic effects may be undone. The stage development perspective provides the leader with some guidelines for making these decisions.

Open or Closed Groups

The preceding discussion of group cohesion, therapeutic factors, and developmental stages emphasizes the importance of using the group environment to maximum advantage. Many operational decisions are connected to the level at which the group is able to operate, and time is an important factor in these decisions. There are some major advantages to using closed groups. The members can move together into deeper interaction, and the therapist can evaluate the progress of each member against that of the others in deciding who or what to encourage, reinforce, or dampen. This is particularly true when using time-limited groups.

There is less need to focus on group development in long-term group psychotherapy, and a slow-open policy is appropriate. It is always wise to admit new members in pairs so that the entry process can be shared. Any change in group membership results in a new social system, and the group must go back to a beginning stage. In ongoing open groups, the group developmental tasks are played out between the older members and the new. If the group has had a well-established working atmosphere, this process may happen quite quickly and the group can get back to its work. The new members can benefit from the established group norms. It is difficult for groups to sustain a major changeover of membership. In circumstances where the new group will be composed of one-half new and one-half old members, it is often wiser to terminate the previous group altogether and begin again.

Therapeutic Strategies

The group therapist must feel comfortable in riding the waves of group interaction without the need to actively control it, particularly in the more intensive groups. Members will experience a strong desire to make the group work and will usually actively dive in if modest guidance and permission are given. Generally, the therapist can lead the group by following the interaction. A lot of therapeutic mileage can be achieved by simply identifying and subtly reinforcing interactions that fit under the list of therapeutic factors. In this way, the group members will see that they themselves are creating a helpful environment. The therapist must be alert that the group is progressing smoothly and that no harmful events are taking place. Above all, the therapist must continuously encourage and, if necessary, direct members to talk to and with each other more than with the therapist.

Therapist Style

Four dimensions of therapist style have been shown to correlate with outcome (Dies 1983, 1985; Lieberman et al. 1973). These four patterns are useful in conceptualizing one's own therapeutic behavior:

1. Therapists who demonstrate a caring and supportive approach tend to have groups in which the members have better outcomes. This is analogous to the effects of a positive therapeutic alliance in individual therapy.
2. Therapists who are interested in promoting an understanding of

group events, in helping members to make sense of them, and in establishing meaning from behavior also tend to have better outcomes.

3. The level of specific control that the therapist exerts in the group is also related to outcome, but in a different manner. Therapists who show few efforts to control the group interaction tend to have poorer outcomes. Therapists who are highly controlling also have poorer outcomes. Thus, more effective group work is associated with moderate levels of control in which the therapist works to guide the group toward the enactment of therapeutic factors and to maintain a working focus without simultaneously assuming stringent control of the group.

4. A similar curvilinear association is found with a dimension of therapist behavior described as emotional stimulation. Therapists who appear uninvolved in the group and show no sense of excitement or interest have groups with the same characteristics. Charismatic leaders who exhort the group to model themselves on therapist behaviors and who may be highly intrusive in their expectations of how strongly members should participate also have poorer overall outcomes. Such therapists tend to have positive results for some members, but also a higher incidence of negative effects. By the force of their personalities, they may pull members to deeper levels of interaction than can be tolerated.

Using the Therapeutic Factors

Earlier in this chapter groups were categorized according to the degree of focus to be placed on interpersonal learning. This dimension is also useful when considering therapeutic strategies. If the group has a largely psychoeducational or supportive function, then the therapist should emphasize therapeutic factors from the supportive cluster. Although these factors tend to be particularly evident in early group interactions, they are at the same time quite powerful. The experience of acceptance and universality is effective in ameliorating anxiety-mediated symptoms and in enhancing self-esteem. For many patients, this allows them to regain a sense of control and self-efficacy that generates a positive cycle of improvement. The effect of learning from others is also a benign influence and often a part of brief groups as well as longer term groups.

Extensive use of factors from the psychological work cluster may interfere with the establishment of early group cohesion. Thus, in the early stages the therapist should interpret material according to themes of commonality, not search for underlying personal meanings or make abstract interpretations. Similarly, the level of self-revelation needs to be monitored as described previously. The therapist should function as a "rate controller" regarding the level of self-disclosure and match this to the objectives and stage of the group. The therapist has a therapeutic responsibility to mold the interaction in a direction that will be most helpful for the group members. The theoretical material in this chapter provides some guidelines that may be useful in this task.

Process Versus Content

The group therapist must be in a position to consider both the content and the process of the group interaction. Although this is true of individual therapy as well, the force of social opinion in a group may make it more difficult. The therapist should practice adopting an observing, distancing position regularly during a group session. Ask the question, "Why is this sort of behavior going on between the members?" Irrespective of the content being discussed, what are these people trying to get from each other?

Therapists who have extensive experience in treating patients with eating disorders may not automatically utilize the group environment. Indeed, experience in individual therapy may work against the recognition of group level events. Behavior may be interpreted primarily from an intrapsychic framework without recognition of its contextual significance in intermember events. Even if the group is conceptualized as primarily an educational process, these group interactional phenomena will be occurring simultaneously. The learning process can be enhanced by actively promoting them. For example, if a member expresses surprise at hearing that some of her own behaviors are shared by others, the therapist can shift out of an educational mode and into a group facilitative mode to encourage broader exploration of the experience of universality amongst the group members. By promoting these sorts of experiences, the therapist will be consolidating and deepening the impact of the educational experience as well.

The most powerful group learning takes place when the members can experience an interaction in the group and then replay it to understand its significance. This idea of using the group interaction as the basis for a "corrective emotional experience" is central to effective group work. It applies to brief educational groups as much as it applies to longer term intensive psychotherapy groups. The difference is only in the nature of the material to be reinforced or examined. The key to successful group therapy is to effectively identify and address with the members what they are experiencing together. For example, asking a member in a psychoeducational group what it was like to hear that others carried out the same sort of purging activities may encourage a powerful normalizing effect that makes mastery of the hidden behavior more likely. Similarly, in a group that is actively exploring interpersonal issues, it might be helpful to ask questions such as "What did it mean to you (or what was your reaction) to being criticized just now? Are these the sorts of events that make you think of bingeing?"

Attention to group process should run in parallel to the clarification of content themes. This applies to all types of groups, from brief supportive programs to longer term intensive psychodynamic formats. The therapist should be continually scanning the group for interactional clues and feeding them into the discussion. When completing group summaries, equal weight should be given to process events as to content material. Drawing a group interaction diagram showing who talked to whom can be helpful in alerting the therapist to process patterns. Supervision can also be balanced between individual content and interactional significance.

Using the Potential of Members

Much of the helpful experience of therapy groups comes not from the therapist but from the members themselves. The expression of concern and support among the members is very helpful in overcoming low self-esteem. The sense of belonging also reinforces self-worth. The group therapist is a much less central figure than the individual therapist. This calls for a change of orientation. The therapist can extend helpful effects by systematically encouraging each group member to act in therapeutic ways. One particularly useful technique is to promote clarification questions: "I didn't quite understand what you meant by that." "Could you say a bit more about the reaction you just had?" This simple technique is quite powerful in promoting a self-exploratory process. It reinforces personal autonomy because the individual must speak for herself. The enhancement of autonomy is particularly important to patients with eating disorders, who frequently experience the need to satisfy the expectations of others. At the same time, as members become skilled in making such interventions, they experience the therapeutic factor of altruism by seeing that their questions are helpful to others.

Therapist Format: Single or Cotherapy

The decision about using a single or cotherapy format should be thoughtfully made. For more intensive groups, it is not recommended that a single male therapist lead a group that is likely to be almost totally made up of female patients. This is asking for a polarization around an authoritarian figure who will be seen as both all-powerful and ultimately depriving. This has nothing to do with the actual person. Eating disorder symptoms have a powerful connection with social stereotypes and expectations regarding gender-specific attitudes and behaviors. A female leader is able to present a role model with whom the patients will find it much easier to align. Parental issues will come to the fore as the group develops but can be addressed on a foundation of goodwill and identification that enhances effective working-through. If a single male therapist is necessary, the role issues need to be addressed early and repeatedly in the group. There would be an advantage for the male therapist to adopt an approach that eschews technical expertise and emphasizes noncontrolling support and interest.

The addition of a cotherapist adds to the complexity of the group system. Even though intermember learning is an important part of the group experience, the role of the leader is a special one and the source of considerable group attention. Adding a second therapist does not just double the opportunities for this. Each therapist will be seen as an individual, but also as part of the leadership subsystem. There will be opportunities to divide the leadership and work one against the other. If the intent is to provide a "parental" image, then the cotherapists should be of opposite sex. If the intent is to provide support for an anxious therapist, then the matter should be reexamined. Cotherapy is a task for the more experienced therapist, not the beginner. It should be chosen for specific reasons, not just as program policy. The empirical literature carries no support for advantages of the cotherapy model and many warnings about its problems.

Cotherapists are best selected voluntarily, not assigned administratively. The nature of the cotherapy function should be regularly reviewed. This requires an open and nondefensive attitude. Common problems revolve around competitive strivings with each trying to have more influence or to get a particular effect. Patients with eating disorders know this territory well and can take full advantage of the circumstances to split the therapists. Sometimes cotherapists use their relationship as a refuge from taking responsibility: "I was going to say something, but I thought you were just going to do it so I held off."

There seems to be little advantage in using two same-gender therapists. Two female therapists will not provide the gender-specific stimulus that justifies doubling the staff involvement; a group led by two male therapists risks extreme danger of polarizing and perhaps shutting down an investigation of female-male relationship issues.

The most logical approach to cotherapy is a female-male pair. This might have some real advantages, but only if the two therapists are comfortable dealing with the nature of their own relationship in the group. For the long-term psychodynamic group, such a cotherapy team has unique advantages in recreating the parental configuration of the primary family and providing a broader array of transference opportunities. In these circumstances, the relationship between the therapists is designed to serve as a parental model for the members, who will certainly be very alert to all the nuances of communication between the two therapists. When group members talk to each other outside of the therapists' presence, it can be guaranteed that the nature of the therapists' relationship will be the source of much speculation. Therefore, the most important prerequisite for coleadership is that the cotherapists are comfortable working together and can maintain a relationship in which support, respect, and complementarity are accentuated. They must be able to demonstrate this in the group, and they cannot remain oblivious to each other's presence in the room. Cotherapists should be able to discuss their reactions to group events in the session, speculate about what is going on, and openly support each other. As the group advances, cotherapists also must be able to model disagreement and the resolution of different perspectives and reactions. There are inherent dangers in a male physician-female nurse team. Role expectations and power dimensions that are extrinsic to the actual relationship between the coleaders will pose problems. If such a pairing is to work effectively, it must be developed carefully and with a willingness to be open about the issues in the group itself.

Supervision

Intensive group therapy with patients with eating disorders is notoriously difficult. By the nature of the disorder, these patients are adept at presenting a helpful and compliant face to the world while covertly sabotaging their successful adaptation to it. They are past masters at managing parental-type relationships to the advantage of their pathology. They are also skillful at testing therapeutic blind spots and will actively or passively challenge the role and power of the therapist. All of these features will emerge during serious group therapy and are enhanced by the pressure of the group system. This underscores the importance for the therapist to have both expertise in conducting interpersonal groups and a solid understanding of eating disorders. It is highly recommended that therapists conducting such groups get systematic supervision, regardless of their level of expertise.

Supervision enables therapists to keep abreast of their reactions and countertransferences to group events. A therapist may find he or she is masking anger at a patient who resists assuming the role of the "good" child. Therapists may overidentify with the patients and lose sight of the dysfunctional nature of their behavior. Competition between the therapists may arise assisted by attempts by the members to split the therapists into "good" parent and "bad" parent. In addition, supervision can help examine the therapist's own personal issues and beliefs surrounding weight and body image. Use of video playback can be particularly helpful. If cotherapy is being used, then special attention must be paid to the nature of that relationship as enacted within the group.

Summary

The selection of therapeutic techniques in groups rests on a careful decision regarding group objectives. In particular, the implications of the group format will determine if the therapeutic milieu should be held in early group mechanisms of support and universalization, or encouraged to move on through more conflictual material into advanced stages of interpersonal work. With both approaches, the therapist should maximize the inherent advantages of a group format by systematically reinforcing intermember learning and validation. This can most effectively be accomplished by subtle guidance of the ongoing flow of group interaction in keeping with guidelines provided by therapeutic factors and group stage development.

References

Bloch S, Crouch E: Therapeutic Factors in Group Psychotherapy. Oxford, Oxford University Press, 1985

Bordin ES: The generalizability of the psychoanalytic concept of the working alliance. Psychotherapy: Theory, Research and Practice 16:252–260, 1979

Bruch H: Anorexia nervosa: therapy and theory. Am J Psychiatry 139:1531–1538, 1982

Budman SH, Demby A, Redondo JP, et al: Comparative outcome in time-limited individual and group psychotherapy. Int J Group Psychother 38:63–86, 1988

Dies RR: Clinical implications of research on leadership in short-term group psychotherapy, in Advances in Group Therapy. Edited by Dies R, MacKenzie KR. New York, International Universities Press, 1983, pp 27–78

Dies RR: Leadership in short-term group therapy: Manipulation or facilitation? Int J Group Psychother 35:435–455, 1985

Docherty JP: The therapeutic alliance and treatment outcome, in Psychiatric Update: American Psychiatric Association Annual Review, Vol 4. Edited by Hales RE, Frances AJ. Washington, DC, American Psychiatric Press, 1985

Garfield SL, Bergin AE: Handbook of Psychotherapy and Behavior Change. New York, John Wiley, 1986

Hendren RL, Atkins DM, Sumner CR, et al: Model for the group treatment of eating disorders. Int J Group Psychother 37(4):589–602, 1987

Lieberman MA, Yalom ID, Miles MB: Encounter Groups: First Facts. New York, Basic Books, 1973

MacKenzie KR: Introduction to Time-Limited Group Psychotherapy. Washington, DC, American Psychiatric Press, 1990

MacKenzie KR, Livesley WJ: A developmental model for brief group therapy, in Advances in Group Psychotherapy: Integrating Research and Practice. Edited by Dies RR, MacKenzie KR. New York, International Universities Press, 1983, pp 101–115

MacKenzie KR, Coleman M, Harper H, et al: Critical Therapeutic Events in the Group Treatment of Bulimia Nervosa. Paper presented at the annual conference of the Canadian Group Psychotherapy Association, Banff, Alberta, October 1985

MacKenzie KR, Livesley WJ, Coleman M, et al: Short-term group psychotherapy for bulimia nervosa. Psychiatric Annals 16:699–708, 1986

Pilkonis PA, Imber SD, Lewis P, et al: A comparative outcome study of individual, group, and conjoint psychotherapy. Arch Gen Psychiatry 41:431–437, 1984

Piper WE, Debbane EG, Bienvenu JP, et al: A comparative study of four forms of psychotherapy. J Consult Clin Psychol 52:268–279, 1984

Piper WE, Perrault EL: Pretherapy preparation for group members. Int J Group Psychother 39:17–34, 1989

Rosman BL, Minuchin S, Baker L, et al: A family approach to anorexia nervosa: study, treatment, outcome, in Anorexia Nervosa. Edited by Vigersly RA. New York, Raven, 1977, pp 341–348

Rutan JS, Stone WN: Psychodynamic Group Psychotherapy. Lexington, MA, Collamore Press, 1984

Strober M: Personality and symptomatological features in young, non-chronic anorexia nervosa patients. J Psychosom Res 24:353–359, 1980

Toseland RW, Siporin M: When to recommend group treatment: a review of the clinical and group literature. Int J Group Psychother 36:171–201, 1986

Yalom ID: The Theory and Practice of Group Psychotherapy, 3rd Edition. New York, Basic Books, 1985

3

Medical Assessment and Management

Sidney H. Kennedy, M.B., F.R.C.P.(C)
Jacqueline Duncan, M.B., M.R.C.Psych.
K. Roy MacKenzie, M.D., F.R.C.P.(C)

◆ ◆ ◆ ◆ ◆ ◆ ◆ ◆ ◆

The medical management of patients with eating disorders in group therapy is critical, given the serious and possibly life-threatening nature of the disorder. Although some group programs are able to assess and monitor the medical needs on an "in-house" basis, others, such as private practice programs, may rely on establishing a medical liaison with an outside medical consultant. Regardless of what arrangement is made, it is imperative that patients with eating disorders be medically screened prior to actual placement in any of the various group treatments. An easily accessed communication network between the group therapist and the attending medical physician and nutritionist also needs to be established at the outset of group treatment. Instances will arise when the medical and/or psychiatric condition of a patient with an eating disorder worsens during the course of group treatment. Circumstances will vary as to whether a member can remain in the group while his or her condition stabilizes or whether a temporary or permanent withdrawal is indicated.—The Editors

The purpose of this chapter is to present a basic framework for assessing and managing the medical needs of patients with anorexia nervosa (AN) and bulimia nervosa (BN) while they are undergoing group treatment. Regardless of the type of group modality, it is critical that patients with eating disorders have their medical and nutritional safety ensured first. This can be a complex process, because the needs and possible medical complications of these patients can vary markedly. For some patients, minimal or no medical/nutritional intervention will be required, whereas for other patients, emergency or ongoing medical/nutritional attention may be in order. Accurate assessment and management of these needs necessitate a complete understanding of the major clinical features of AN and BN as reviewed in Chapter 1 and as detailed elsewhere (see Garfinkel and Garner 1982; Johnson and Connors 1987).

Early Recognition

Often family and friends of a person with an eating disorder are oblivious to the gradual changes in behavior and appearance that may occur over months or even years. With AN there is often a narrowing of food choices, with a preference for "diet foods," avoidance of red meats, sauces, desserts, and other "high-calorie foods." The anorexic patient may become increasingly absent from family dining, offering excuses that she "has already eaten" or "will eat later." Visits to the bathroom become prolonged and may be associated with vomiting and abuse of laxatives or diuretics. Excessive exercise is common, often pursued with an obsessive determination: it is no longer a sociable activity, and is seen solely as a means of burning off calories. There may also be a withdrawal from social activities, particularly those involving eating or drinking. Apart from weight loss, early changes in appearance may include a deterioration in the texture of scalp hair, hair loss, dry or pigmented skin, and cold extremities.

Clinical Assessment

History Taking

The standard psychiatric inquiry needs to be expanded to include information about recent and past eating habits, especially food restriction, practices of weight control, binge eating, and methods of purging. Asking a patient to review a typical day during the past few weeks helps to put eating behavior in context. Details should be obtained of current weight including actual weighing, previous highest and lowest weights and weight over the range of developmental periods: preschool, elementary school, puberty, early adulthood, and so on. Similar attention should be paid to weight fluctuations since the eating disorder began. Particular attention should be paid to weight during periods when normal eating, activity, and menstrual function occurred in order to gain an idea of that individual's "set point." It is also helpful to inquire about the patient's perceived "ideal weight" and about any particular "phobic weight" criteria—for example, never to weigh more than 99 pounds.

Because of the frequent comorbidity of depression and substance/alcohol abuse, particularly among patients with BN, exploration of these areas should also be routine. Because about 30% of patients treated in the Toronto Program during recent years disclose a history of childhood sexual abuse, it is important to facilitate such disclosure during preliminary assessment (DeGroot et al., in press). A variety of characterologic features are associated with the eating disorders and a survey of Axis II syndromes should be conducted. Impulsive, obsessive, and avoidant features are particularly relevant.

Physical and Laboratory Examinations

Most abnormal physical and laboratory findings occur as a result of starvation and metabolic disturbances. Discernible clinical or laboratory abnormalities are likely to occur in those individuals who have lost more than 20% average body weight (Kaplan and Woodside 1987) and in those indulging in daily vomiting practices.

Fluid and electrolyte imbalance give rise to concern in both AN and BN patients. Life-threatening potassium loss with hypokalemia may result from restricted intake, vomiting, and diuretic or laxative misuse. Cardiac conduction disturbances, hypokalemic nephropathy, and smooth or skeletal muscle paralysis can also occur. Bradycardia and hypokalemic arrhythmias are the commonest cardiac abnormalities and can prove fatal.

Common physical complaints of starvation include cold intolerance, constipation, and abdominal pain. Amenorrhea occurs in most cases and generally follows weight loss. Gastrointestinal complications include a delay in the rate of gastric emptying, particularly for solid foods, and an elevation of liver enzymes. Anemia, leukopenia, and thrombocytopenia may all be associated with the starved state. Thyroid indices (T3, T4, and TSH) may also be decreased in association with elevated levels of reverse T3. Generalized cerebral and cerebellar atrophy associated with ventricular enlargement have also been reported in AN patients.

Although fewer studies have been reported involving patients with BN, there are several physical complications associated with the act of repeated binge eating and vomiting. Common findings include facial puffiness, parotid gland enlargement, dental enamel erosion and accompanying toothache, abdominal pain, menstrual irregularities, and callus formation on the back of the hand (Fairburn 1990). Less common complications of binge eating include pancreatitis, dehydration, epileptic seizures, renal damage, abdominal dilation, and gastric rupture. Purgative misuse may lead to steatorrhea, edema, and finger clubbing. The persistent misuse of emetics such as ipecac to induce vomiting after bingeing may result in cardiomyopathy, which may be fatal (Johnson and Connors 1987).

Exhaustive laboratory investigations are not indicated in the diagnosis or management of AN or BN. Routine testing might include complete blood count; serum electrolyte levels; and thyroid, renal, and liver function tests, as well as electrocardiography. These should be followed over time as indicated. Serum amylase levels may provide an index of vomiting, whereas elevation of creatinine kinase may occur following ingestion of ipecac. The principal medical complications of the eating disorders are summarized in Table 3–1.

Neuroendocrine and Neurotransmitter Abnormalities

Most biological disturbances in patients with AN and BN appear to be secondary to the consequences of starvation and metabolic imbalances (Garfinkel and Kaplan 1985). These include disturbances of the hypothalamic pituitary axes to the thyroid, adrenal, and gonadal organs. These are reviewed in greater detail in Kennedy and Garfinkel (1987).

The noradrenergic (NE) and serotonergic (5HT) neurotransmitter systems have been the focus of extensive research for two reasons. First, animal studies have directly implicated these systems in mediating eating behavior (Liebowitz 1983; Morley and Levine 1983). Increased intrasynaptic norepinephrine is associated with an increase in food consumption, whereas an increase in intrasynaptic serotonin tends to reduce food consumption. Second, these are the systems in which consistent abnormalities have been reported in different groups of psychiatric disorders, including depression, obsessive-compulsive disorder, and eating disorders (Crow and Deakin 1985). In patients with BN, residual abnormalities of both systems have persisted beyond weight restoration, raising the question of a trait rather than a state-related abnormality (Kaye et al. 1984, 1990b). At the neuroendocrine level, recent work suggests that a disturbance of central nervous system corticotropin releasing hormone (CRH) is likely to be responsible for hypercortisolemia in AN and BN patients (Kaye et al. 1989).

The importance of this work is not yet clear. Some of the reported changes could be related to nutritional status, stress, high activity level, or electrolyte disturbance. The available studies are essentially correlational in nature and the etiological significance of the changes is unknown.

Comorbidity With Other Psychiatric Disorders

Depression

The relationship between eating disorders and mood disorder, particu-

Table 3–1.   Complications of anorexia nervosa and bulimia nervosa

Complication	Cause	Treatment
Cardiovascular system		
Peripheral cyanosis	Starvation	Weight and fluid restoration
Bradycardia	Starvation	Weight and fluid restoration
Hypotension	Starvation	Weight and fluid restoration
Arrhythmias	Starvation/hypokalemia	May need potassium supplements
Cardiomyopathy	Starvation/ipecac abuse	Weight restoration/stop ipecac
Metabolic		
Hypokalemia	Vomiting, diarrhea	Correct starvation and dehydration
Hyponatremia	Laxative abuse, diuretic abuse	May need potassium supplements
Increased serum amylase	Usually secondary to vomiting	Stop bingeing and purging
Edema	Starvation, bingeing, refeeding	Weight and fluid restoration
Increased blood urea nitrogen	Dehydration	Weight and fluid restoration
Gastrointestinal		
Dental caries	Acid from vomitus	Dental consultation
Parotitis	Bingeing and vomiting	Stop bingeing and purging
Bloating/early satiety	Starvation	Domperidone 10–20 mg tid
Constipation	Starvation	Use diet; try to avoid laxatives
Diarrhea	Laxative abuse	Gradually reduce laxatives
Esophageal or gastric dilation or rupture	Very rare: results from severe bingeing, vomiting, or rapid refeeding	Medical emergency
Pancreatitis	Secondary to large binges or starvation	
Endocrine		
Amenorrhea	Low weight, emotional stress, chaotic eating	Restore weight to 90% of average
Hypothermia	Starvation	Restore weight to 90% of average
Increased growth hormone levels	Starvation	Restore weight to 90% of average
Increased cortisol levels	Starvation	Restore weight to 90% of average
Decreased T3, T4	Starvation	Restore weight to 90% of average
Musculoskeletal		
Delayed bone maturation	Starvation	Refeeding
Reduced stature		Increased calcium intake
Osteoporosis		
Hematologic		
Mild anemia	Starvation	Weight restoration
Low white blood cell count		Balanced diet
Low erythrocyte sedimentation rate		May need iron supplement
Neurologic		
Seizures	Secondary to metabolic abnormality	Correct abnormality Neurologic evaluation
Dermatologic		
Dry skin and nails	Starvation	Weight restoration
Thinning scalp hair	Starvation	Weight restoration
Lanugo (downy hair)	Starvation	Weight restoration
Carotene pigmentation	Starvation	Weight restoration
Callus formation on hands	Repeated induction of vomiting	Stop bingeing and vomiting
Irritation at corners of mouth	Repeated induction of vomiting	Stop bingeing and vomiting

larly depression, has been considered extensively (Kennedy and Walsh 1987; Strober and Katz 1988) and has important treatment implications. Although there is substantial evidence to argue against a simple shared diathesis model linking eating disorders and mood disorders, the longitudinal course of people with both AN and BN emphasizes considerable overlap. Over 50% of people with AN or BN have lifetime diagnoses of mood disorders, and following remission of eating disorder symptoms, there is a high prevalence of recurrent depression (Toner et al. 1986).

Recent studies have found that normal weight bulimic patients have lowered cerebrospinal fluid (CSF) and plasma norepinephrine concentrations. Just the reverse is true in depression. In addition, antidepressants reduce the frequency of binge eating in nondepressed bulimic patients. These findings suggest that normal weight bulimia is not a subtype of depressive disorder but a separate illness with its own unique neurobiological profile (Kaye et al. 1990a).

Obsessive-Compulsive Disorder (OCD)

Similarities also exist between OCD and eating disorders with regard to such symptoms as feeding rituals, compulsive exercise, and preoccupation with body image (Solyom et al. 1982). Family histories (Dilsaver and White 1986) and neuroendocrine abnormalities (Hollander et al. 1990) are also found in common. Kaye and colleagues (1990c) found elevated levels of 5-HIAA, the major brain serotonin metabolite, in weight-restored anorexic patients. This suggests a trait-related condition and is similar to the disturbance in serotinin activity that has been implicated in the pathogenesis of OCD. Clinical response is found in both conditions to pharmacotherapy with serotonin-uptake inhibitors such as fluoxetine and clomipramine (Solyom et al. 1989; Weltzin et al. 1990). The relationship has also been supported by demonstrating comorbidity in the opposite direction. Kasvikis and colleagues (1986) and Rasmussen and Eisen (1988) reported that 10% and 17%, respectively, of OCD patients had "an eating disorder," although this was not confirmed in a study by Joffe and Swinson (1987), who examined only current eating disorder symptoms.

Personality Disorder

A third area of comorbidity related to AN and BN involves personality disorder. According to DSM-III-R (American Psychiatric Association 1987) Axis II, three clusters are recognized: an eccentric or odd group (paranoid, schizoid, and schizotypal); an impulsive or dramatic group (borderline, narcissistic, histrionic, and antisocial); and an anxious or fearful group (avoidant, dependent, compulsive, and passive-aggressive).

When AN patients were categorized according to the presence or absence of bulimic symptoms, those with the combined AN+BN diagnosis showed more impulsive features, including substance abuse, self-harmful behavior, and sexual promiscuity (Garfinkel and Garner 1982). Piran and colleagues (1988) have also reported a high rate of the impulsive disorders among AN+BN subjects; 55% had borderline personality disorder. The same authors reported a high rate of anxious disorders in the AN group; 60% met criteria for avoidant personality disorder. However, recent findings indicate a significant reduction in most personality disorder diagnoses when a self-report measure (The Millon Clinical Multiaxial Inventory [MCMI]) was administered to hospital patients with AN or BN before and after treatment (Kennedy et al., in press). Personality disorder considerations are hampered by controversy over diagnostic approaches and measurement instruments with only modestly adequate psychometric properties.

Principles of Medical Management

Treatment approaches must take into account medical problems, eating behaviors, and psychological issues. During the last decade, the Program for Eating Disorders in Toronto has developed treatment interventions along a spectrum of intensity ranging from intensive day hospital and inpatient treatments to psychoeducation and cognitive group psychotherapy on an outpatient basis to intensive longer term psychotherapy (see Figure 3–1). Such group treatment interventions are addressed in other chapters of this book. First priority must be paid to the "track one" issues of nutritional stabilization and the correction of medical complications when they are present.

Starvation

Most patients with AN are able to start treatment on an outpatient basis. The effects of starvation on a person's thinking, emotions, and behavior need to be corrected before the factors that initiated or helped to maintain the fear of gaining weight can be addressed. A program of regular meals supervised by family members may be tried. When weight loss continues or increases, admission to hospital is indicated. One guideline is persistent maintenance of weight below 70% of a previous healthy body weight. Elective inpatient treatment for AN generally involves refeeding, weight restoration, and reintegration into "normal" life patterns. The average length of stay is about 12 weeks.

Even patients who appear to have been surviving on minimal quantities of food before admission to a hospital are able to consume a 1,500-calorie diet on admission. Refeeding edema, if it occurs, should be carefully monitored but rarely requires specific treatment. "Health food" diets, in-cluding vegetarianism, are regarded as an expression of anorexic thinking and are not permitted. The aim is to facilitate a weight gain of 1 to 1.5 kg (2 to 3 lb) per week, which can be achieved by increasing caloric intake grad-ually, in increments of 300 calories. Liquid supplements are to replace food not taken at regular mealtimes, and may also be preferable when patients require more than 3,000 calories per day to continue gaining weight. There is no absolute certainty about the correct target weight for each patient, but it is reasonable to aim for a premorbid weight at which normal menstrual function occurred in the absence of excessive weight or body shape preoc-cupation. This should provide a body mass index greater than 20. Patients should stay in hospital for at least 2 weeks after they reach the target weight range.

Food refusal can pose a major challenge. It also has the effect of limit-

Figure 3–1. Overview of eating disorder programs at the Toronto Hospital (1990)

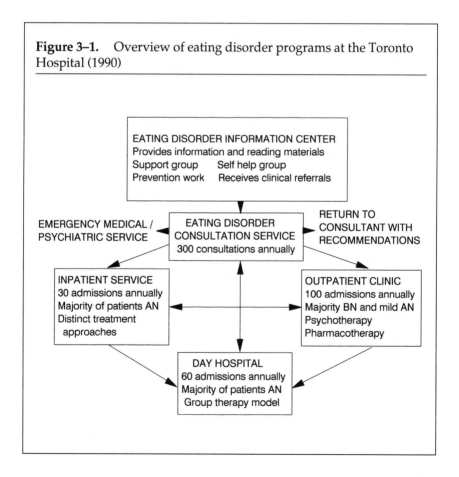

ing interventions by staff in other areas of treatment, such as family or group psychotherapy. On the rare occasion when nasogastric tube feeding is considered necessary, clear goals of tube feeding should be stated in advance. For example, a contract can be made stating, "the tube is to be inserted and used up to a weight of 38 kg (84 lb); it will then remain in situ but normal meals will be offered, and only if meals are not completed will the tube be used to give supplementation. At 41 kg (90 lb) the tube will be removed." This circumvents recurrent battles around the removal of the tube before the patient is able to demonstrate control over eating.

Breaking the Binge and Purge Cycle

A variety of approaches have been shown to improve bulimic symptoms significantly. In addition to the above described standard techniques of refeeding and nutritional stabilization, it can be helpful to offer small amounts of binge foods under supervised conditions using an "exposure with response prevention" technique. Anxiety symptoms become less severe after each exposure. This behavioral technique has the effect of breaking the association between a particular food and uncontrolled eating. This can be useful in developing a normalized eating pattern. Keeping a diary of food intake as well as of purges, associated mood states, and daily events may help point out behavior patterns that are likely to trigger binge eating. Self-monitoring helps patients take measures to master difficulties they previously regarded as outside their control.

Patients are encouraged to follow a rigid "three meals a day" plan and to avoid missing meals even if they have binged. They are advised to increase the daily intake gradually to include a wide range of foods and to allow their bodies to find a body weight "set point" that can be maintained without dieting or bingeing activities. The rationale for this is based on increasing evidence that dietary restraint can perpetuate bulimic behavior.

Emergency Admissions

The most common reason for emergency admission is an acute metabolic crisis. This usually involves a dangerously low potassium level due to an increased rate of vomiting. This responds quickly to oral replacement. It is best to limit treatment to management of the immediate crisis as the impulsive quality to such events is often made worse by inpatient care. The same approach can be taken to impulsive suicidal behavior unless it occurs in the context of a positively diagnosed major depression.

For example, a 22-year-old female BN patient was in her fourth week of an outpatient psychoeducational group when she complained of severe dizziness and muscle cramping. Upon questioning, the patient admitted to increased vomiting episodes over the week, ranging from 3 to 5 times per day, as well as laxative and alcohol abuse. A medical consult was arranged for the following day and she was hospitalized with hypokalemia (potassium level of 2.4 mmole/l). During her brief hospitalization, the patient's electrolyte balance was restored and she was weaned off laxatives. She continued to attend the group sessions during her hospitalization.

Most individuals with BN can be treated as outpatients or day patients. However, admission to an inpatient unit may be necessary and beneficial when serious medical complications are present (see Table 3–1). Admission may also be indicated when patients are very depressed or suicidal, if further assessment and observation are necessary to clarify the diagnosis, or if outpatient treatment has failed and an admission is necessary to interrupt the binge-purge cycle. The following case is an example.

> A 28-year-old single male with borderline personality features, a past history of obesity, and a 7-year history of AN+BN required brief hospitalization midway through his involvement in a day hospital eating disorder program. This patient became very distraught at the rate of his weight restoration. He started to engage in self-mutilation (i.e., burning and laceration of arms), voiced feeling very depressed, started to experience suicidal ideation, had no social support network in the city, and did not regard his home environment as providing him enough safety. He was subsequently hospitalized for 1 week during which time his suicidal ideation abated and he was able to refrain from self-harm behaviors. Following his inpatient discharge, the patient was able to resume his group treatment in the day hospital program.

Pharmacotherapy

There are no specific "anti-anorexia nervosa" agents. Nevertheless, anxiety and depression are common in people who have AN. For the occasional patient for whom anxiety before meals is a major obstacle to progress, short-acting benzodiazepines taken half an hour before meals can have a beneficial effect.

Patients who have an overwhelming urge to exercise or pace around the ward may benefit from a neuroleptic given in small doses for a limited period of time. In both instances, the potential hazards of these agents must be balanced against their beneficial effects. For some, a gastrokinetic agent, such as Domperidone, given about 30 minutes before meals, can alleviate the sense of gastric bloating experienced after eating. The issue of when to prescribe antidepressants to patients with AN is complex. In general, it would be reasonable to wait until the effects of acute starvation are no longer apparent and offer antidepressants only when neurovegetative symptoms persist in association with a depressed mood (Goldbloom et al. 1989). Because of the hypothesized association between AN and serotonin metabolism, it would be reasonable to initiate treatment with serotonin-uptake inhibitors such as fluoxetine or clomipramine.

There is evidence of at least short-term benefit from antidepressants among outpatients with BN, whether or not they have a concurrent depressive illness. In controlled trials, tricyclics such as imipramine or desipramine (Agras et al. 1987; Hughes et al. 1986; Pope et al. 1983), as well as the monoamine oxidase (MAO) inhibitors phenelzine and isocarboxazid (Kennedy et al. 1988; Walsh et al. 1988), have been found beneficial in decreasing bulimic symptoms. Fluoxetine has also been shown to have "antibulimic" effects (Fluoxetine Bulimia Nervosa Collaborative Study Group, in press).

Desipramine and fluoxetine are usually drugs of first choice for BN. Contrary to expectations, bulimic patients do not seem to have carbohydrate craving or significant weight gain secondary to antidepressants. A typical regimen for desipramine would start with 50 mg at night, increasing every 2 to 4 days as tolerated until a therapeutic dosage is reached (usually 200 mg at bedtime). Plasma levels are particularly valuable for desipramine in determining therapeutic levels in bulimic patients. Fluoxetine dose begins at 20 mg and can be slowly raised, bearing in mind that stable blood levels are not achieved for 4 to 5 weeks. The main guide, as always, is the patient's clinical response to the medication, which should be evident within 3 to 4 weeks for desipramine and 4 to 5 weeks for fluoxetine. If patients respond well, the drug should be maintained for 4 to 6 months.

Outcome Studies

Despite a better understanding of risk factors and the role of starvation in perpetuating AN, morbidity and mortality rates remain alarmingly high (Theander 1985; Toner et al. 1986). Keeping people who have a chronic form of the disorder alive and providing effective follow-up treatment for them are important challenges for clinicians. Once life-threatening emaciation is under control, it is reasonable to offer an intensive psychotherapeutic course, preferably in a group format. For those severe anorexic patients who have not responded to these measures, a low-demand, supportive, long-term approach seems most helpful (see Chapter 13).

The more severe forms of BN do not appear to be a short-lived disorder (Abraham et al. 1983; Swift et al. 1987) and it is important that patients learn strategies to prevent relapse. This may involve recognizing "at risk" times, planning alternative activities, and restructuring their time. Psychotherapeutic approaches can help patients manage emotions and interpersonal relationships in more functional ways. Both professional and social support may be required for months or years.

The natural history of the eating disorders is not well understood and it remains uncertain which factors influence prognosis. Large fluctuations in weight, high impulsivity, a history of associated substance abuse or affective disorder, poor psychosocial adjustment, high levels of suspiciousness and distrust, and low self-esteem have all been cited as predictors of lower response to treatment. A lengthy history also predicts poor outcome. This might indicate that vigorous treatment at an early point in the course may prevent further deterioration. Longer term outcome studies are required to confirm this point.

Measuring Clinical Change

The process of change with psychotherapy is complex and involves a number of dimensions and viewpoints, ranging from the highly subjective to the specifically objective. There is general agreement that the measures selected to document clinical change should tap a range of symptoms, various areas of functioning, and different viewpoints, and include both behavioral and subjective measures. It is useful to solicit data from the patient, the therapist, and the clinical record. For more elaborate studies, trained raters might be used and information sought from significant others in the patient's outside world. The type of information desired usually includes psychiatric symptoms, social functioning, target goals, and a general measure of adaptation. For the eating disorder population it would be useful to obtain measures specific to eating behaviors and attitudes as well as an assessment of interpersonal functioning. The following short list of available instruments is offered as an introduction to the possibilities (Table 3–2).

Clinical Record

Age, sex, and marital status are standard demographic measures. Social class can be calculated from education level and occupation category. All of these may be relevant variables in assessing treatment effectiveness. Health statistics provide a "hard" measure of service utilization and the medical record provides an accessible source. These might include days in hospital, outpatient visits, and visits to the emergency room. It is interesting to compare such measures in the 6 months before treatment and in a comparable period after it has ended.

Symptom Checklist (SCL-90-R).   The SCL-90-R is a standard self-report symptom inventory. Results are expressed on a number of symptom dimensions, such as depression and interpersonal sensitivity. A Global Severity Index gives an overall measure of symptom status (Derogatis 1977).

Table 3–2.   Change measures battery

Type of information	Source of information		
	Patient	Therapist	Clinical record
Demographics/ statistics			Data sheet Service utilization
Symptoms	SCL-90-R		
Social functioning	SAS		
Interpersonal functioning	IIP		
Individual measure	TG	TG	
General functioning		GAFS	
Eating behavior	EAT/EDI		

Source. SCL-90-R = Symptom Checklist (Derogatis 1977); SAS = Social Adjustment Scale (Weissman and Bothwell 1976); IIP = Inventory of Interpersonal Problems (Horowitz et al. 1988); TG = Target Goals; GAFS = Global Assessment of Functioning Scale; EAT/EDI = Eating Attitudes Test/Eating Disorder Inventory (Garner and Garfinkel 1979; Garner et al. 1983).

Social Adjustment Scale (SAS).   The SAS is a 60-item self-report instrument that taps behavior and satisfaction in a range of social functions such as work, family, and leisure activities (Weissman and Bothwell 1976).

Target Goals (TG).   A simple TG form can be completed by both the patient and the therapist. This helps to establish some direction for treatment and creates a collaborative approach to problems the patient sees as important.

Global Assessment of Functioning Scale (GAFS).   The GAFS is included as Axis V of the DSM-III-R multiaxial system. It is a simple way to record overall clinical judgment regarding how the patient is functioning.

Inventory of Interpersonal Problems (IIP).   The IIP is a relatively new instrument designed as a companion to the SCL-90-R, but taps issues concerning relationships such as sociability, assertiveness, and control (Horowitz et al. 1988).

Eating Attitudes Test (EAT).   The EAT is a short scale that measures symptoms of anorexia and is useful for identifying abnormal eating patterns (Garner and Garfinkel 1979).

Eating Disorder Inventory (EDI).   The EDI is a 64-item self-report instrument. It is more specific than the EAT and focuses on cognitive and behavioral dimensions that may be used to meaningfully differentiate subgroups of patients (Garner et al. 1983). The EDI contains the following scales:

1. Drive for thinness
2. Bulimia
3. Body dissatisfaction
4. Ineffectiveness
5. Perfectionism
6. Interpersonal distrust
7. Interoceptive awareness
8. Maturity fears

This battery of measures can be easily implemented in a clinical setting. All of the instruments have clear relevance to the therapeutic issues involved in treating eating disorders and "make sense" to patient and clinician alike.

Measuring Group Process

It is more difficult to measure the group process. The most accessible dimension has to do with the patients' perceptions of the cohesiveness of the group. This global concept has the best correlation with positive outcome and meshes nicely with the idea of the group as a stabilizing focus for the patient with an eating disorder.

Group Climate Questionnaire (GCQ).   This is a short 12-item instrument that yields a score on three dimensions: Engaged, Conflict, and Avoidance of Personal Responsibility. It is coupled with a Critical Incident form that provides interesting information about the patient's perceptions of the group process (MacKenzie 1983).

Group Environment Scale (GES).   This is a longer scale of 90 items that is clinically useful but too long for regular use in a clinical setting. It does contain a 10-item Cohesion subscale that could be used by itself (Moos 1974).

Summary

Treatment of patients with eating disorders represents a challenge to the clinician. In addition to the identification and management of complex psychodynamic issues, comorbidity with other disorders, and often significant character pathology, the clinician must be prepared to identify and treat the complex physical consequences of the behaviors engaged in by these patients. The use of standard measures can serve as an additional source of information regarding the progress of treatment.

References

Abraham SF, Mira M, Llewellyn-Jones D: A study of outcome. International Journal of Eating Disorders 2:175–180, 1983

Agras WS, Dorian B, Kirkley BG, et al: Imipramine in the treatment of bulimia: a double-blind placebo controlled study. International Journal of Eating Disorders 6:28–38, 1987

American Psychiatric Association: Diagnostic and Statistical Manual of Mental Disorders, 3rd Edition, Revised. Washington, DC, American Psychiatric Association, 1987

Crow TJ, Deakin JFW: Neurohumoral transmission, behavior and mental disorder, in Handbook of Psychiatry 5. Edited by Sheperd M, Zangwill OL. Cambridge, Cambridge University Press, 1985

DeGroot J, Kennedy SH, McVey G, et al: Sexual abuse: prevalence and impact on psychological profiles in anorexia nervosa and bulimia nervosa. Can J Psychiatry (in press)

Derogatis LR: SCL-90 administration, scoring and procedures manual—I. Baltimore, MD, Johns Hopkins University Press, 1977

Dilsaver SC, White K: Affective disorders and associated psychopathology: a family history study. J Clin Psychiatry 47:162–169, 1986

Fairburn CG: Bulimia nervosa. BMJ 300:485–487, 1990

Fluoxetine Bulimia Nervosa Collaborative Study Group: Fluoxetine in the treatment of bulimia nervosa: a multicentre placebo-controlled double blind trial. Arch Gen Psychiatry (in press)

Garner DM, Olmsted MP, Polivy J: Development and validation of a multi-dimensional eating disorder inventory for anorexia nervosa and bulimia. International Journal of Eating Disorders 2:15–34, 1983

Garner DM, Garfinkel PE: The eating attitudes test: an index of the symptoms of anorexia nervosa. Psychol Med 9:1–7, 1979

Garfinkel PE, Garner DM: Anorexia Nervosa: A Multidimensional Perspective. New York, Brunner/Mazel, 1982

Garfinkel PE, Kaplan AS: Starvation based perpetuating mechanisms in anorexia nervosa and bulimia. International Journal of Eating Disorders 4:651–665, 1985

Goldbloom DS, Kennedy SH, Kaplan AS, et al: Recent advances in pharmacotherapy: anorexia nervosa and bulimia nervosa. Can Med Assoc J 140:1149–1154, 1989

Hollander E, DeCarira C, Stein D, et al: Serotonin and eating dysregulation in obsessive compulsive disorder. Paper presented at the annual meeting of the American Psychiatric Association, New York, May 1990

Horowitz LM, Rosenberg SE, Baer BA, et al: Inventory of Interpersonal Problems: psychometric properties and clinical applications. J Consult Clin Psychol 56:885–892, 1988

Hughes PL, Wells LA, Cunningham CJ, et al: Treating bulimia with desipramine: a double blind placebo-controlled study. Arch Gen Psychiatry 43:182–186, 1986

Joffe RT, Swinson RP: Eating attitudes test scores of patients with obsessive compulsive disorder (letter). Am J Psychiatry 144:1510–1511, 1987

Johnson C, Connors ME: The Etiology and Treatment of Bulimia Nervosa: A Biopsychosocial Perspective. New York, Basic Books, 1987

Kaplan AS, Woodside DB: Biological aspects of anorexia nervosa and bulimia nervosa. J Consult Clin Psychol 55:645–653, 1987

Kasvikis YG, Tsakiris F, Marks IM, et al: Past history of anorexia nervosa in women with obsessive-compulsive disorder. International Journal of Eating Disorders 5:1069–1075, 1986

Kaye WH, Ebert MH, Gwirtsman HE, et al: Differences in brain serotoninergic metabolism between non-bulimic and bulimic patients with anorexia nervosa. Am J Psychiatry 141:1598–1601, 1984

Kaye WH, Berrettini WH, Gwirtsman HE, et al: Contribution of CNS neuropeptides (NPY, CRH, beta endorphin) alterations to psychophysiological abnormalities in anorexia nervosa. Psychopharmacol Bull 25:433–438, 1989

Kaye WH, Ballenger JC, Lydiard RB, et al: CSF monoamine levels in normal-weight bulimia: evidence for abnormal noradrenergic activity. Am J Psychiatry 147:225–229, 1990a

Kaye WH, Gwirtsman HE, George DT, et al: Disturbances of noradrenergic systems in normal weight bulimia: relationship to diet and menses. Biol Psychiatry 27:4–21, 1990b

Kaye WH, Weltzin TE, Hsu LK, et al: New evidence links anorexia nervosa to OCD. Paper presented at the annual meeting of the American Psychiatric Association, New York, May 1990 (1990c)

Kennedy SH, Garfinkel PE: Disorders of eating, in Handbook of Clinical Psychoneuroendocrinology. Edited by Nemeroff C, Loosen PE. New York, Guilford, 1987

Kennedy SH, Walsh BT: Drug therapies for eating disorders: monoamine oxidase inhibitors, in The Role of Drug Treatments for Eating Disorders. Edited by Garfinkel PE, Garner DM. New York, Brunner/Mazel, 1987

Kennedy SH, Piran N, Warsh JJ, et al: A trial of isocarboxazid in the treatment of bulimia nervosa. J Clin Psychopharmacol 8:391–396, 1988

Kennedy SH, McVey G, Katz R: The effect of treatment on self report measures of personality disorder in anorexia nervosa and bulimia nervosa. J Psychiatr Res 24(3):259–269, 1990

Liebowitz SF: Hypothalamil catecholamine systems controlling eating behavior: a potential model for anorexia nervosa, in Anorexia Nervosa: Recent Developments in Research. Edited by Darby PL, Garfinkel PE, Garner DM, Coscina DV. New York, Alan R. Lisa, 1983

MacKenzie KR: The clinical application of a group climate measure, in Advances in Group Psychotherapy: Integrating Research and Practice. Edited by Dies RR, MacKenzie KR. New York, International Universities Press, 1983

Moos RF: Evaluating Treatment Environments. New York, John Wiley, 1974

Morley JD, Levine AS: The central control of appetite. Lancet 1:398–401, 1983

Piran N, Lerner P, Garfinkel PE, et al: Personality disorders in anorexic patients. International Journal of Eating Disorders 7:470–475, 1988

Pope HG Jr, Hudson JI, Jones MM, et al: Bulimia treated with imipramine: a placebo-controlled double blind study. Am J Psychiatry 140:554–558, 1983

Rasmussen S, Eisen J: Clinical and epidemiological findings of significance in neuropharmacological trials in obsessive-compulsive disorder. Psychopharmacol Bull 24:465–469, 1988

Solyom L, Freeman R, Miles J: A comparative psychometric study of anorexia nervosa and obsessive neurosis. Can J Psychiatry 27:282–286, 1982

Solyom L, Solyom C, Ledwidge B: Trazodone treatment of bulimia nervosa. J Clin Psychopharmacol 9:287–290, 1989

Strober M, Katz JL: Depression in the eating disorders: a review and analysis of descriptive, family and biological findings, in Diagnostic Issues in Anorexia Nervosa and Bulimia Nervosa. Edited by Garner DM, Garfinkel PE. New York, Brunner/Mazel, 1988

Swift WJ, Ritholz M, Kalin NH, et al: A follow-up study of thirty hospitalized bulimics. Psychosom Med 49:45–55, 1987

Theander S: Outcome and prognosis in anorexia and bulimia: some results of previous investigators compared with those of a long-term study. J Psychiatr Res 19:493–508, 1985

Toner BB, Garfinkel PE, Garner DM: Long-term follow-up of anorexia nervosa. Psychosom Med 48:520–529, 1986

Walsh BT, Gladis M, Roose SP, et al: Phenelzine vs. placebo in 50 patients with bulimia. Arch Gen Psychiatry 45:471–475, 1988

Weissman MM, Bothwell S: Assessment of social adjustment by patient self-report. Arch Gen Psychiatry 33:1111–1115, 1976

Weltzin TE, Kay WHI, Hsu LKG, et al: Fluoxetine improves outcome in anorexia nervosa. Paper presented at the annual meeting of the American Psychiatric Association, New York, May 1990

4

Cognitive-Behavioral Group Treatment for Bulimia Nervosa: Integrating Psychoeducation and Psychotherapy

Ron Davis, Ph.D., C.Psych.
Marion P. Olmsted, Ph.D., C.Psych.

♦ ♦ ♦ ♦ ♦ ♦ ♦ ♦

A psychoeducational component forms an integral part of most treatment formats for eating disorders. Specific incorrect beliefs are almost universal in patients with eating disorders. These are best addressed directly in conjunction with whatever other techniques are also employed. The psychoeducational program described here for patients with bulimia nervosa is based on a cognitive-behavioral model of eating disorders and is specifically designed for a group modality. It represents one of the least intrusive treatment approaches. For most bulimia nervosa patients, this sort of group will serve as an adjunctive component of their overall treatment. For a substantial minority, it may be sufficient without the need for additional treatment. This is particularly true for patients who have a recent onset of an eating disorder and exhibit less psychopathology. A psychoeducational group provides an excellent opportunity to assess a patient's suitability for more intensive psychotherapy.—The Editors

This chapter outlines several therapeutic principles and practical considerations in applying cognitive-behavioral (CB) psychotherapy to the group treatment of bulimia nervosa (BN). A brief overview of the current status of research on CB psychotherapy is provided and a CB model of the eating disorders is presented. A detailed description of a brief group psychoeducation program follows along with an overview of some of the issues involved in the integration of group psychoeducation and CB psychotherapy.

Current Status of Cognitive-Behavioral Psychotherapy

There is currently no empirical evidence to suggest that group CB psychotherapy is more efficacious in the treatment of BN than other psychosocial or physical treatments. Controlled comparative studies regarding the efficacy of CB psychotherapy in BN are not available. It is therefore left to clinical judgment to select the approach that makes most sense. No single approach is suited to the needs of all patients. This chapter presents one approach that may serve to broaden the range of therapeutic options available for those suffering from BN.

Research on the treatment of BN has burgeoned in the last few years; however, our knowledge in this area remains at a rudimentary stage. Virtually all of the published reports concerning the psychosocial treatment of BN have included cognitive and/or behavioral techniques in their psychotherapeutic approaches. This emphasis on CB treatment has several origins. Many of the early reports concerning therapeutic effects for BN used such techniques. They provided detailed descriptions of the treatment, thereby permitting replication at different centers (Fairburn 1985). The emergence of interest in BN occurred coincidentally with a "cognitive zeitgeist" in the broader field of mental health treatment (Fairburn 1988). It has also been suggested that CB principles are particularly appropriate to the treatment of patients with eating disorders because such individuals engage in clearly aberrant eating behaviors, and because their psychopathology appears to be rooted in specific cognitions and distortions related to body weight and shape (Garner et al. 1987).

A parallel bias toward group over individual CB therapy also characterizes the BN treatment literature. Cox and Merkel (1989) identified twice as many studies of group treatment as of individual treatment in their recent review. Yet, to date there has been only one direct comparison of individual and group modalities (Freeman et al. 1988), and conclusions regarding their relative efficacy would be premature. However, utilizing a meta-analytic approach, Garner and colleagues (1987) found that group treatments had twice the rate of dropouts compared to individual treatment studies. The bias toward group treatments for BN may be related to the prevalence of studies based on individuals who are recruited through the media, often from university campuses, to participate in research. The provision of group treatment may be viewed as sufficient for these individuals (Garner et al. 1987). Alternatively, in busy treatment centers, the ratio of patient demands to treatment resources may dictate the use of a group approach.

There have been several recent reviews of the BN treatment literature and for present purposes only four issues will be highlighted. First, despite the many methodological problems inherent in the current treatment research, it appears that symptom control does not spontaneously occur without treatment. There is substantial variability in outcomes across CB treatment studies, with abstinence rates in eating symptoms ranging from impressively high to abysmally low. Garner and colleagues (1987) reported a median posttreatment abstinence rate for vomiting of 33% in their review of 19 CB treatment studies. Second, while there is a consensus among recent reviewers that CB treatment for BN does generally seem to be effective, it is also clear that mechanisms responsible for change have not yet been identified (Cox and Merkel 1989; Fairburn 1988; Garner et al. 1987; Wilson and Smith 1987).

A third and related point concerns the tremendous variability across CB studies both in the relative emphasis on specific techniques and in the theoretical rationale for matching technique to the psychopathology of the individual patient. Cognitive-behavioral psychotherapy represents a hybrid of therapeutic techniques designed to effect change in cognition, affect, and behavior (Dobson 1988). In connection with BN, CB therapy does not denote one specific approach or set of techniques but, rather, refers to many different compositions drawn from the pool of cognitive and behavioral treatment strategies. Some of the more commonly employed techniques in the current CB treatments for BN include self-monitoring, stimulus control methods, psychoeducation, cognitive-restructuring, training in problem solving, developing coping skills, assertiveness training, and exposure with response prevention (see Garner et al. 1987). In some cases, CB techniques have been combined with psychodynamic or experiential features, while in other published studies there has been a more exclusive adherence to CB psychotherapy. Finally, in many reports the treatment has not been described in sufficient detail and, as Fairburn (1988) has noted even for specific CB procedures, there is no standard form of delivery.

A Cognitive-Behavioral Model of the Eating Disorders

The detailed description of a group psychoeducation program for BN that follows is firmly rooted in a cognitive-behavioral model of the eating disorders. The model is illustrated in Figure 4–1, which depicts three distinct layers of pathology. Each pathology is predicated on the one below. Dietary and biological chaos refers to the patient's chief and presenting complaint; namely, the symptoms of binge eating, compensatory behaviors of forced vomiting, laxative abuse, vigorous exercise, extreme dieting, and the attendant physical and psychological sequelae. The compensatory behaviors are understood to be rooted in the patient's body image disturbances of distortion and disparagement, which represent the middle layer of the pathology pyramid. Body image disturbance, in turn, is predicated upon the patient's deficiencies in self-concept, most notably a severely constricted range of self-definition and self-evaluation in which the body becomes objectified as the primary means of maintaining a faltering semblance of self-worth (see Appendix; Garner and Davis 1986). This is revealed in the ego-syntonic attitudes about controlling weight and shape reported by individuals with BN (see Table 4–1).

According to this pathology pyramid, different modalities of treat-

Figure 4–1. A model of the layers of psychopathology of the eating disorders.

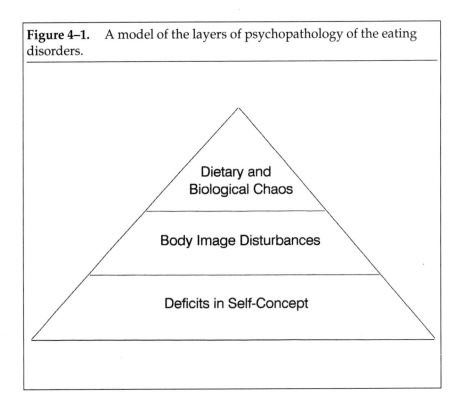

ment will have different ports of entry into the recovery process. Behavior therapies such as exposure with response prevention, stimulus control techniques, and physically based treatments such as nutrition therapy and pharmacotherapy enter from the top of the pyramid. They focus on the remission of eating symptoms or on the physical sequelae resulting from a nutritionally deprived and semistarved state. Psychodynamic modes of psychotherapy enter the recovery process from the bottom layer of the pyramid. They focus on difficulties with interpersonal relatedness and such intrapersonal issues as identity formation, object relations, and personality issues of perfectionism and impulse control. Multimodal approaches like CB psychotherapy simultaneously enter into the recovery process from all three layers, although it is important to note that in the early stages of treatment it is the top layer of the pyramid that becomes the principal focus of the CB therapeutic work. This is because psychological factors associated with the disorder may not be meaningfully assessed or addressed until the bulimic symptom pattern is brought under some degree of control (Garner and Davis 1986; Garner et al. 1990).

Table 4–1. Ego-syntonic nature of attitudes about weight and shape

% Agreement	Attitude
74	I have never felt better than when I lose weight.
65	Being at a low weight is the most important part of my identity.
60	My desire to be thin is the most important thing in my life.
58	Weight control is more important than anything else in my life.
54	If treatment means weight gain, I am not interested.
45	Restricting my food intake makes me feel special.
32	I would prefer to have all of my current problems than to gain weight.

Note. The data refer to the percentage of 95 patients who endorsed agreement with the item prior to participating in group psychoeducation. Patients met diagnostic criteria for bulimia nervosa or its subsyndromal variant.

Group Psychoeducation for Bulimia Nervosa

In their review of CB treatment studies, Garner and associates (1987) found that psychoeducation was an integral aspect of many CB treatments for BN. A psychoeducational program provides information about the nature of a disorder for the purposes of fostering attitudinal and behavioral change in the recipient. It is a didactic process whereby the practitioner thoughtfully distills and summarizes relevant scientific information to address questions such as "Why did I develop this problem?" and "What can I do to get better?" Most importantly, it involves the compassionate provision of advice and recommendations for self-care, which logically follow from the conceptual framework and scientific information provided by the practitioner.

Psychoeducation appears well suited to the treatment of eating disorders for a variety of reasons. There now exists a body of scientific literature supporting a multidetermined model of BN, which implicates sociocultural, psychological, and biological factors both in the development and perpetuation of the disorder. Patients with BN are invariably perplexed and distressed about certain core eating symptoms and associated sequelae. They seek concrete answers so that they can understand their own psychological and biological experience. BN patients are generally young and educated; many are still in school or have recently graduated. Most are not strangers to the quest for knowledge through the didactic process of formal learning.

Since 1986, we have been running brief psychoeducation groups for patients meeting diagnostic criteria for BN or its subsyndromal variant. The initial rationale for offering such treatment was based upon the clinical observation that a significant minority of BN patients responded well to information about the disorder and to specific recommendations for self-care without the clinical need for further treatment. We adopted a stepped-care model of treatment based on the philosophy that the least intrusive form of treatment should be attempted first, with more intensive treatments subsequently offered to meet the clinical needs of the patient (Garner et al. 1986). The psychoeducation group was conceived as being the first step in this sequencing of treatments for bulimic patients. We were also aware of another group of BN patients who were unable to readily engage in the therapeutic process. For some, ego-syntonic attitudes about the disorder resulted in panic and premature termination of therapy at the thought of change. Others exhibited borderline personality features that interfered with their ability to engage in the therapeutic relationship. For many of these patients, the psychoeducation group served as a benign introduction to the treatment process, which prepared them for more traditional psychotherapy.

The advantages of utilizing group psychoeducation as a first stage intervention are many. The didactic and brief nature of the group enables the therapist to conduct groups of virtually any size since the group process itself is not used as a major therapeutic factor. Thus, patients do not have to wait for a limited number of treatment spots. Patients are given the opportunity to learn about their disorder and strategies for self-care without the threat of having to self-disclose in the early stages of treatment. Finally, psychoeducation is a cost-effective first stage of treatment that is associated with symptom remission for a significant minority of patients. Intensive psychotherapy, which draws more heavily on treatment resources, can be reserved for individuals who do not respond well to brief group psychoeducation and who appear motivated for more challenging psychotherapeutic work.

Psychoeducation groups may vary both in the number of sessions and in the number of participants. Our groups have included 6 to 18 participants, and the number of sessions have ranged from 5 to 8. The program has evolved into a highly structured format consisting of 7 consecutive weekly meetings, each 1½ hours long. All patients referred to the program undergo a pretreatment assessment and preparatory meeting with the group leaders. The assessment utilizes semistructured interviews and self-report instruments designed to assess the extent and severity of specific eating pathology and associated psychopathology such as depression, personality features, and comorbidity of psychiatric diagnosis (Davis 1988; Davis et al. 1990). Patients who are acutely suicidal or in medical crisis are excluded. In addition, those who suffer from anorexia nervosa are considered inappropriate for group psychoeducation. The first two exclusion criteria generally apply to outpatient care. Patients with anorexia nervosa require more intensive treatment than that afforded by group psychoeducation, although they too will need to learn about their disorder.

Patients are informed that the purpose of the group is to help them to work toward a normalized relationship with food as the first essential step in their recovery process. They are explicitly told that the group is not designed to help them to achieve weight loss but, rather, to achieve biological and psychological stability, which for some may ultimately involve an increase in body weight. The following elements of a verbal therapeutic contract are discussed with each patient in the preparatory meeting: 1) to make a personal commitment to attend all of the meetings, 2) to complete and turn in weekly symptom self-monitoring forms, 3) to apprise their family physician of their enrollment in the program and that the family physician is responsible for monitoring their medical status, and 4) not to seek any form of concurrent treatment for their eating difficulties or for related psychological problems until the conclusion of the group psychoeducation program.

Each psychoeducation group meeting is highly structured. In essence, group leaders present a lecture to the participants, the topic of which follows a specific format. The lectures are paralleled by a participants' manual entitled *The Road to Recovery* (see Appendix). This manual is given to participants during the preparatory meeting and they are expected to read the corresponding sections in the manual prior to each meeting. Group leaders solicit opinions and comments from participants from time to time depending upon the topic under consideration, but in no instance do they explicitly ask participants to disclose personal information about themselves. Group leaders convey information and advice in a compassionate, professional manner that is often balanced with humor and identification with patient issues where appropriate—for example, the sociocultural pressures on women to be thin. When opinions are solicited from participants, group leaders accept them as being genuine beliefs held by the people. Challenging individuals about their ego-syntonic attitudes within this particular therapeutic context is avoided as it would only serve to alienate the patient and invite premature termination. However, challenging beliefs is an integral part of group CB psychotherapy to be discussed later in this chapter.

Each meeting is introduced by a list of organizing themes or topics to be covered by group leaders. These may be presented visually with a projector, chalkboard, or flipchart, or summarized in a handout. Most of the topics represent chapter or section headings from *The Road to Recovery*, which serves as an orientation for both participants and leaders.

Meeting 1: Overview of the Eating Disorders

◆ Orientation to the group
◆ Core features of the eating disorders
◆ Eating disorders and emotional distress
◆ Physical complications
◆ The fluctuating course of the eating disorders

Orientation to the group: From the moment they enter the group room, participants are seeking verification of the therapeutic contract and there should be no surprises. For example, if a group leader stated in the preparatory meeting that participants would not be expected to self-disclose, then it would be inappropriate to start the meeting by having participants introduce themselves or reveal personal agendas for being in the group. Similarly, the group setting must be arranged in the manner promised. In our group, the seating arrangement is intended to maximize the didactic process between leaders and participants, and at the same time to minimize the potential for group process among participants. Specifically, the lighting is dimmed to focus attention on the visual slides, and chairs are arranged facing the front of the room so that participants are in full view of the projector screen, chalkboard, and the group leaders who typically stand when addressing the group. If one wishes to foster a greater balance between didactic and group process, then seating might be arranged in the more conventional, circular manner to promote interaction among participants.

In the early minutes of the first meeting, group leaders review aspects of the therapeutic contract including the purposes and goals of the group, and issues of attendance, confidentiality, self-monitoring, and concurrent treatment. Leaders present a cognitive framework to participants that allows them to understand the function of the group and the manner in which they may use the experience to maximize personal benefit. This is an important issue to attend to as participants invariably wonder "Will the group help me?" We describe the group to participants as a catalyst for personal change rather than as an agent of personal change. Participants are told that the meetings are designed to inform them about a number of issues relevant to the process of recovery from an eating disorder, and that it is the information and the group setting that stimulate personal change. For any one participant, we cannot predict ahead of time how beneficial the experience will be, but we do give participants some suggestions that might increase their potential to benefit. We expect them to attend all of the meetings, to read the participants' manual, and to try and relate what they learn to their own situation. Self-knowledge is emphasized as a key aspect of personal change. We ask them to consider the period of time that they are involved in the group as a personal experiment, a period of time in which they should allow themselves to keep an open mind about what they learn and what they can do to facilitate their own recovery. This is particularly important, because some of the things that they will learn run counter to their ego-syntonic attitudes regarding weight, shape, and food. Finally, we encourage participants to be "risk takers" and to confront their beliefs and fears in a calculated way, yet at a pace that is comfortable for them.

Leaders must convey an attitude of patience and acceptance of the fact that each participant is different in her ability and readiness to apply strategies learned or to implement change. Participants are encouraged to try the suggestions that group leaders make and to observe what happens in as objective a manner as possible. We encourage participants to take personal credit for any changes they make in eating behavior and in the manner in which they view themselves. After all, changes come about through their own persistent efforts in examining beliefs about food, weight, shape, and any underlying issues that may serve to perpetuate their eating disorder. Most of this work occurs *outside* the psychoeducation group.

Core features of the eating disorders.   Participants are reminded that they are unique individuals with their own sets of strengths, life experiences, and goals for the future. Yet, by virtue of having an eating problem, each participant experiences certain issues common to other participants in the group. One set of issues involves the core features of anorexia nervosa and bulimia nervosa, which have been outlined in detail elsewhere (Davis 1988; Fairburn and Garner 1986; also see Appendix). The purpose of reviewing these features is to provide the participants with a framework within which they may begin to understand the interconnections among seemingly disparate affective, cognitive, behavioral, and biological difficulties that they face.

The first core feature is extreme concern about weight and shape that is a hallmark of both anorexia nervosa and bulimia nervosa. Concerns about weight and shape are by no means unique to individuals who have eating disorders, but appear widespread among North American women who live in a society that places a premium on their slenderness. Yet for the individual with an eating disorder, weight and shape are of such fundamental importance in determining self-worth as to render most, if not all, other pursuits secondary to achieving thinness. We ask participants to try thinking about why they feel uncomfortable with their body size. Body dissatisfaction is often a clue that there are deeper feelings of personal distress, a theme to be continued in Meeting 6. It is essential for leaders to convey the idea that weight control will not help participants to sort out inner emotional turmoil or to permanently raise self-worth. On the contrary, dieting serves to perpetuate the eating disorder and to distract the participant from meaningfully addressing any underlying psychological issues that may exist.

Extreme practices of weight control are the second hallmark of the eating disorders. Table 4–2 displays the frequency with which patients presenting to our center engage in various practices for weight control. Caloric restriction and forced vomiting are the most common methods of weight control in BN patients, and both are linked to the third core feature—binge eating. The body is equipped to handle short-term caloric restriction without much difficulty. Sustained restriction is, however, met with many biological and psychological consequences, one of which can be binge eating. Participants are informed that bingeing is a natural consequence of caloric deprivation, and the bingeing symptom is most likely to persist as long as the individual continues to diet. Regarding vomiting, participants are informed that it typically begins as a way of regaining control after bingeing but soon results in even greater breakdown in control since the vomiting "legitimizes" the binge (Garner et al. 1985). Participants are informed about the dangers of habitual vomiting, laxative and diuretic abuse, and vigorous exercise (see Physical Complications). The ineffectiveness of laxative and diuretic abuse for weight control is also described.

Maintenance of a low body weight is the fourth core feature of the eating disorders. While it is a diagnostic feature of anorexia nervosa, many individuals with bulimia nervosa are also below their "set point" or healthy natural body weight, even though they are at a statistically normal weight. Some individuals will not experience relief from acute caloric deprivation and the urge to binge until they achieve a healthier weight. Others are close to their natural weight, but fail to recognize this because of their chaotic relationship with food. While periods of restricted intake between binge episodes cause them to experience the effects of semistarvation, their binge eating allows their bodies to maintain a weight that is, in many cases, near or even above their natural weight range. In overcoming the eating disorder, participants are told that it is essential not to focus on weight change. The emphasis should be on normal eating and getting well. It is important to stress that eating is not an indulgence to feel guilty about or afraid of; it is a basic requirement of life.

As all members of the group experience episodes of binge eating, considerable attention is paid to a discussion of this symptom. An episode of binge eating is one in which the individual consumes an excessive amount

Table 4–2.   Practices of weight control in the eating disorders

Practice	Anorexia nervosa ($n = 79$–101) %	Bulimia nervosa ($n = 279$–304) %
Vomit[a]	48	75[*]
Abuse laxatives[a]	30	30
Exercise[a] vigorously	49	56
Reduce calories[b]	70	74
Restrict sweets[b]	71	71
Restrict fats[b]	80	69[*]
Skip meals[b]	67	57
Fast[b] completely	27	18
Go on fad diets[b]	16	27[*]

[a] Percentage of sample who engage in this practice on a weekly or more frequent basis.
[b] Percentage of sample who endorse "often" or "always" engaging in this practice on the Diagnostic Survey for Eating Disorders.
[*] Groups significantly different at $P < .05$.

of food in an uncontrolled manner, after which she feels self-disgust, guilt or anxiety about possible weight gain. The speed of eating and type and quantity of food eaten are all experienced as beyond one's control. Binges typically involve calorie-dense carbohydrates that are avoided at other times. The eating is almost always done in secrecy and often ends only at the point of running out of food, being interrupted by others, or becoming painfully full with abdominal distention. The binge eating may be preceded by strong food cravings, particularly for high calorie food mainly in the form of carbohydrate such as sweets, bread, ice cream, pastry, or salty snacks. The binge may also be preceded by such emotions as anxiety, depression, frustration, or boredom. These emotions may be the result of an unpleasant experience such as an argument with someone, doing poorly on some task, or finding it difficult to fill unstructured time. During the binge, one may be distracted from these unpleasant thoughts or emotions, but they invariably return when the binge has ended.

Most participants in the group are perplexed and guilt-ridden about their chaotic eating behavior. Many regard themselves as "emotional eaters" and view their binges as temporary lapses in rigid self-control over food intake that occur when they are upset. Indeed, BN patients frequently experience a worsening of mood just prior to binge eating (Davis et al. 1985, 1988). On the basis of this association between mood and binge eating, many participants have come to construe their binge eating as a method of coping with distressing thoughts and feelings. In many cases, this is a misconception of the mechanisms that underlie binge eating. Negative moods tend to trigger a binge *only* if the person is a chronic dieter. In a nondieter, even the most stressful situation or intense feeling will not lead to an episode of binge eating.

Binge eating is a natural response to chronic dieting and sustained efforts to maintain a lower body weight. Individuals who engage in this symptom are avid dieters. They attempt to restrict both the quantity and type of food in their pursuit of thinness or avoidance of fatness. The individual typically begins the day with a strong resolve to be a "good dieter" in terms of how much food she will consume, but as the day progresses, mounting hunger and food cravings lead to increased preoccupation with food. This eventually gives way to uncontrolled eating in the form of a binge if circumstances permit. Participants are informed that this vicious cycle of undereating and overeating becomes self-perpetuating. Their attempts to control weight and compensate for previous binges by undereating set the stage for subsequent binge episodes. Consequently, they are encouraged to begin thinking about normalizing their intake as the first step in overcoming their eating disorder.

Eating disorders and emotional distress. It is difficult to imagine a

Table 4–3.   Symptoms of emotional distress in the eating disorders

Symptom	Anorexia nervosa (n = 93) %	Bulimia nervosa (n = 300) %
Anxiety	68	65
Irritability	65	61
Tiredness	61	62
Extreme sadness	61	58
Wide mood fluctuations	58	67
Early insomnia	48	34*
Crying episodes	33	27

Note. The data refer to the percentage of sample who endorse "often" or "always" experiencing this symptom on the Diagnostic Survey for Eating Disorders.
* Groups significantly different at $P < .05$.

practitioner experienced with eating disorders who has not been struck by the sheer magnitude of emotional distress with which many sufferers present. The literature documenting the comorbidity of other psychiatric disorders and psychosocial dysfunction in eating disorders is controversial (Bulik 1987; Goldbloom and Garfinkel 1988; Hatsukami et al. 1986; Norman and Herzog 1986; Pope and Hudson 1989; Pope et al. 1989). What is clear is that patients with eating disorders also experience concomitant emotional distress. Table 4–3 displays the frequency with which patients who present to our center experience such symptoms as anxiety, irritability, wide mood fluctuations, and extreme sadness.

Group leaders should engage in a frank discussion of the association between eating disorders and emotional distress, in particular highlighting the fact that the nature of the association is presently unknown but that the emotional distress is recognized as a very real part of the participants' current psychological state. For example, for some people a clinical depression precedes the onset of their eating disorder. For others, depression occurs and persists following weight loss or the onset of chaotic eating patterns. For some, depression is a sign of demoralization, which the individual experiences in relation to the chronicity of her eating disorder. Participants need to know that depression is also a common by-product of semistarvation that often improves when weight is restored and eating is normalized (Fairburn et al. 1985; Garner et al. 1990; Laessle et al. 1988b).

It is also instructive for participants to know that emotional distress may be a sequela of acute biological changes resulting from a deprived nutritional state. For example, research indicates that diet-induced depletion of serum tryptophan produces a rapid lowering of mood and increased selective attention to dysphoric stimuli in healthy subjects (Spring et al. 1987; Young et al. 1985). Other data indicate that lowered blood sugar levels are associated with impaired cognitive performance, adverse emotional states, and transient somatic symptoms (Cameron et al. 1988; Hale and Rabak 1981; Taylor and Rachman 1988). Impaired glucose tolerance is an indicator of starvation and carbohydrate restriction and it has been found in bulimic individuals (Schweiger et al. 1987). The point is that participants need to be aware of the relationship between nutritional status and acute changes in emotional state, with the implication that proper nutrition may attenuate their risk of experiencing acute lability in mood.

Physical complications.   A frank discussion of the multiple physical sequelae of the eating disorders is critical as participants need to know what has happened, or what can happen, to their physical well-being. A review of the complications is presented in the following references. Patients may have read extensively regarding this subject, perhaps erroneously, so it is important for therapists to familiarize themselves with the literature before imparting this information (Kaplan 1988; Kaplan and Woodside 1987; Mitchell 1986a, 1986b; Mitchell et al. 1987, 1988; Palla and Litt 1988). Such a discussion provides the rationale for previous advice given by group leaders that participants need to be followed by a physician to ensure that their medical needs are being met.

Pregnancy is an issue that is important to many participants, most of whom are at a developmental stage, physically and psychologically, to be at least contemplating having children. Little is known about the course of pregnancy in women with eating disorders or of the health of their offspring. Pregnancy can be a psychologically traumatizing experience for the woman who is already concerned about her weight and shape. For those who conceive while their eating behavior is still chaotic, there is greater risk for complications of pregnancy and delivery, and the health of the infant can be jeopardized as reflected in lower birth weight and lower Apgar scores (Brinch and Tolstrup 1988; Stewart et al. 1987). Consequently we strongly recommend that pregnancy be delayed until the eating disorder is in remission.

Impaired perception of satiety or fullness has been documented in eating disorder patients and this may be a biological factor that contributes to the perpetuation of the bingeing symptom for some individuals (Owen et al. 1985). Although controversial, the literature documents that at least some sufferers experience a delay in gastric emptying (Domstad et al.

1987; Robinson et al. 1988; Shih et al. 1987) and this has also been implicated in the act of binge eating (Strickler 1984). We suggest to participants that impaired perception of hunger and satiety can have a biological basis that is likely to improve with continued efforts at normalized eating and stabilization of weight, a theme continued in Meeting 4.

The fluctuating course of the eating disorders. The literature on the long-term course of anorexia nervosa suggests that a substantial minority of individuals remain chronically ill while others recover after years of biopsychosocial disability (Herzog et al. 1988a; Theander 1985; Tolstrup et al. 1985; Toner et al. 1986). Follow-up studies of bulimia nervosa have been of comparatively shorter duration, yet a similar picture emerges in which outcome varies considerably with the passage of time (Drewnowski et al. 1988; Herzog et al. 1988b; Keller et al. 1989; Mitchell et al. 1986a, 1986b; Norman and Herzog 1986; Swift et al. 1987; Yager et al. 1987, 1988). Most of this literature is based on the study of individuals who present to specialized treatment facilities and may therefore be a biased view about the natural history of BN. For example, the rate of spontaneous remission and recovery in individuals who do not present themselves for treatment is not known. From the studies based on treatment-seekers, the eating disturbance tends to wax and wane over time, with many individuals experiencing both periods of quiescence in their eating disturbance and periods of exacerbation, particularly during times of stress.

Patients should know that, while eating chaos can remit, underlying psychological issues, if they exist, may make the individual vulnerable to recurrence or exacerbation of symptoms. This point nicely prepares them for the second and third meetings in which perpetuating factors of the eating disturbance are discussed; in particular, the maintaining influence of extreme attitudes and behaviors related to issues of food, weight, and shape. A frank discussion of this issue also helps participants to begin to address personal questions such as "Why have I had this problem for so long?" and "How long is it likely to last?"

The contents of the first meeting of the psychoeducation group have been discussed in considerable detail. Many of the issues will become recurring themes throughout the series of meetings and group leaders are only able to touch upon them in the first meeting as a preview for issues to be raised again in subsequent meetings. If one were to prioritize the issues to cover in the first meeting, most of the time and attention should probably be paid to the orientation to the group and the physical complications; the latter issue typically evokes the greatest interest and number of questions and concerns from participants. As in the closing minutes of all meetings, we summarize the most important points raised and encourage participants to ask questions or comment on the issues arising from the meeting and relevant sections from the participants' manual. It is important that the group leaders respond to questions in an open and honest manner, noting their own limits in knowledge of the disorder. We may on occasion tell participants that we will attempt to find answers to their questions and report back at the beginning of the next meeting.

Meeting 2: The Multidetermined and Self-Perpetuating Nature of the Eating Disorders

♦ Predisposing, precipitating, and perpetuating factors
♦ Where do I begin?

Predisposing, precipitating, and perpetuating factors. It is generally accepted that anorexia nervosa and bulimia nervosa are both multi-determined and self-perpetuating disorders that develop and persist as a result of the interplay between and among sociocultural, psychological, and biological factors (Agras and Kirkley 1986; Crisp 1981; Fairburn 1982; Garfinkel and Garner 1982; Slade 1982). This model is depicted in Figure 4–2, which we show to participants. Our discussion of this model is strongly prefaced by remarks from the group leaders that the developmental path and maintaining influences are not identical for all participants, and that some factors may be more or less relevant, or indeed completely irrelevant to some participants. We suggest to participants that they reflect upon their own developmental background as they consider this model in order to begin to come to some personal understanding about their own disorder.

The discussion of predisposing factors begins with the sociocultural context. This is generally regarded as a significant influence in the development of body image problems that are common to many women in contemporary society. A number of issues relevant to this particular factor are reviewed in the group, including 1) society's pressures on women to be thin, 2) the historical changes in the aesthetic ideal of beauty, 3) the implications of the way the female body is used in advertising, 4) the changing roles for women, 5) the glorification of eating disorders, and 6) the prejudice against obesity (Boskind-White and White 1986; Garner et al. 1985; Silverstein et al. 1986a, 1986b; Striegel-Moore et al. 1986). This consciousness-raising effort is designed to instill a degree of righteous indignation among participants so they may begin to combat their overwhelming feelings of powerlessness to resist social pressure to conform. Participants are encouraged to consider themselves as agents and doers, rather than as passive objects valued mainly for their appearance. Examination of the sociocultural context is achieved through the use of visual slides depicting the unrealistic, aesthetic images of beauty in the contemporary media, and charts and graphs of data depicting the arbitrariness in the changing ideals of beauty over the past several decades. The group leaders maintain a running commentary about the implications these issues have for women.

The individual and familial risk factors are mentioned only briefly. Generalized statements are avoided as they may be quite irrelevant to some participants. These factors apply in a more unique manner to each individual and often become a major focus in ongoing psychotherapy where they may be dealt with in a more meaningful and personalized manner with the participant.

There are often precipitating factors that lead the predisposed person to develop an organized system of beliefs about the importance of controlling weight and shape as the principal means of maintaining a semblance of self-worth. The following is a list of the frequency of life events reported by 296 BN patients at our centre that have coincided with the onset of their eating disorder: teased about appearance (57%), prolonged period of dieting (59%), family problems (54%), problems in a romantic relationship (51%), leaving home (31%), failure at work or school (28%), and a difficult

Figure 4–2.   The multidetermined and self-perpetuating nature of the eating disorders.

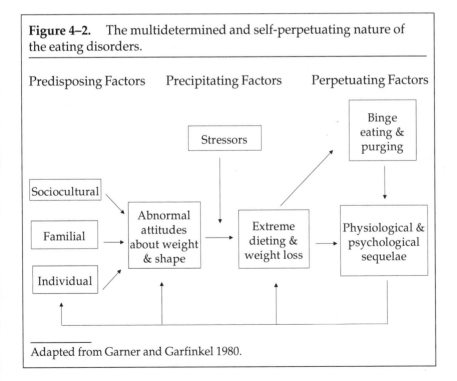

Predisposing Factors   Precipitating Factors   Perpetuating Factors

Adapted from Garner and Garfinkel 1980.

sexual experience (25%). We also briefly introduce some of the possible perpetuating factors, particularly the physiological and psychological responses to starvation (see Meeting 3).

Where do I begin?   To understand the development of their disorder, participants are instructed to "read" Figure 4–2 from left to right. To overcome their eating disorder they must read from right to left. Participants are encouraged to deal in the here and now with the goal of overcoming their specific eating disturbance. In doing so, their current psychological state is likely to change, enabling them to begin to sort out which psychological issues are primary (i.e., causally related) and which are secondary elaborations of a serious eating disorder (Garner et al. 1990). Participants are given clear direction for their focus on recovery. This is important to the many who have come to believe that deep-seated psychological issues from the past must be unraveled before they will be free of eating symptoms. We suggest to participants that working on symptom reduction through nondieting is the essential first step in the recovery process, after which intrapersonal or interpersonal issues can be more meaningfully addressed, if they indeed exist.

Meeting 3: The Regulation of Body Weight and the Consequences of Dieting

◆ Effects of starvation
◆ The notion of set point.

Effects of starvation.   The psychological and physiological responses to starvation are carefully reviewed. It is emphasized that simple food deprivation can make even the healthiest and most psychologically robust of individuals vulnerable to a number of symptoms like those that they themselves are experiencing. To bring this point home, participants are asked to imagine themselves placing a close female friend on the same dietary regimen as they themselves follow, and to consider how that person might feel both physically and emotionally.

The notion of set point.   The biological basis of energy balance and the notion of "set point" are introduced along with human and animal literature that supports the idea that the body vigorously defends a predetermined amount of fat, and that movement away from the set point is strongly resisted at a biological level (Bennett and Gurin 1982). Permanent and significant weight loss of the proportions most participants aspire to achieve is virtually impossible because of our homeostatic propensity to resist weight change (Bennett and Gurin 1982; Garner et al. 1985). In their attempts to achieve weight control, participants have developed the symptom of binge eating that is likely to persist as long as they continue to diet. This is a frightening prospect for most participants, particularly the one in three of the patients who were premorbidly obese. It is essential for all to understand that while the pursuit of happiness is a natural human endeavour to be encouraged, attempting to achieve it through weight and shape manipulation is destined to failure. Of all the issues raised in the psychoeducation group, none are more contentious and emotionally charged for participants than these. In our experience, the vast majority of participants are skeptical about these points, and understandably so, given the generally accepted view in society that weight control is both positive for aesthetic and medical reasons *and* achievable (Polivy and Herman 1988).

The group leaders must be well versed in the literature pertaining to set point, the inheritability of body weight, basal metabolic rate, and the physical and psychological consequences of dieting (see Bennett and Gurin 1982; Devlin et al. 1990; Garner et al. 1985; Keesey 1986; Perkins et al. 1987; Polivy and Herman 1985; Price 1987; Schweiger et al. 1988; Smoller et al. 1987; Thompson and Blanton 1984; also see Appendix). Group leaders, like the participants, are socialized by prevailing cultural attitudes and they too must undergo a fundamental shift in their thinking about the issue of weight control. For those who are unable to do so, acting as a group leader is strongly discouraged as this would only serve to collude with one of the participants' most important therapeutic issues: the need to relinquish dieting and the pursuit of thinness.

Meeting 4: Developing a Healthy Relationship With Food

♦ The nondieting approach
♦ Coping strategies for the washout phase

The nondieting approach. Up to this point participants have been repeatedly encouraged to work toward normalized eating as the most crucial, first step in the recovery process. This meeting is devoted to a detailed explanation of how they may proceed, and is eagerly anticipated by participants. Timing of this meeting is important. It is purposely delayed until group leaders have had sufficient opportunity to give participants a rationale as to why relinquishing their drive for thinness is critical to recovery. Encouraging and instructing participants to normalize eating without first providing a rationale can result in panic and premature termination of treatment. The idea of relinquishing dieting is antithetical to the belief held by all that the pursuit of thinness is of paramount importance, and that giving it up signals personal failure and incompetence. Group members have learned by this point about the perpetuating influence that dieting has on chaotic eating symptoms, and that with normalized eating comes the reasonable expectation that the eating chaos will diminish and that physical and psychological health will improve.

Concepts such as "nondieting" and "mechanical eating" are carefully defined and operationalized using some concrete examples of mealplans (see Appendix). Participants are shown pictures of meals considered to be examples of dieting and nondieting intakes. They find this very instructive; not because they are unaware of what is healthy nutrition (Laessle et al. 1988a), but because it seems to give them "permission" to eat in a way that they have perhaps avoided since childhood or early adolescence. Some basic nutritional information is reviewed, in particular the biological necessity and functions of fat, carbohydrate, and protein, and the recommended dietary allowances (Food and Nutrition Board Committee on Dietary Allowances 1980). Although a contentious and often hotly debated issue in the group, we firmly encourage participants to work toward three balanced meals per day. These should gradually and systematically incorporate "forbidden" foods in a planned manner. The total daily intake should never be less than 1,500 calories and an intake of 2,000 calories is recommended. Participants are informed that nondieting will protect them from overeating and undereating; both outcomes are framed by the group leaders as being equally negative for recovery.

Coping strategies for the washout phase.   Participants are forewarned that many will experience physical discomforts, continued bouts of binge eating, and psychological difficulties in the early stages of their nondieting efforts. This is due, in part, to the fact that they haven't yet learned to respond to fullness cues or to cope with the physical and psychological discomfort associated with resuming a normalized eating pattern. We refer to this early period of the recovery process as the washout phase. We provide participants with several specific coping strategies that they may invoke to help them continue to adhere to their nondieting program (see Appendix). These strategies are grounded in CB therapy, graded exposure and response prevention, stimulus control strategies, cognitive reframing, and coping self-statements. Details of these can be found in one of the basic texts that describe such procedures (e.g., Dobson 1988; Garfield and Bergin 1986; Kendall 1983).

Meeting 5: Attitudes About Weight, Shape, and Dieting as Impediments to Recovery

◆ Binge eating as a coping mechanism
◆ Problem solving
◆ Challenging troublesome attitudes

Binge eating as a coping mechanism.   Those suffering from BN frequently note a close, temporal association between negative mood states and the onset of a binge episode (Cooper and Bowskill 1986; Davis et al. 1985, 1988; Johnson and Larson 1982). These observations have led some to speculate that bingeing and purging serve to regulate internal tension states that are not managed in more adaptive ways (Goodsitt 1983; Johnson et al. 1984; Swift and Letven 1984). A theoretical analysis of the stress process (Cattanach and Rodin 1988) and the mechanisms of conditioning (Booth 1988) does support an association between mood and food for the sufferer of BN. Several authors have advocated teaching individuals alternative methods of self-nurturance and problem-solving skills to cope more adaptively with antecedent mood states and triggering events of a binge episode (Fairburn 1985; Johnson et al. 1987; Lehman and Rodin 1989).

Problem solving.   Part of this meeting is devoted to reviewing with participants the steps to effective problem solving (see Fairburn 1985; Goldfried and Goldfried 1975) so that they may utilize these procedures when faced with a triggering condition for a binge. This typically involves negative interpersonal events, experiences of loss or failure, or negative mood states such as anxiety, anger, or loneliness. It is critically important that group leaders do not unwittingly communicate the idea that the participants only have to learn new ways to cope with old problems that trigger a binge. Such coping strategies are *only useful* as long as the participant is simultaneously working toward becoming a nondieter. Changed eating behavior attenuates the diet-induced "biological" component of the urge to binge. This leaves the "emotional" component to be more effectively dealt with over succeeding months of nondieting by invoking newly learned coping strategies when circumstances warrant.

Challenging troublesome attitudes.   Cognitive restructuring techniques are discussed that can be used to identify, evaluate, and supplant faulty cognitions about the self. These can be replaced with more adaptive, realistic ones (Garner and Davis 1986). Cognitive processes are intimately involved in the coping process (Cattanach and Rodin 1988; Lazarus and Folkman 1984; Moos and Billings 1982), particularly when one is dealing with vigilance over dietary restraint (Polivy and Herman 1988) or the prevention of relapse into symptomatic behavior (Brownell et al. 1986; Kirschenbaum 1987). Participants are only introduced to the very important notion that personal beliefs influence the way we feel and behave. Subjecting such beliefs to objective scrutiny can lead to changes in behavior and the enhancement of self-concept. This material becomes the principal therapeutic task in group CB psychotherapy discussed later in this chapter.

Meeting 6: Developing a Healthy Relationship With Your Body

- ♦ Common body image problems
- ♦ The notion of displacement
- ♦ Escaping the cycle

Common body image problems. Body image distortion represents a bona fide inability to accurately perceive one's body size, while body image disparagement represents the affective and attitudinal components of body image. Deficiencies in self-concept are connected to dietary chaos through the mechanism of overconcern about weight and shape as shown in Figure 4–1.

Displacement. In this meeting, participants are introduced to the notion of displacement by which the body has become the object to which all disparaging feelings about the self are attributed. The body has become a metaphor for mood and feelings about one's self.

Escaping the cycle. The reciprocal nature of the relationship between body and mood may be illustrated as follows: "I am a loser because I am fat," and "I am fat because I am a loser." The intent of this meeting is to heighten participants' awareness of the connection between affect and attitudes. They may then begin to redress negative feelings about the self in more adaptive ways than through the pursuit of thinness (Cooper and Taylor 1988; Wooley and Kearney-Cooke 1986; also see Appendix).

Meeting 7: The Road to Recovery

The purpose of this meeting is to bring the therapeutic experience to closure for the participants. They are reminded of the dieting-bingeing connection and it is stressed that they should continue with their nondieting efforts for at least the next 6 months. The 6 months are framed as a personal experiment in nondieting. Only at the end of the experiment should the participants attempt to evaluate the costs and benefits of nondieting. If at that point she decides that she prefers her old pattern of dieting and the likely consequences of bingeing, that avenue is still open. The following points about the recovery process are reviewed (see Appendix): 1) recovery takes time; 2) each day should be treated as a new day; 3) reinforce one's self for progress made; 4) one's body may lag behind one's behavior; and 5) resume planning and monitoring eating behavior if one is slipping back into old eating patterns.

Cognitive-Behavioral Psychotherapy for the Eating Disorders

Psychoeducational material may be easily integrated into a longer series of group therapy meetings in which there is greater attention to group process. For this, the seating is arranged in the conventional circular manner to encourage engagement. The psychoeducational approach is expanded to include an array of techniques designed to promote greater consolidation and application of the material. Our clinical experience indicates that participants are generally very enthusiastic about participating in such group work at this juncture of their treatment.

These techniques were originally described for individual CB psychotherapy, but they are readily applicable to the group situation. Indeed, there is some advantage to conducting CB psychotherapy in the group setting where patients learn to challenge each other's beliefs and where the veracity of one's beliefs can be tested in the presence of others. Table 4–4 displays several therapeutic components of CB psychotherapy for the eating disorders that can be added to the psychoeducational material presented earlier in this chapter. More detailed discussion of these methods can be found in regard to the treatment of anorexia nervosa (Garner and Bemis 1985) and bulimia nervosa (Fairburn 1985).

Cognitive-behavioral psychotherapy is a strategic therapy rather than a series of techniques or maneuvers. Therapists who operate within a purely technical mode without regard to guiding principles or strategies will find their therapy sessions degenerating into a confusing dialogue between therapist and patient (Beck and Emery 1985; Fairburn 1985). An understanding of basic cognitive strategies is essential (Beck 1976; Beck and Emery 1985; Beck et al. 1979; Guidano and Liotti 1983). The principles may be summarized as follows (Garner and Davis 1986):

1. Cognitive-behavioral psychotherapy is designed to teach the patient to monitor her own thinking and to heighten awareness of that thinking. This involves extracting core aspects of dysfunctional beliefs that must be articulated over the course of therapy. Maladaptive thinking processes (Beck 1976) and consequent dysfunctional beliefs about food, body shape, and weight are pathogenic features of BN that need to be modified over the course of treatment (see Table 4–1).

2. The patient is helped in therapy to recognize the connection between these dysfunctional beliefs and their maladaptive affective and behavioral consequences.

3. The essence of CB psychotherapy involves teaching patients to examine the validity of their beliefs on a moment-to-moment basis (Garner and Bemis 1985). The implications of certain attitudes or beliefs about

---

Table 4–4.   Components of cognitive-behavioral psychotherapy for eating disorders

Behavioral methods

- ◆ Self-monitoring
- ◆ Meal planning
- ◆ Stimulus control
- ◆ Problem solving

Cognitive methods: Testing and challenging beliefs

- ◆ Understanding the relationship between beliefs, affect, and behavior
- ◆ Reframing body image disturbances
- ◆ Examining the connection between self-worth and physical appearance
- ◆ Examining the adaptive/functional value of beliefs
- ◆ Distancing of beliefs
- ◆ Examining available evidence for beliefs
- ◆ Testing beliefs prospectively
- ◆ Determining realistic consequences
- ◆ Searching for alternative explanations
- ◆ Developing realistic beliefs

Adapted from Olmsted et al. 1988: Tape rating instrument for psychotherapy of eating disorders. Toronto, The Toronto Hospital, unpublished manuscript.

---

food, weight, and body shape should be followed to their logical conclusion in therapy meetings. Patients can then collect and examine the evidence for the beliefs between therapy meetings.

4.   Cognitive-behavioral psychotherapy encourages the patient to substitute more realistic interpretations based upon the evidence accumulated.

5.   The ultimate goal is the modification of the underlying assumptions (Beck 1976), deep knowledge structures (Guidano and Liotti 1983), or self-referent schemata (Hollon and Kriss 1984) so that the patient can break the self-perpetuating cycle of BN.

Group Psychoeducation Versus Cognitive-Behavioral Psychotherapy

Table 4–5 compares the features of group psychoeducation and CB psychotherapy, both individual and group formats. Although all three treat-

Table 4–5. Comparison of group psychoeducation and cognitive-behavioral psychotherapy

Feature	Group psychoeducation	Cognitive-behavioral psychotherapy	
		Group	Individual
Domains of focus			
Dietary and biological chaos	+++	++	++
Body image disturbances	+	++	++
Deficits in self-concept	+	+++	+++
Parameters of the treatment			
Duration	+	+++	+++
Group size	++	+	—
Therapist activity	+++	++	++
Participant activity	+	++	++
Homogeneity of membership	+	++	—
Therapeutic focus			
Imparting information	+++	++	++
Instillation of hope	+	++	+
Universality	+	++	—
Altruism	+	++	—
Group cohesiveness	+	++	—
Interpersonal learning	+	++	—
Corrective emotional experience	+	++	++
Efficacy			
Immediate therapeutic response	+	++	++
Cost-effectiveness	+++	+	—
Long-term outcome	?	?	?

Note.   — = Not applicable
    + = Minimally present
  ++ = Moderately present
 +++ = Maximally present
  ? = Unknown

ments have the same domains of focus, group psychoeducation places relatively more emphasis on the patient's dietary and biological chaos whereas CB psychotherapy is more able to focus on body image disturbances and deficits in self-concept. These differences are partly an artifact of the parameters of the treatment. Specifically, CB psychotherapy is of considerably longer duration (i.e., 12 to 24 sessions), and it involves a much higher degree of participant activity, which invites self-disclosure on the part of the patient. Therapeutic change related to body image disturbances and deficits regarding self-concept is definitely facilitated through self-disclosure of personal beliefs over a period of time. In doing so, the patient begins to articulate her beliefs and is able to challenge them within a supportive therapeutic context.

Regarding the constituency of the group, psychoeducation is able to accommodate many more participants than is group CB psychotherapy and, obviously, individual CB psychotherapy. Indeed, the more participants there are in the group psychoeducation, the more purely psychoedicational it is because a large group of 12 or more facilitates the didactic process and discourages group process. In CB psychotherapy one needs to attend to homogeneity of group membership more so than in group psychoeducation. MacKenzie (1990) has described a number of relative contraindications for group work that are more pertinent to CB psychotherapy where group process is essential (e.g., marked paranoid, antisocial, and borderline personality features). Such personality features are less of a contraindication for group psychoeducation, particularly when self-disclosure and interpersonal exploration occur infrequently.

Perhaps the greatest distinctions between and among the three treatments involve what Yalom has described as the therapeutic factors operating in group psychotherapy (Vinogradov and Yalom 1989). When patients self-disclose in the presence of others, they are able to benefit from such factors as the instillation of hope, universality, altruism, group cohesion, and interpersonal learning. Most of these therapeutic factors are maximally present in group CB psychotherapy, only moderately present in group psychoeducation, and largely absent or quite attenuated in individual CB psychotherapy. Participants in group psychoeducation benefit somewhat from these factors by virtue of being in the same room as others and by sharing some of their feelings and opinions. The high degree of self-disclosure that is typical of group CB psychotherapy enhances the potential for participants to benefit from these therapeutic factors.

The three forms of treatment may also be compared in terms of efficacy. There is a sizeable body of data that suggests that all three are likely to produce clinically significant change for some patients at least in the short term. In their review of CB treatment studies, Garner and colleagues (1987) reported a median of 33% of patients were abstinent from vomiting at the end of treatment, with no clear advantage for individual over group treatment. In our original group psychoeducation program, which involved only five 90-minute meetings, 21% of BN patients were symptom free in the month following treatment (Davis et al. 1990; Olmsted et al., in press). Clinically significant changes in dysfunctional attitudes and psychological distress were also associated with this treatment. A direct comparison of our brief psychoeducational group with longer individual CB psychotherapy indicated that the benefits obtained with psychoeducation are slightly smaller than those found with individual CB psychotherapy, but group psychoeducation is dramatically more cost-effective (Olmsted et al., in press). The longer-term efficacy of all three treatments is not yet well established, but the available initial reports appear promising (Garner et al. 1987).

Where treatment resources are constantly outstripped by patient needs, both cost-effectiveness and the rational matching of patients to treatments are essential. Work at our center has shown that patients who vomit more frequently and report higher levels of depression benefit less from group psychoeducation (Davis et al., in press). When compared with individual CB psychotherapy, group psychoeducation was equally effective for the two-thirds of patients who were vomiting the least frequently. Individual CB psychotherapy was significantly more effective for the one-third of patients who were initially vomiting most frequently (Olmsted et al., in press). These findings support the utility of a stepped care model of treatment for patients with BN in which nonresponders to group psychoeducation would then be offered more intensive treatment.

Summary

The goals of group psychoeducation are to promote healthy attitudes and behaviors for self-care which the patient may engage in without the need for protracted involvement in treatment. Psychoeducation differs from CB psychotherapy not in terms of the goal but, rather, in terms of the manner in which it is carried out. Psychoeducation as we have described it in this chapter is highly directive and brief. Although other systems of therapy share these features (e.g., behavior therapy), psychoeducation is relatively unique in its reliance on the didactic provision of information and advice as the principal activity of the therapist. In its pristine form, group psychoeducation does not involve self-disclosure on the part of the patient. By contrast, in group CB psychotherapy one of the more important therapeutic activities is to promote group cohesiveness so that the patient may engage in self-discovery through self-disclosure over a period of time. The role of the leader, the expectations for the participant, and the resulting therapeutic relationship distinguish group psychoeducation from CB psychotherapy.

By way of analogy, an actor learns her role in a play by actively rehearsing with the cast and director and by receiving corrective feedback regarding her performance. The observer in the audience also learns about the play but through a more vicarious instructional experience. Similarly in group CB psychotherapy, the individual actively participates with others and, through this interpersonal experience, "learns" about her own modes of thinking and feeling. In group psychoeducation, the participant processes the information with the expectation that continued learning will take place outside the therapy room. Depending upon their level of dietary chaos and psychological distress, some individuals with BN are able to benefit from group psychoeducation as the sole intervention. For others, the addition of group psychotherapy will be necessary to help them to engage in self-care. In this way, psychotherapy picks up where psychoeducation leaves off. However, the artful integration of psychoeducation and psychotherapy is undoubtedly necessary for many individuals to overcome their difficulties.

References

Agras WS, Kirkley BG: Bulimia: Theories of etiology, in Handbook of Eating Disorders. Edited by Brownell KD, Foreyt JP. New York, Basic Books, 1986

Beck AT: Cognitive Therapy and the Emotional Disorders. New York, International University Press, 1976

Beck AT, Emery G: Anxiety Disorders and Phobias: A Cognitive Perspective. New York, Basic Books, 1985

Beck AT, Rush AJ, Shaw BF, et al: Cognitive Therapy of Depression. New York, Guilford, 1979

Bennett W, Gurin J: The Dieter's Dilemma: Eating Less and Weighing More. New York, Basic Books, 1982

Booth DA: Culturally corralled into food abuse: the eating disorders as physiologically reinforced excessive appetites, in The Psychobiology of Bulimia Nervosa. Edited by Pirke KM, Vandereycken W, Ploog D. Berlin, Springer-Verlag, 1988

Boskind-White M, White WC: Bulimarexia: a historical-sociocultural perspective, in Handbook of Eating Disorders. Edited by Brownell KD, Foreyt JP. New York, Basic Books, 1986

Brinch M, Tolstrup K: Anorexia nervosa and motherhood: reproduction pattern and mothering behavior of 50 women. Acta Psychiatr Scand 77:611–617, 1988

Brownell KD, Marlatt GA, Lichtenstein E, et al: Understanding and preventing relapse. Am Psychol 41:762–782, 1986

Bulik CM: Drug and alcohol abuse by bulimic women and their families. Am J Psychiatry 144:1604–1606, 1987

Cameron OG, Buzan R, McCann DS: Symptoms of insulin-induced hypoglycemia in normal subjects. J Psychosom Res 32:41–49, 1988

Cattanach L, Rodin J: Psychosocial components of the stress process in bulimia. International Journal of Eating Disorders 7:75–88, 1988

Cooper PJ, Bowskill R: Dysphoric mood and overeating. Br J Clin Psychol 25:155–156, 1986

Cooper PJ, Taylor MJ: Body image disturbance in bulimia nervosa. Br J Psychiatry 153:32–36, 1988

Cox GL, Merkel WT: A qualitative review of psychosocial treatments for bulimia. J Nerv Ment Dis 177:77–84, 1989

Crisp AH: Anorexia nervosa at normal body weight—the abnormal normal weight control syndrome. Int J Psychiatry Med 11:203–233, 1981

Davis R: Clinical assessment of the eating disorders, in Current Update: Anorexia Nervosa and Bulimia Nervosa. Edited by Garfinkel PE. Kalamazoo, MI, Upjohn, 1988

Davis R, Freeman R, Solyom L: Mood and food: an analysis of bulimic episodes. J Psychiatr Res 19:331–335, 1985

Davis R, Freeman RJ, Garner DM: A naturalistic investigation of eating behavior in bulimia nervosa. J Consult Clin Psychol 56:273–279, 1988

Davis R, Olmsted MP, Rockert W: Brief group psychoeducation for bulimia nervosa: assessing the clinical significance of change. J Consult Clin Psychol 58(6):882–885, 1990

Davis R, Olmsted MP, Rockert W: Brief group psychoeducation for bulimia nervosa, II: prediction of clinical outcome. International Journal of Eating Disorders (in press)

Devlin MJ, Walsh T, Kral JG, et al: Metabolic abnormalities in bulimia nervosa. Arch Gen Psychiatry 47:144–148, 1990

Dobson KS: Handbook of Cognitive-Behavioral Therapies. New York, Guilford, 1988

Domstad PA, Shih WJ, Humphries L, et al: Radionuclide gastric emptying studies in patients with anorexia nervosa. J Nucl Med 28:816–819, 1987

Drewnowski A, Yee DK, Krahn DD: Bulimia in college women: incidence and recovery rates. Am J Psychiatry 145:753–755, 1988

Fairburn CG: Binge-eating and bulimia nervosa. SK+F Publications 1(4):1–20, 1982

Fairburn CG: Cognitive-behavioral treatment for bulimia, in Handbook of Psychotherapy for Anorexia Nervosa and Bulimia. Edited by Garner DM, Garfinkel PE. New York, Guilford, 1985

Fairburn CG: The current status of the psychological treatments for bulimia nervosa. J Psychosom Res 32:635–645, 1988

Fairburn CG, Garner DM: The diagnosis of bulimia nervosa. International Journal of Eating Disorders 5:403–419, 1986

Fairburn CG, Cooper PJ, Kirk J, et al: The significance of the neurotic symptoms of bulimia nervosa. J Psychiatr Res 19:135–140, 1985

Food and Nutrition Board Committee on Dietary Allowances. Recommended Dietary Allowances, 9th Edition. Washington, DC, National Academy of Sciences, 1980

Freeman C, Barry F, Dunkeld-Turnbull J, et al: Controlled trial of psychotherapy for bulimia nervosa. BMJ 296:521–525, 1988

Garfield S, Bergin AE (eds): Handbook of Psychotherapy and Behavior Change. New York, John Wiley, 1986

Garfinkel PE, Garner DM: Anorexia Nervosa: A Multidimensional Perspective. New York, Brunner/Mazel, 1982

Garner DM, Bemis KM: Cognitive therapy for anorexia nervosa, in Handbook of Psychotherapy for Anorexia Nervosa and Bulimia. Edited by Garner DM, Garfinkel PE. New York, Guilford, 1985

Garner DM, Davis R: Principles of cognitive-behavioral therapy for bulimia nervosa. American Mental Health Counselors Association Journal 8:185–192, 1986

Garner DM, Garfinkel PE: Socio-cultural factors in the development of anorexia nervosa. Psychol Med 10:647–656, 1980

Garner DM, Rockert W, Olmsted MP, et al: Psychoeducational principles in the treatment of bulimia and anorexia nervosa, in Handbook of Psychotherapy for Anorexia Nervosa and Bulimia. Edited by Garner DM, Garfinkel PE. New York, Guilford, 1985

Garner DM, Garfinkel PE, Irvine MJ: Integration and sequencing of treatment approaches for eating disorders. Psychother Psychosom 46:67–75, 1986

Garner DM, Fairburn CG, Davis R: Cognitive-behavioral treatment of bulimia nervosa: a critical appraisal. Behav Modif 11:398–431, 1987

Garner DM, Olmsted MP, Davis R, et al: The association between bulimic symptoms and reported psychopathology. International Journal of Eating Disorders 9:1–15, 1990

Goldbloom DS, Garfinkel PE: Psychiatric morbidity and outcome, in Current Update: Anorexia Nervosa and Bulimia Nervosa. Edited by Garfinkel PE. Kalamazoo, MI, Upjohn, 1988

Goldfried MR, Goldfried AP: Cognitive change methods, in Helping People Change. Edited by Kanfer FH, Goldstein AP. New York, Pergamon, 1975

Goodsitt A: Self-regulatory disturbances in eating disorders. International Journal of Eating Disorders 2:51–60, 1983

Guidano VF, Liotti G: Cognitive Processes and the Emotional Disorders: A Structural Approach to Psychotherapy. New York, Guilford, 1983

Hale F, Rabak D: Postprandial hypoglycemia and "psychological" symptoms. Biol Psychiatry 17:125–130, 1981

Hatsukami D, Mitchell JE, Eckert ED, et al: Characteristics of patients with bulimia only, bulimia with affective disorder, and bulimia with substance abuse problems. Addict Behav 11:399–406, 1986

Herzog DB, Keller MB, Lavori PW: Outcome in anorexia nervosa and bulimia nervosa: a review of the literature. J Nerv Ment Dis 176:131–143, 1988a

Herzog DB, Keller MB, Lavori PW, et al: Short-term prospective study of recovery in bulimia nervosa. Psychiatry Res 23:45–55, 1988b

Hollon SD, Kriss MR: Cognitive factors in clinical research and practice. Clinical Psychology Review 4:35–76, 1984

Johnson C, Larson R: Bulimia: an analysis of moods and behavior. Psychosom Med 44:341–351, 1982

Johnson C, Lewis C, Hagman J: The syndrome of bulimia: review and synthesis. Psychiatr Clin North Am 7:247–273, 1984

Johnson C, Connors ME, Tobin DL: Symptom management of bulimia. J Consult Clin Psychol 55:668–676, 1987

Kaplan AS: Medical aspects of anorexia nervosa and bulimia nervosa, in Current Update: Anorexia Nervosa and Bulimia Nervosa. Edited by Garfinkel PE. Kalamazoo, MI, Upjohn, 1988

Kaplan AS, Woodside DB: Biological aspects of anorexia nervosa and bulimia nervosa. J Consult Clin Psychol 55:645–653, 1987

Keesey RE: A set-point theory of obesity, in Handbook of Eating Disorders. Edited by Brownell KD, Foreyt JP. New York, Basic Books, 1986

Keller MB, Herzog DB, Lavori PW, et al: High rates of chronicity and rapidity of relapse in patients with bulimia nervosa and depression. Arch Gen Psychiatry 46:480–481, 1988

Kendall PC (ed): Advances in Cognitive-Behavioral Research and Therapy, Vol 2. New York, Academic, 1983

Kirschenbaum DS: Self-regulatory failure: a review with clinical implications. Clinical Psychology Review 7:77–104, 1987

Laessle RG, Schweiger U, Daute-Herold U, et al: Nutritional knowledge in patients with eating disorders. International Journal of Eating Disorders 7:63–73, 1988a

Laessle RG, Schweiger U, Pirke KM: Depression as a correlate of starvation in patients with eating disorders. Biol Psychiatry 23:719–725, 1988b

Lazarus RS, Folkman S: Coping and adaptation, in Handbook of Behavioral Medicine. Edited by Gentry WE. New York, Guilford, 1984

Lehman AK, Rodin J: Styles of self-nurturance and disordered eating. J Consult Clin Psychol 57:117–122, 1989

MacKenzie KR: Introduction to Time-limited Group Psychotherapy. Washington, DC, American Psychiatric Press, 1990

Mitchell JE: Anorexia nervosa: medical and physiological aspects, in Handbook of Eating Disorders. Edited by Brownell KD, Foreyt JP. New York, Basic Books, 1986a

Mitchell JE: Bulimia: medical and physiological aspects, in Handbook of Eating Disorders. Edited by Brownell KD, Foreyt JP. New York, Basic Books, 1986b

Mitchell JE, Davis L, Goff G, et al: A follow-up study of patients with bulimia. International Journal of Eating Disorders 5:441–450, 1986a

Mitchell JE, Hatsukami D, Pyle RL, et al: The bulimia syndrome: course of the illness and associated problems. Compr Psychiatry 27:165–170, 1986b

Mitchell JE, Seim HC, Colon E, et al: Medical complications and medical management of bulimia. Ann Intern Med 107:71–77, 1987

Mitchell JE, Pomeroy C, Huber M: A clinician's guide to the eating disorders medicine cabinet. International Journal of Eating Disorders 7:211–223, 1988

Moos RH, Billings AG: Conceptualizing and measuring coping resources and processes, in Handbook of Stress: Theoretical and Clinical Aspects. Edited by Goldberger L, Breznitz S. New York, Free Press, 1982

Norman DK, Herzog DB: A 3-year outcome study of normal-weight bulimia: assessment of psychosocial functioning and eating attitudes. Psychiatry Res 19:199–205, 1986

Olmsted MP, Davis R, Rockert W, et al: Efficacy of a brief group psychoeducational intervention for bulimia nervosa. Behav Res Ther 29(1):71–83, 1991

Owen WP, Halmi KA, Gibbs J, et al: Satiety responses in the eating disorders. J Psychiatr Res 19:279–284, 1985

Palla B, Litt IF: Medical complications of eating disorders in adolescents. Pediatrics 81:613–623, 1988

Perkins KA, McKenzie SJ, Stoney CM: The relevance of metabolic rate in behavioral medicine research. Behav Modif 11:286–311, 1987

Polivy J, Herman CP: Dieting and binging: a causal analysis. Am Psychol 40:193–201, 1985

Polivy J, Herman CP: Diagnosis and treatment of normal eating. J Consult Clin Psychol 55:635–644, 1988

Pope HG, Hudson JI: Are eating disorders associated with borderline personality disorder? A critical review. International Journal of Eating Disorders 8:1–9, 1989

Pope HG, Hudson JI, Yurgelun-Todd D: Depressive symptoms in bulimic, depressed, and non-psychiatric control subjects. J Affective Disord 16:93–99, 1989

Price RA: Genetics of human obesity. Annals of Behavioral Medicine 9:9–14, 1987

Robinson PH, Clarke M, Barrett J: Determinants of delayed gastric emptying in anorexia nervosa and bulimia nervosa. Gut 29:458–464, 1988

Schweiger U, Poellinger J, Laessle R, et al: Altered insulin response to a balanced test meal in bulimic patients. International Journal of Eating Disorders 6:551–556, 1987

Schweiger U, Laessle RG, Fichter MM, et al: Consequences of dieting at a normal weight, in The Psychobiology of Bulimia Nervosa. Edited by Pirke KM, Vandereycken W, Ploog D. Berlin, Springer-Verlag, 1988

Shih WJ, Humphries L, Digenis GA, et al: Tc-99m labelled triethelene tetraamine polysterene resin gastric emptying studies in bulimic patients. Eur J Nucl Med 13:192–196, 1987

Silverstein B, Perdue L, Peterson B, et al: The role of the mass media in promoting a thin standard of bodily attractiveness for women. Sex Roles 14:519–532, 1986a

Silverstein B, Peterson B, Perdue L: Some correlates of the thin standard of bodily attractiveness for women. International Journal of Eating Disorders 5:895–905, 1986b

Slade P: Towards a functional analysis of anorexia nervosa and bulimia nervosa. Br J Clin Psychol 21:167–179, 1982

Smoller JW, Wadden TA, Stunkard AJ: Dieting and depression: a critical review. J Psychosom Res 31:429–440, 1987

Spring B, Chiodo J, Bowen DJ: Carbohydrates, tryptophan, and behavior: a methodological review. Psychol Bull 102:234–256, 1987

Stewart DE, Raskin J, Garfinkel PE, et al: Anorexia nervosa, bulimia, and pregnancy. Am J Obstet Gynecol 157:1194–1198, 1987

Strickler EM: Biological basis of hunger and satiety: therapeutic implications. Nutr Rev 42:333–340, 1984

Striegel-Moore RH, Silberstein LR, Rodin J: Toward an understanding of risk factors for bulimia. Am Psychol 41:246–263, 1986

Swift WJ, Letven R: Bulimia and the basic fault: a psychoanalytic interpretation of the binging-vomiting syndrome. Journal of the American Academy of Child Psychiatry 23:489–497, 1984

Swift WJ, Ritholz M, Kalin NH, et al: A follow-up study of thirty hospitalized bulimics. Psychosom Med 49:45–55, 1987

Taylor LA, Rachman SJ: The effects of blood sugar level changes on cognitive function, affective state, and somatic symptoms. J Behav Med 11:279–291, 1988

Theander S: Outcome and prognosis in anorexia nervosa and bulimia: some results of previous investigations compared with those of a Swedish long-term study. J Psychiatr Res 19:493–508, 1985

Thompson JK, Blanton PE: The effects of dieting and exercise on metabolic rate. Behavioral Medicine Abstracts 5:v-viii, 1984

Tolstrup K, Brinch M, Isager T, et al: Long-term outcome of 151 cases of anorexia nervosa. Acta Psychiatr Scand 71:380–387, 1985

Toner BB, Garfinkel PE, Garner DM: Long-term follow-up of anorexia nervosa. Psychosom Med 48:520–529, 1986

Vinogradov S, Yalom ID: Concise Guide to Group Psychotherapy. Washington, DC, American Psychiatric Press, 1989

Wilson GT, Smith D: Cognitive-behavioral treatment of bulimia nervosa. Annals of Behavioral Medicine 9:12–17, 1987

Wooley SC, Kearney-Cooke A: Intensive treatment of bulimia and body-image disturbance, in Handbook of Eating Disorders. Edited by Brownell KD, Foreyt JP. New York, Basic Books, 1986

Yager J, Landsverk J, Edelstein CK: A 20-month follow-up study of 628 women with eating disorders, I: course and severity. Am J Psychiatry 144:1172–1177, 1987

Yager J, Landsverk J, Edelstein CK, et al: A 20-month follow-up study of 628 women with eating disorders, II: course of associated symptoms and related clinical features. International Journal of Eating Disorders 7:503–513, 1988

Young SN, Smith SE, Pihl RO, et al: Tryptophan depletion causes a rapid lowering of mood in normal males. Psychopharmacology 87:173–177, 1985

5

Interpersonal Group Psychotherapy

Heather Harper-Giuffre, B.N., B.Sc., M.Sc.
K. Roy MacKenzie, M.D., F.R.C.P.(C)
Denise Sivitilli, M.A.

◆ ◆ ◆ ◆ ◆ ◆ ◆ ◆

Numerous psychodynamic and developmental formulations have been proposed regarding the development of eating disorders. The theoretical perspective described in this chapter has been developed from the perspective of self psychology. This self psychological application deviates from the more orthodox psychoanalytic position by advocating that food and weight related issues be acknowledged and explored and that the therapist adopt a more directive role, integrating an amalgam of cognitive-behavioral and psychodynamic therapeutic techniques. The longer duration of this particular group modality is well suited to identifying and working through the variety of intrapsychic and interpersonal issues so common to patients with eating disorders. This group treatment entails a more intrusive perspective and, as such, it would be instituted only after the patient has achieved significant weight and nutritional stabilization.—The Editors

This chapter describes the use of longer term interpersonal groups for the treatment of eating disorders. This usually takes place in an outpatient setting. The management of such groups for the nutritionally stabilized patient with an eating disorder resembles that for other intensive group formats. A central thesis throughout this book is the importance of achieving control over eating behaviors as the first step in treatment. Thus most patients will begin with a management approach that emphasizes psychoeducational, cognitive-behavioral, and pharmacological strategies. For the majority of patients presenting with mild eating symptoms, these forms of treatment will be adequate.

Longer term group psychotherapy is indicated for the more difficult anorexia nervosa (AN) or bulimia nervosa (BN) patients. These are patients with a history of eating symptoms going back many years, accompanied by greater intensity and frequency of symptoms and more interference with general functioning. The eating behavior itself must be seen in the context of these general problems of adaptation. Most such patients will exhibit significant characterological difficulty, often with narcissistic and borderline features accompanied by passive or passive-aggressive qualities. Because the maladaptive difficulties are so pervasive, it is unrealistic to expect significant response from brief treatment. Intensive work with these patients calls for advanced skills in group psychotherapy.

An Integrated Psychodynamic and Cognitive-Behavioral Framework

Various theories derived from the psychoanalytic tradition have been used to provide explanatory hypotheses for these complex disorders. One of the more useful approaches has been the use of a central linking mechanism that connects many of the eating features to underlying deficits in the perception of self. This deficit model contrasts with conflict or object-relations models. A more complete discussion of these three theoretical approaches is found in Goodsitt (1985).

The deficit model suggests that the patient with a severe eating disorder has experienced difficulties in internalizing basic control functions relating to self-regulation. These include the capacity to provide one's own sense of stability, to regulate tension states, and to maintain positive self-esteem. The person with such deficits will continually try to compensate by seeking external relationships that can supply the missing integration. When such resources are not available, the person is likely to experience a sense of inner fragmentation and helplessness, or emptiness and boredom. Because the expectations of what others can supply is unrealistic, the patient will experience most relationships as unsatisfactory. These relationships turn into situations where she feels excessively influenced and perhaps exploited without any sense of satisfaction.

The eating behavior may be seen as a defense to cope with these underlying feelings of inadequacy, ineffectiveness, and lack of a cohesive sense of self. The management of food and weight serves as a displacement focus to contain anxiety and provide a sense of identity. This is one area where it appears that self-control can be maintained. This approach works most effectively for the AN patient. There is continuity between the desire for control and the successful attainment of an emaciated state. The patient with

BN is likely to be less satisfied with the result. Bingeing and purging behaviors are seen as loss of control without the "reward" of weight loss. This leaves the patient caught between the desire to control food and weight and the realization that binges are lapses of control. The ego-dystonic nature of BN probably accounts for the greater receptivity to treatment approaches. From this perspective, the eating disorder itself may be seen as an adaptive strategy, albeit laden with unfortunate side effects. Some of the eating disorder symptoms, such as binge eating, may become secondarily autonomous. They operate independently of the precipitating conflicts for which the symptom was originally intended. It is important in assessing patients with eating disorders to carefully investigate both aspects of the presentation: eating behavior and psychological distress. When the latter is minimal, there is a higher likelihood of early response to treatment techniques focused primarily on the eating behavior.

Another way of conceptualizing patients with eating disorders stems from the cognitive-behavioral theoretical tradition that is concerned primarily with maladaptive thinking patterns. Interventions derived from cognitive-behavioral approaches used to treat depression and neurotic disorders have been modified for use with these patients (Beck et al. 1979; Fairburn 1985; Garner and Bemis 1982). These cognitive formulations of eating disorders are quite compatible with psychodynamic models that focus on the importance of developmental issues in the etiology of eating disorders.

There are a number of maladaptive thinking patterns commonly found in the eating disorders. These have been discussed in Chapter 4, particularly those surrounding attitudes and ideas about food and body image. In addition to these eating-specific ideas, patients with eating disorders characteristically show maladaptive thinking in a more general sense.

It is common to find a dichotomous "black-or-white" thinking style. Reactions, particularly reactions about interpersonal events, are polarized into extremely positive or negative categories. Persons are seen as all good or all bad. This manner of thinking prevents an integrated view of relationships or results in overidealization with subsequent disappointment, and arbitrary condemnation without chance for repeal. The same absolute evaluative style is applied to the self. This results in a curious combination of self-condemnation coupled with a sense of entitlement and conviction. Unrealistic and irrational standards for self-appraisal are commonly found. Perfectionistic and perhaps overtly obsessional features may develop in an attempt to satisfy the high expectations. These are bound to be unsuccessful, and, as the eating disorder progresses, a vicious spiral may be created of increasingly self-critical appraisals associated with frantic attempts to appease them through higher levels of performance regarding work, social duties, and eating control.

Another pervasive attitude concerns personal ineffectiveness and powerlessness. This leads to a belief in the futility of attempting change. Personal needs are discounted or denied. This may be accompanied by a high need for approval from others but a strong inclination to deny or qualify any positive comments that are received.

Intensive Interpersonal Group Therapy for Eating Disorders

Psychotherapy has been described as the cornerstone of treatment for AN and BN (Garfinkel and Garner 1982). It provides an empathic context in which the segments of the underdeveloped self can be revealed, understood, and mastered. The goal is to foster a corrective emotional experience that repairs underlying conceptual distortions and associated difficulties with self-regulation, identity, and autonomy. It is anticipated that this will result in improvements with regard to social isolation, fear of intimacy, and self-esteem. The group environment is a particularly powerful format for promoting a sense of personal empowerment.

Reports of longer term interpersonal eating disorder groups have begun to appear in the literature (Barth and Wurman 1986; Hendren et al. 1987; Laube 1990; MacKenzie et al. 1986; Roth and Ross 1988; Roy-Byrne et al. 1984; Yellowlees 1988). Longer term customarily refers to groups that run for more than about 25 sessions. These may be in a strictly time-limited and closed format, or open to a slow turnover of membership. The term interpersonal is adopted from the general model of group psychotherapy most closely identified with Yalom (1985). It is designed to treat a variety of nonpsychotic psychological disorders and is variously called interactional, experiential, or psychodynamic. Over time, it has evolved into an eclectic approach using an amalgam of techniques from various theoretical backgrounds.

Interpersonal groups can be regarded as learning laboratories in which patients have the opportunity to work through internal and interpersonal difficulties. Such groups are particularly well suited to resolving self deficits. The group functions as a transitional object that sustains the patient during the course of change. Unlike individual therapy, group therapy provides multiple and diverse relationship possibilities (Barth and Wurman 1986). A unique holding environment is created that fosters the development of self-care, connectedness, and accountability (Laube 1990).

The unstructured "here-and-now" format of an interpersonal group promotes the expression and identification of significant affects that otherwise may remain camouflaged behind the "false self" that predominates in many patients with eating disorders. The process of sharing these affects allows the development of a social microcosm in which the members will begin to interact with one another in a manner similar to the way they interact with people outside of the group. It is this interactional milieu that fosters changes in the nature of interpersonal relationships. For example, during the beginning phase of a group, a member may identify one of her interpersonal difficulties as an inability to express any negative emotions, coupled with a tendency to assume caregiving roles contributing to superficial and nonintimate relations. With time, she will start to exhibit the same maladaptive mode of relating to others in the group setting. She may, for instance, deny or avoid the expression of any differences or hostility toward members and assume an active role of attending to the needs of other members. Hence, the group will no longer need to be told about this part of herself, as they will witness it in their interactions with her. The emergence of this problem in the here-and-now context of the group affords the member an opportunity to reexperience this process in a context in which it can be actively discussed.

For such phenomena to be meaningful, they must occur in a cohesive group where the connections among the members have deepened into important relationships. This can take place in brief groups (Budman and Gurman 1988). However, because patients with eating disorders are generally well defended in regard to interpersonal problems, the process of group formation is often slow. It is important that sufficient time be allowed for the group culture to mature in order to provide a corrective emotional experience for the members. Then the group can move beyond the "supportive" and "learning from others" therapeutic factors discussed in Chapter 2 to apply the "psychological work" factors in more depth. It is not unusual for members to require 1 or 2 years to maximize this process (MacKenzie et al. 1986).

Conceptualizing the work of the psychotherapy group within a developmental stage framework provides a clinically effective means to address the psychopathology of patients with AN and BN (MacKenzie 1990; MacKenzie et al. 1986; Roy-Byrne et al. 1984). Understanding group development can help the therapist focus attention on the formation of therapeutic norms and tasks, on those elements considered necessary to promote engagement in group work, and on group resistances. In addition, understanding of stage phenomena coupled with a careful formulation of each patient's conflicts and personality structure enables the therapist to predict when difficulties are most likely to be encountered by each member.

Patient Selection and Group Composition

Systematic screening for suitability helps to reduce the rate of dropouts in a given group and to maximize the therapeutic effectiveness for both the individual and the entire group. A number of successive steps are involved in the selection process. First, a diagnostic and psychodynamic assessment is essential. This is best achieved through administration of an interpersonally oriented clinical interview, a self-report test battery, a physician-conducted medical examination, and a screening laboratory workup. A thorough discussion of the assessment process is found in Chapter 3. If the patient meets the criteria for an eating disorder and is deemed appropriate for an outpatient setting, one is then in a position to assess the patient's suitability for an interpersonal group.

The timing of placing a patient into a long-term psychodynamic group is a critical factor. Psychodynamic groups do not lend themselves well to the management of the first phase of treatment that deals with issues surrounding eating, weight, and physical health. These treatment issues are more effectively managed through individual psychotherapy, psychoeducational groups, a day hospital program, and (in certain instances) a course of inpatient hospitalization. Such group approaches are dealt with in other chapters of this book.

As a general rule, patients function optimally in a psychodynamic group if they have first achieved substantial resolution of their eating behavior and physical health. By selecting patients who have achieved some symptom relief around eating, the way is cleared for group members to focus on psychological and interpersonal problems. Severe emaciation, starvation, or extremely chaotic eating patterns are unquestionably contraindications to an intensive outpatient group therapy setting. Often patients may be involved concurrently in individual psychotherapy, family therapy, nutritional counseling, or pharmacotherapy. In these instances it is important that the group therapist maintain a good liaison with the other caregivers to maintain continuity and consistency of treatment and minimize the potential of splitting.

Exclusion Criteria

As a general guideline, patients with eating disorders are poor candidates for an outpatient intensive therapy group if they exhibit the following:

1. Current major substance abuse
2. Active psychosis
3. Severe depression
4. Moderate to severe suicidal ideation
5. Major current situational crisis
6. Major risk of assuming a deviant group role

These criteria are not specific to eating disorders and have been identified by Yalom (1985) as applicable to most outpatient intensive therapy groups. Patients with these sorts of problems are at high risk for therapeutic failure because of their inability to take part in the principal task of the group—that is, the attainment of a group culture characterized by closeness, acceptance, introspection, openness, and empathy. Their tendency to assume interpersonal roles that are deleterious to both themselves and the group make such patients high dropout risks. Note that all of these criteria refer to severe problems leaving a substantial grey zone for clinical judgment.

Think of the patient who adamantly de-emphasizes or denies the internal and interpersonal issues surrounding her eating disorder and manifests no curiosity about her inner life. Not only would this patient be unlikely to benefit from a psychodynamic approach, but she also runs a high risk of becoming a deviant member in the eyes of the group. Group deviancy leads to an increased likelihood of premature termination, of being harmed by the group experience, and of impeding the progress of the group (Lieberman et al. 1972).

Personality Disorders

Personality disorders are commonly diagnosed in patients with eating disorders, most notably narcissistic and borderline features. These patients manifest problems in object constancy and integration (Leszcz 1989). They demonstrate impulsivity and chronic feelings of emptiness alternating with a desire for, and fear of, attachment and acceptance. When severe, such features may preclude effective participation.

It is important for the therapist to make a judgment about how the patient's interpersonal style will be applied in an intensive group setting. For instance, one severe borderline patient may obtain some help from a group but at the same time may have a deleterious influence on the progress of other group members due to her inability to share the therapist and her low ability to tolerate any ambiguity. Conversely, another borderline patient's propensity to be less influenced by societal inhibitions and her ability to recognize subtle psychological nuances may have a beneficial effect on the group process by steering the group into a more candid and intimate climate (Yalom 1985). Hence, it is the responsibility of the therapist to attempt to weigh whether or not the individual's behavior is likely to be accepted and tolerated in the group. Some groups may seem better able to cope with borderline behavior than others.

Perhaps the critical decision regarding character disorder is not whether certain patients should be included in a group, but how many patients should be integrated in each group and with what level of severity. Restricting the number of patients with severe personality disorders to one or two members is recommended. Exceeding this criterion can be counterproductive to the group functioning, endangering its stability and cohesiveness.

The distinctive benefits of group therapy in the treatment of patients with character disorders have been clearly established (Horwitz 1980; Leszcz 1989; Wong 1980). Clinical experience suggests that these group advantages also apply to those patients with eating disorders manifesting personality disorders. It can be helpful to assess these patients in a preceding psychoeducational or support group. This may allow a more objective measure of the patient's ability to use the group environment. The therapist's personal feeling toward the personality disordered patient can be an important factor when making a decision about group suitability. Should the therapist experience a clear and intense aversion toward a particular patient and anticipate difficulty working through these negative feelings, the likelihood of successful engagement is seriously jeopardized.

Motivation and Psychological Mindedness

The patient's motivation for interpersonal group therapy cannot be overemphasized. It is crucial that patients want help for themselves and can acknowledge that they have difficulties, regardless of the level of resolution of eating behavior. Prior individual psychotherapy or involvement in a brief time-limited psychoeducational group can serve as a useful therapeutic trial to assess the level of motivation and ability to deal with the interpersonal issues that will arise in a longer term group. The prospective member must convey a desire for personal change and a willingness to assume responsibility for addressing interpersonal issues in the group.

Patients selected for group will have varying levels of insight surrounding their difficulties. Interpersonal problems commonly cited by patients during assessment include social withdrawal and isolation; loneliness; difficulty establishing and/or maintaining close, meaningful relationships; fears of rejection, assertiveness, and dependency; hypersensitivity to criticism; avoidance of conflict; extreme competitiveness; and difficulty identifying and/or expressing affect. Some patients may have difficulty identifying any explicit interpersonal problem. Some may show a marked degree of alexithymia, or difficulty in identifying affective states. Instead, they talk vaguely about their world seeming empty and void, as if something is missing. Such symptoms usually have interpersonal underpinnings. Clearly major insight is unrealistic for such patients at the beginning, but they need to be able to acknowledge that there might be internal issues worth exploring.

Commitment to Time

A vital criterion for inclusion in an intensive longer term group is the patient's willingness to commit herself for at least 1 year. In addition, the patient must agree to attend the first 12 sessions. Absences during this critical forming stage interfere with the opportunity of members to experience the benefits of group membership and greatly impede the development of cohesiveness. There should be no hesitation in postponing a scheduled starting date of a group for a week or two to accommodate all members. This reinforces the importance of attendance. For many patients, these stipulations may initially sound far too onerous, particularly for those with impulsive tendencies or those whose past eating behavior has interfered with their ability to be reliable and keep commitments. But it is these very patients who need the most help in cementing the structural foundation needed to enter into therapeutic work. For high school and college students, the time criterion can be modified in accordance with the academic schedule. In these groups patients are expected to maintain full attendance while the academic term is in progress, with scheduled holiday and spring breaks.

Consider the patient whose business traveling would necessitate a group absence every 4 to 6 weeks, or the patient who is awaiting confirmation of her spouse's pending work transfer, or the patient whose work hours are likely to conflict with the group meeting time and result in repetitive lateness. Given that regular and stable attendance is critical for the development of a cohesive group (Yalom 1985), inclusion of such patients with potential time commitment difficulties is ill-advised. This underscores the importance for a therapist to make rigorous inquiries about possible conflicts with work scheduling, potential geographic moves, or any major pending change in the person's life during the pregroup screening.

By making attendance mandatory for acceptance into the group, the therapist imparts a very powerful message that the group experience is expected to take precedence over other factors, such as time conflicts with work, school, or vacation plans. If, for instance, a patient indicates that she was planning to be away on vacation 1 month after the group begins, she would have the following alternatives: 1) cancel her vacation plans or reschedule them for a later time, 2) be placed on the waiting list for another group, or 3) consider an alternative therapeutic modality. The majority of patients opt for the first alternative. For groups that are time-limited and closed, a definite ending date may be helpful for some patients by forcing a decision to make a yearlong commitment. In postgroup follow-up evaluations, patients frequently cite these time requirements as having played an important role in establishing their commitment to therapeutic work (MacKenzie et al. 1985a).

Homogeneous Group Composition

Once a series of patients have been deemed suitable for a longer term psychodynamic modality, the next task of the therapist is to compose the actual group. There is a general clinical sentiment that group composition influences the nature and process of eating disorder groups (Hendren et al. 1987; MacKenzie et al. 1986; Roy-Byrne et al. 1984; Wooley and Wooley 1985). A number of composition criteria have emerged largely through clinical trial and error.

It is the traditional view that psychodynamically oriented groups that are homogeneous for diagnosis are not as likely to be effective as heterogeneous groups (Yalom 1985). The common symptomatology characterizing homogeneous groups may interfere with the development of the working phase needed for interpersonal change.

This rationale has been challenged for eating disorder groups. Clinical experience suggests that there are significant advantages to homogeneous eating disorder groups (see Chapter 2) and that they are able to move beyond a superficial level. The first impact of homogeneity is during the engagement stage of the group. Having members with common eating experiences is a great help in breaking down the veil of secrecy that commonly surrounds the eating behavior. Later in the working stages of the group, members are able to detect and challenge subtle efforts to sabotage the therapeutic enterprise because they can recognize the techniques being used. The therapist will need to be alert that the members do not collude in resistant maneuvers rather than identifying problematic behaviors with which they themselves are familiar. On balance, the advantages of homogeneity appear to outweigh the potential disadvantages.

There is also general agreement that combining AN and BN patients in the same group is not contraindicated, providing there are at least two patients with the same diagnosis so as to prevent the creation of a group isolate (Hendren et al. 1987; Neuman and Halvorson 1983). A discussion of this composition feature is found in Chapter 2.

Another factor for consideration in group composition is age. Psychodynamic eating disorder groups seem to function best when the adolescent and adult populations are separated. This enables members to address age-specific concerns surrounding sexuality, emerging independence, and the implications of individual and family developmental tasks. For instance, the majority of adolescents are still living at home. Common group themes among members of an adolescent group include concerns surrounding preparation for separation from family, emerging sexuality and dating, establishing friendships, and dealing with competition among peers, as well as confused and ambivalent personal and social values and future school or career interests. Young adult patients in the 18-to-25 age range may also be grouped separately to focus on age-appropriate issues surrounding education, career options, the approach to intimate relations, and adjustment to separation from the family home. Older adult groups characteristically address such matters as evaluation of career and relationships, adaptation to changing family circumstances, difficulties with assertiveness and low self-esteem, and more general existential issues such as the realization that one must assume ultimate responsibility for the way one lives and conducts one's life.

Despite homogeneity for age and diagnosis, considerable heterogeneity will still exist in the eating disorder groups. Although groups will be predominantly female, male members need not be excluded, though attempts should be made not to have a single male. A male cotherapist is also helpful. Groups comprise members with different marital statuses; from diverse professional, educational, and socioeconomic levels; with various interpersonal needs; with varying levels of psychological-mindedness and awareness; from different family backgrounds; and with a spectrum of personality traits. The general rule is to try to circumvent the possibility of group isolates on any of these features.

Although following these guidelines for group selection and composition will not guarantee the prevention of all group dropouts, it will go a long way to ruling out those most at risk and to increasing the likelihood of a successful therapeutic experience for all the patients.

Group Structure

Several considerations regarding the group format and structure need to be addressed before the group commences. The specific format chosen for the psychodynamic groups described in this chapter is characterized by the following features:

1. Closed membership
2. Group size limited to no more than 8 members
3. Minimum span of 1 year or a full academic term
4. Weekly meetings
5. 90-minute sessions with pre- and postgroup discussion for the leaders
6. Private room setting, free from distraction

Establishing a closed membership of 7 or 8 suitable members who agree to attend the group regularly for a minimum duration of 1 year is the recommended format. The therapist should also be committed for the entirety of the group or with a similar minimal 1-year commitment. Should the group have a cotherapy team, both therapists should commit for the entire span of the group. If this is not possible, the use of cotherapy needs to be questioned. If it is designed to facilitate an educational experience, then an observer role might be considered for the student. A stable group format provides the members with a secure environment with clear external boundaries—an environment that lends itself to establishing a group identity and to fostering intermember interaction.

Although either a time-limited or an open-ended group approach may be used effectively for interpersonal eating disorder groups, there are some advantages to a time-limited approach. Group members are allowed a greater sense of control, autonomy, and accomplishment (MacKenzie 1990), and their fantasies of timelessness and distorted sense of reality can be effectively challenged by the structural clarity of a time-limited approach (Leibovich 1983). Knowing that a group will not go on forever can help the patients prioritize and maintain focus on their major presenting issues.

One or two group dropouts are not uncommon for interpersonal groups (Yalom 1985), and this frequency should be anticipated for psychodynamic eating disorder groups as well. The addition of new members may be necessary if the group size is reduced to fewer than five members. Excessively small groups tend to have problems with establishing an interactive climate and are less productive (Fulkerson et al. 1981). The timing of admitting new members into an ongoing group is critical and should not take place when the group is in the midst of a crisis or entering into a new stage of development.

As with most outpatient psychotherapy groups, the sessions are scheduled weekly for 90 minutes. Therapist pregroup and postgroup meetings are important, preferably immediately before and after the session. Pregroup meetings review the previous week's session and the current issues confronting the group. Postgroup meetings provide a forum for catharsis for the therapists, allow observers an opportunity for questioning and feedback, and enable the therapists to review the content and process of the session, including any critical incidents that may have arisen. Cotherapy issues should always be addressed and plans developed for the following session. A written summary of each group is completed by the therapists at this time for their future reference.

The physical setting should be free of any distractions and provide privacy. Chairs are arranged in a circle in order that all members can have eye contact with one another. It is recommended that no central barriers, such as coffee tables, be present. If a two-way mirror or videotaping is to be utilized for supervision purposes, the patients must be fully informed at an early point in the selection process and sign authorization forms before the group convenes. Live supervision is a decided advantage in groups that pose the difficulties commonly encountered in eating disorder groups.

The sessions are nonstructured and experiential in nature, with considerable emphasis on the here-and-now interaction. Often a member is encouraged to experiment and carry out interpersonal tasks in between group sessions, in order that treatment extends beyond the therapy room and promotes a generalization of change.

Pretherapy preparation is discussed in Chapter 2. It is particularly important in the type of outpatient groups being discussed in this chapter. The primary purpose of preparation is to facilitate early group cohesion. This is particularly pertinent to eating disorder groups, where premature termination is a commonly reported problem (Hall 1985; Oesterheld et al. 1987; Roy-Byrne et al. 1984).

Managing the Group

Management strategies will change as the work of the group advances. A useful way of conceptualizing this is with the language of group developmental stages. The general principles of group development have been introduced in Chapter 2. In the following discussion, these will be applied in more detail as they apply to the qualities that are commonly present in patients with eating disorders. The discussion will focus particularly on the tasks of both the leader and the members as they evolve over time.

The Engagement Stage

The chief concerns at the beginning of the group are acceptance, approval, and commitment to the group. The initial disclosures in an eating disorder group typically center on the members' identification of their eating behaviors and symptoms. One advantage of a homogeneous group is that the engagement process tends to be accelerated because members manifest common symptoms and difficulties. During the first group session, one or two members will typically take the initiative in divulging the type of eating disorder they have along with some of their eating and weight concerns, such as preoccupation with body image. Other members tend to readily follow suit and openly relate to these disclosures that are so similar to their own. A process of mutual identification and consensual validation ensues that fosters rapid cohesiveness.

Because matters dealing with eating provide excellent material for the experience of universalization, it is useful to promote a detailed discussion. This has an additional advantage. In the early anxiety and enthusiasm for group acceptance, considerable information may be revealed about the eating pathology. This not only identifies the extent of the problem, but also constitutes an acknowledgment by the patient to herself that these issues need to be addressed.

Some group members will have historically abided by a self-imposed vow of secrecy surrounding their eating disorder. Divulging their disorder to nonprofessionals for the first time can thus be a very powerful experience. Discovering that one is no longer totally alone in problems and that others possess similar shameful thoughts, behaviors, and feelings can provide great relief. This promotes a sense of belonging and triggers the operation of the important early therapeutic factor of instillation of hope.

Once all the group members have disclosed their eating disorders, they are generally more receptive to proceed to a sharing of information about other sensitive interpersonal concerns that have brought them to the group. Personal characteristics commonly shared among members include a high need for approval, a tendency to overaccommodate in relationships, perfectionistic self-expectations, and hypersensitivity to criticism and perceived rejection. They will describe lack of assertiveness, impulsivity, difficulty establishing close relationships, and difficulty in expressing affect. As these topics emerge, the therapist can keep in mind that the important process is one of identifying themes that will be addressed in more depth as the group progresses. At this point, it is of primary importance to continue the process of universalization, not of developing deep insight; excessive interpretive probing will shut down the process.

Some groups may exhibit resistance to making the switch to deeper self-revelations without the aid of the therapist's direction, whereas other groups will enter into this transition quite readily with minimal prompting. Permitting a group to become exclusively preoccupied with the topic of eating behaviors and symptoms may lead to potentially dangerous repercussions. The group could end up developing a comfortable and supportive milieu that maintains a symptom focus free from the therapeutic challenges essential to promote change. The group could become "jelled" or fixated in a restrictive focus combining features of psychoeducational groups with those of cognitive-behavioral techniques for managing eating behavior. Most patients who are accepted into longer term interpersonal groups have been through these experiences already. The expectation for a shift in attention onto psychological issues must be maintained.

Case 1

> For example, during the fifth session in an outpatient group, Eileen, a 38-year-old single professional engineer with a 17-year history of BN, reflected how strange she felt having finally divulged so many intricacies surrounding her eating disorder with someone other than her long-term individual therapist. Although she had read a lot of material on eating disorders and could relate to many of the cited personal accounts, she described always believing that in person these afflicted individuals would somehow look and act totally different from herself. She was surprised that some of the other members had similar lengthy eating disorder histories and that they too had become masters in deception and had hidden from view their intense feelings of loneliness and low self-esteem.

Working predominantly with males, she added that she was not accustomed to relating to females, that she regarded herself as superior to them, and that in the past she had always held the general belief that females were "flighty, catty, and mistrustful" (an issue explored in considerably more depth during a later phase of the group development). These revelations triggered other members to reflect both on their initial personal disclosures and on their perceptions of the group. Throughout this discussion, many members introjected their relief that members were so understanding and accepting and that the group was beginning to feel safe for them.

Eileen then helped accelerate the group's task of deeper self-disclosure by relating that although part of her was also beginning to feel a sense of belonging and acceptance, she also was aware that the group had only "scratched the surface" of her despair and misery. She still felt very wary about letting the group get to know some of the other, more troubled facets of her, fearing they would not only dislike her but would also regard her as crazy. This comment elicited nods from nearly all members along with heightened anxiety that momentarily seemed to freeze the group. The therapist picked up on this, validated the members' anxiety, and helped them make the shift to the identification of other sensitive personal issues.

Members may begin to reveal information about family dynamics. Preliminary, but not excessive, revelations of this type provide an opportunity for members to compare their experience in the group to that of outside situations. With patients who have eating disorders, this usually entails the need to present a pleasing social facade (MacKenzie et al. 1986). Once again, this information should be used for the purpose of establishing common themes, not for detailed working through. The acknowledgment and identification of problems in other aspects of their lives leads the members to realize that the issues of food, weight, and appearance are not the sole evidence of their difficulties. As members begin to perceive the group as applicable to their personal needs and a place where they can engage in meaningful psychotherapeutic work, the external boundaries of the group are further reinforced and cohesion deepens.

Patients with eating disorders are particularly susceptible to the universal fear upon entering a group that they will be deemed unacceptable by others. The lack of structure of the group can be very threatening, particularly for those members with controlled and orderly personality features. With no structure to follow and no behavioral exercises to perform, members are unsure how to be the desired "good" patient. The therapist may need to provide general encouragement without taking over the process. A discussion about the difficulties of being in a group and a restatement of the importance of individual initiative will be helpful. The leaders must accept the marked dependency and idealization that members will feel toward them during this initial stage. This is readily evidenced by members constantly glancing over at the therapist in search of direction and approval. This is best addressed not by critical or interpretive remarks but by constant efforts to have the members talk to each other and not the therapist. This gives the message that the impetus of the group is expected to come from the members, not the leader.

At the same time, it is imperative that the therapist assume an active role in this initial stage. One of the most basic and important therapist responsibilities is to ensure that all members have the opportunity to participate. Starting with the first group session, the therapist will strive to have every member share some personal information or take part in the group at some level. Silent members must actively be drawn in. Spontaneous expressions along with appropriate intermember interactions should be verbally supported and reinforced by the therapist. If the group moves into a flexible discussion of relevant issues, the therapist can remain silent and let the process unfold. It is a sign of increasing group competence when members initiate more interaction with one another of their own accord without waiting for the therapist's direction and no longer attempt to talk through the therapist. It is similarly a positive sign when active listening and clarification replaces the advice-giving or advice-seeking that is common in the early sessions.

The therapist must also be watchful and prepared to intervene if members start to talk excessively or make premature self-disclosures of sensitive information that they may later regret. Usually this talkativeness reflects initial anxiety about joining and being accepted in the group. The therapist must ameliorate the level of anxiety and help contain the talkative group members (Hall 1985). Normalizing patients' anticipatory anxiety can be very reassuring to the members and often activates a discussion about what it was like coming to and becoming part of the group. Lengthy silences or conflict between members can threaten the group integrity at this stage. It is the therapist's obligation to ensure that these situations are not allowed to develop. Collectively, these therapist interventions function to shape the therapeutic process and to deter the development of norms that may impede the development of a constructive learning environment.

As with other beginning groups, eating disorder groups may experience difficulty putting closure on a group session without the aid of the therapist. Approximately 10 minutes before the end of a session, the therapist may alert the group on the time remaining and, if required, actively assist the members in wrapping up the session. Particularly when the affect has been intense, it is helpful to ask the members what it will be like leaving today and whether anyone has any concerns about any other member. Members may be worried that the group is ending when it is obvious that a certain member is still very upset or has not had sufficient time to explore a specific issue. Often such concerns have their origins in questions as to whether the therapist is concerned or available. It is useful for the group to explore its concerns with the involved member who usually is less worried about them than the other members. Ways of managing the distress may be discussed. The therapist can also acknowledge the importance of continued exploration of an issue and encourage the member or group to bring it up at the start of the next session. By following through with the responsibility of ending the group on time, the therapist reinforces the importance for members to raise issues early in the group, conveys the message that concerns will not be resolved in the short term, and demonstrates realistic limit setting.

The activities of the engagement stage have direct relevance to the nature of the eating disorders. By assuming an active role, the therapist is providing reassurance that the group is in good hands. At the same time, encouragement for the members to talk mainly to one another develops an expectation that they will be able to control the process. An understanding and supportive stance that avoids direct interpretations creates a positive and nonthreatening atmosphere. All of these strategies are designed to create a holding atmosphere that will serve to contain the patients' needs and expectations. This validates their experiences and helps to begin the process of identifying the inner aspects that constitute a sense of self. In individual therapy, this function is provided by the therapist directly. In group psychotherapy, it is achieved through the development of a cohesive group atmosphere.

The therapist must be careful not to underestimate the level of anxiety the patients are experiencing. They are highly skilled simulators and will attempt to portray a facade of competence. The therapist needs to be sure that the meaning of the group for the members is continually explored and reinforced. The members should be encouraged to respond to the tension each is experiencing and, by acknowledging it, help each other to regulate it. The source of tension should not be explored early in the group; management of it is the goal.

A lot of information is provided in the early sessions about eating behaviors, attitudes toward food and body image, self-esteem, and relationship concerns. As this material is brought out, the therapist can take an active role in making sure it is thoroughly discussed and that no important statement goes without a response from the group. The purpose of this is to constantly validate the individual's experience. This directly addresses the problems in self-definition characteristic of this clinical population. By clarifying what the person is experiencing and validating it as understandable, the group is promoting internal self-organization. The members need to learn to attend to each other's affective states and to seek to understand the nature of the tension. This promotes an integration between external behavior and inner states and decreases the discrepancy between the "true self" and the "false self." During the early stages of the group, a nondirective empathic stance is more helpful in facilitating this process than an interpretive mode.

The presence of gross distortions and misinterpretations of interpersonal events and about self provides material for cognitive-behavioral techniques. The style of thinking can be clarified and opened for discussion by the members. Customarily members will judge the reactions of others far more accurately than they will their own. This "double standard" offers an opportunity to examine the validity of long-held beliefs. This must be handled in a neutral manner that does not involve a blaming component. It is a process that is generally more acceptable when it comes from other members than from the leader. Once a belief system has been exposed, the therapist can help the group to track it over time for reoccurrence or modification.

The engagement stage is accomplished when all members have taken part in personal self-disclosure and are committed to participate. The group is now primed to shift into the next phase of development equipped with a cohesive interactive climate and a sense of solidarity among members. These are essential elements needed to manage the emergence of individual differences and conflicts among group members. Bearing in mind that each group moves at its own pace, most outpatient weekly eating disorder groups take 2 to 3 months to master the task of engagement.

The Differentiation Stage

The group task in the second stage is to develop a way of tolerating and incorporating different viewpoints among the members. This process establishes a milieu characterized by greater confrontation and questioning. Former assumptions of similarity are now challenged, and the group's core concerns shift to issues surrounding dominance, control, and power, leading to a temporary drop in group cohesion (Yalom 1985). It is characteristic for these issues to be polarized and couched in exaggerated and stereotyped statements. Expectations concerning the way the group operates are commonly challenged and at times altered, leading to the development of more explicit and solidified group norms. This process is in sharp contrast to that witnessed in the engagement stage, where the norms regarding the way the group should function are governed predominantly by the therapist.

The differentiation stage poses a particular dilemma in groups for patients with eating disorders. Although this is an important stage in all psychodynamic groups, the personality features characteristic of many patients with eating disorders form a distinctive resistance to the development of differentiation (MacKenzie et al. 1986). Many of these patients experience extreme anxiety with the very notion of dealing openly with negative affects. They commonly hold catastrophic beliefs that it is dangerous to differ and that disagreement with others will result in rejection, humiliation, or loss of control. Because of this difficulty in dealing with conflict and differences, the members will predictably attempt to avoid the emergence of the Stage II process. Groups that succeed in avoiding this stage will either remain fixated in the stage of engagement or eventually fragment because of a sense of futility.

Case 2

For example, Susan began arriving consistently late during the third month of the group. Immediately upon her exhibitionistic entrance into the room, she would interrupt the group with lengthy apologies along with detailed accounts of the reasons for her lateness. On many of these occasions the group would delay commencing work on any issues until after Susan's arrival and increasingly began to allow her to direct the content of the session. Not only did members refrain from challenging Susan with this behavior, they denied sharing any of the therapist's concerns about punctuality and instead offered full support and understanding of Susan's seemingly valid excuses. During one session, another member's tearful disclosure was interrupted and disregarded due to Susan's late entrance. The group then seemed to shut down, dealing only with superficial issues. Midway through the group session, the therapist wondered what the members would be experiencing if the session were to end at this moment. One member responded that she had been preoccupied and concerned for the member who was interrupted, yet was reluctant to voice these concerns or refocus the content in fear of upsetting her or possibly offending Susan. Another member acknowledged that she too was concerned for the member who was interrupted, adding that she was starting to feel angry about Susan's lateness and wondered why the group was granting her special status when many others in the group had to make a concerted effort to ensure they arrived on time. Two other members went to Susan's unsolicited rescue while another member attacked the therapist for failing to take total responsibility in rectifying the lateness issue. Some of the members voiced that they were able to identify and acknowledge their anger only after hearing other members disclose this feeling first. Furthermore, many thought they didn't really have the right to question or confront Susan, particularly when she was always so apologetic.

Over the next several sessions, the group dealt with the norm of punctuality and arrived at their own guidelines as to how deal with this situation in the event it should arise. For instance, the group decided that lateness would not be condoned and that members would have to phone in advance to leave a message. The group also began to confront and explore the nature and meaning of Susan's lateness, helping her arrive at a preliminary understanding that this behavior was related to her fear and avoidance of conflict. In the later working phase of the group development, Susan's lateness in the group along with her perpetual tardiness and absenteeism in outside group events were explored within the context of her personality features.

The individual members must learn to tolerate and deal with differences, conflict, and anger both in themselves and others. They struggle over the extent to which they should abide by and assert their own ideas and beliefs versus the extent to which they should go along with the collective opinion of the group. Inherent in this struggle is the threat of being negatively judged either as different or as compromising oneself for the sake of the social system (MacKenzie and Livesley 1983). Early attempts at more assertive postures may be met by waves of guilt and self-condemnation for allowing such reactions to show.

Once members are able to deal openly with negative affects and learn that anger is not inevitably destructive, it is common for them to express an increased sense of self-esteem and self-control. For those patients whose bulimic symptoms have not yet resolved, many will report a decrease in symptomatology once they achieve the task of differentiation. It appears that they are more capable of relinquishing their bulimic symptoms when they can distinguish their feelings from those of others, affirm their own boundaries, and engage in more assertive behavior.

Cognitive therapy is particularly effective in helping individual members explore their various distorted interpersonal beliefs, such as the belief that one should always strive to please other people or the belief that it is wrong to openly verbalize anger toward people, particularly parental or authority figures. Systematic examination of distorted beliefs permits the members to test them against reality, first within the group setting and then in situations external to group.

The task of the therapist is first to facilitate the identification and expression of differences and anger, and second, to promote the exploration of these differences among members, along with their perceptions of the events. The therapist needs to ensure that the intensity of affect does not transcend the patient's or group's tolerance level. It is of utmost importance that the therapist take an active role in moving the group beyond the initial phase of ventilating anger and hostility. The ensuing cognitive component involving the members' understanding of the experience is vital for the achievement of conflict resolution. The therapist can direct the discussion to an exploration of what it is like to assert different beliefs and opinions, to experience anger, and to deal with anger in themselves and others. These types of therapist interventions should be frequent but brief and focused. The intent is to enhance members' responsibility for the content of the session. MacKenzie and Livesley (1983) caution that if this cognitive work is neglected, the affect affiliated with it either goes underground or stays elevated and unresolved; both situations pose a potential threat to group integrity and increase the risk of dropouts.

Case 3

For example, Andrea, a 21-year-old hotel management student who was the youngest child in a large, enmeshed immigrant family, presented to the group with borderline personality features and a 5-year history of AN+BN. Her past history revealed sexual abuse from a paternal uncle, periodic episodes of alcohol abuse, some self-mutilation (cutting of extremities), and one charge for shoplifting. Andrea had been seen in individual therapy for 3 years and during this time was hospitalized on 3 occasions, twice for severe emaciation and once for a suicide attempt in which she attempted to overdose on her mother's antidepressants. A series of family therapy sessions were integrated during two of these hospitalizations. Her course in individual therapy, albeit turbulent, had nevertheless been quite effective. For the year prior to Andrea's referral to the group, she had abstained from alcohol, she was functioning adequately in her college program, and her weight, although below the 85th percentile of normative values for weight, had stabilized. Given the nature and multitude of interpersonal conflicts in her life, the individual therapist thought Andrea would benefit from a group involvement. Plans were for her to continue receiving individual therapy concurrently with her group. In spite of misgivings concerning Andrea's suitability for an intensive group, the male-female cotherapists accepted her into the group.

Entering the group recapitulated Andrea's position in her family. Although there were two other members close to her in age, Andrea seemed considerably younger in emotional maturity. As the group moved into the stage of differentiation, Andrea became increasingly unsettled. She either withdrew and remained on the periphery in what seemed to be her attempts to be a good girl, or she consumed the group's focus by staging temper tantrums and a host of other disruptive behaviors, becoming the bad child that she had been in her own family. Although the therapists were successful in circumventing the group's two attempts to scapegoat Andrea, they were unsuccessful in their attempts to help Andrea manage and work through her hostility and differences on an emotional or cognitive level. The intensity of Andrea's negative affect exceeded her tolerance level as well as that of the group. During one such episode, Andrea sighed and rolled her eyes in response to another member's sensitive disclosure, creating considerable discomfort for the members who witnessed this. When confronted by one of the members with the comment that it seemed she had something to say, she suddenly became very upset, screamed a few obscenities at the confronting member, accused the group of being out to get her, and tearfully stormed out of the room. Two members spontaneously followed her out and after several minutes coaxed her into returning to the session. For the remainder of the session, Andrea refused to speak about the episode or anything else, although in response to the members' voiced concerns, she nodded that she would return for the next session and that she would not harm herself over the next week.

Andrea did not attend the next session. Most of the session in which she was absent was centered on the members' concern for Andrea's well-being and safety and their worry that they were responsible for her absence. When Andrea returned the following week and nonchalantly commented that she had forgotten all about the session until it was well in progress and that it had been silly of them to sit and waste the previous session worrying about her, the group became distraught and wondered with her what she would have expected them to do. Andrea yelled out that she knew she shouldn't have come to the session, bolted up from her chair toward the door, but was persuaded by other members to remain. At this point, she refused to discuss the matter any further, threatening that if any attempts were made to do so she would leave the session. The group members failed in their attempt to shift the focus and came to realize this was only escalating the acute tension in the room. With the therapists' direction, they then began to process the event and address the dilemma facing them. One of the members commented that the current turmoil in the group was similar to her chaotic home life with a younger rebellious sibling, and that perhaps Andrea would be of help to her in learning more effective ways to cope with these situations. Andrea did not reply to this statement until just before the group's closing. She angrily volunteered that she couldn't possibly see how she could be of help and added that she didn't come to this group to be used. When the member tried to clarify that perhaps she had not made herself clear and that she had not meant her comments to be viewed as criticism, Andrea bolted out of her chair, bellowed that she had made herself quite clear, and exited the group. In her weekly individual psychotherapy session, Andrea announced to her therapist that she was dropping out of the group. She refused to contact the group therapists to inform them of her intentions and refused to return to the group to say goodbye.

During the therapists' review of this case, it became clear that they had not given enough attention to their selection process. They recollected how they had been eager to fill the last placement in order to get the group under way, that they had conducted a hasty screening interview with Andrea but had nevertheless been impressed by her voiced enthusiasm, and that, in retrospect, they were also influenced by the request of their fellow colleague to seriously consider accepting Andrea.

The task of differentiation deals directly with concerns that are central to the pathogenesis of eating disorders. It is therefore incumbent on the therapist to monitor the process of the group to ensure these concerns are adequately explored. Achieving this task in an eating disorder group generally requires more time and active work on the part of the therapist than most psychotherapy groups. Moreover, there is an artistry involved on the part of the therapist to maintain a safe, holding environment while the group is in the midst of a temporary loss of cohesion. Members generally find it much easier to interact with one another in a "there-and-then" context rather than a "here-and-now" framework. They will try to avoid the present group context unless directed by the therapist, who must desensitize the members to examining the here and now.

It is customary for group members to first challenge the therapist before risking intermember challenge. These confrontations often center on the group norms or aspects of the leadership role. Such confrontations should be regarded by the therapist as a positive signal that the group is progressing in its development. The therapist is now in a position to model the interpersonal skills of receiving feedback and dealing with differences. This receptivity to confrontation plays an integral role in establishing the norm of interpersonal honesty and emotional expression. For many patients with eating disorders, this experience represents the first time that they have dealt openly with conflict regarding an authority figure.

These challenges may be uncomfortable for a group therapist. Ongoing supervision plays an important function in helping the therapist tolerate the directed hostility and distinguish between attacks on the role of the therapist versus attacks on the therapist's personhood. Groups will avoid dealing directly with negative feelings toward the therapist if they sense the therapist is threatened by conflict or in need of protection. In these instances, the group may resort to developing maladaptive means of conflict resolution such as the scapegoating of a member or subsequent suppression of any negative feelings toward the therapist and other members.

In groups with a male cotherapist, the leadership challenge often centers on the ineptitude of men in understanding women. Roy-Byrne and colleagues (1984) and Inbody and Ellis (1985) note the protest directed toward the male cotherapist and the considerable group time consumed on the theme of shortcomings of men. The issue of hostility toward men, like other conflict stage themes, tends to be polarized and framed in the context of gender role stereotypes. Nonetheless, this work represents important preparation for in-depth exploration of male/female issues later in the group's life. Although these matters regarding men will surface whether or not a male cotherapist is present, in postgroup interviews members have generally placed significant value on having had the opportunity to work this through with both a male and a female therapist present (MacKenzie et al. 1985b).

The work of this stage is directly relevant to separation-individuation issues. It marks a shift from using the group as a supportive environment to considering it a testing ground for autonomous behavior. Patients with eating disorders may experience profound guilt for undertaking such tasks. It goes against a lifetime of obedience, obligation, and appeasement. The idea of having a separate identity invokes a reaction that they are abandoning those they love. The open emergence of negative affect threatens the tight defenses that have been employed and creates a fear that there will be total loss of control. The therapist needs to be prepared to expose these concerns through the members. If they are not addressed, the group may relapse back into the safer waters of universalization or begin to suffer dropouts as members choose to avoid the issues in the air. This work continues in a largely noninterpretative manner. The goal is definition and clarification more than understanding.

Case 4

For example, Judy, a 30-year-old patient who had a lengthy history of AN+BN dating back to her early teens, was able to verbalize her feelings of anger toward the therapist in reaction to the therapist's line of questioning toward another patient. Judy perceived the therapist as being unduly confrontational and added that had this been directed at her, she personally would have felt singled out and embarrassed. Along with other members, Judy proceeded to acknowledge how difficult it was to feel and express anger toward the therapist and other authority figures in her life, a situation she typically would have gone to great lengths to avoid. A few days following the session, Judy placed a call to the therapist wondering whether the group was still scheduled for the upcoming week.

Judy appeared extremely anxious in the subsequent session, assuming a head-down, nonparticipatory position. In response to the group members' attention to this, Judy uttered softly that she felt "very ashamed—like a fool" for expressing her anger toward the therapist in the previous week's session and proceeded to attempt to undo her feelings, apologetically claiming she didn't know what had gotten into her and that she must have been overtired. Judy expounded that she became progressively more upset by her behavior as the week went on and began to fear that the therapist would somehow retaliate or perhaps ask her to leave the group. In response to her mother's query as to her apparent upset, Judy stated that for the first time since the group's inception, she discussed with her what had transpired in the session. Her mother, whom Judy described as having a passive, inferior, and meek nature similar to her own, reacted to the story in alarm. She agreed with Judy's concern that she had "stepped out of line" and advised that she should retract her comments. Judy had worked herself up to such a frenzy that she became convinced the therapist would hate her and she contemplated dropping out of the group. However, when Judy phoned to cancel the session, she noted that for some unknown reason she couldn't follow through with this option and rather found herself fumbling and finally questioning whether the group was still scheduled for this week.

The therapist and group members reinforced Judy's decision to return to the group and not act on her inclination to drop out. Over the next several sessions Judy was able to further process this critical event and explore her distorted catastrophic beliefs of expressing negative affect. In spite of her continued feelings of discomfort and guilt at expressing negative affect, she eventually realized that she could cope with these feelings and indeed feel better than when she kept them hidden inside.

The stage of differentiation approaches resolution when a cooperative means of conflict resolution is achieved and when all of the members have participated in the assertion of individual ideas and beliefs. As each member's uniqueness becomes known, the group is in a position to recognize and appreciate the different roles members may assume in the group. Group norms become consolidated as members arrive at a consensus regarding the way the group should operate. This process is accompanied by members accepting more personal responsibility for therapeutic change and by a resurgence in group cohesion.

The work on conflictual issues may take a long time in eating disorder groups—often several months. Because the thematic material is so important for these patients, it is important that the therapist not try to rush this process. Repeated review of the same themes as they emerge from different perspectives within the group is necessary. Successful mastery of the tasks of engagement and differentiation prepares the group to look more closely at interpersonal issues.

The Interpersonal Work Stages

The working phase of group development is centered around three major themes: individuation, intimacy, and mutuality. These build naturally on each other. The transition zone between these substages is less distinct than the earlier developmental stages, and the content themes often appear in varying mixtures. The term "interpersonal work" is used in the sense of the group now focusing particularly on the meaning of the interactions between and among the members.

The eager therapist who jumps too quickly into intensive interactional material runs the risk of stalling or fragmenting the group. This is particularly likely in eating disorder groups, where lengthy preparation is required to equip the members to deal openly with both negative interactions and greater intimacy. As the group matures, it begins to resemble other longer term groups and the pace of change may quicken. The identification of cognitive distortions and components of self-image that began in the two earlier stages can now be applied more intensely to the real relationships emerging among the group members.

Individuation.   In this substage, the task for the individual member is to become increasingly receptive to psychological exploration in order to develop greater insight and acceptance of the complexity of self. Although this stage may be intense and painful for the individual, it is generally considered to be more satisfying than the work of the preceding stage. A part of this process concerns understanding the connections between psychological events and eating behavior. This is an important progression because patients with eating disorders often derive their sense of personal identity and self-worth from their perceptions of their eating habits and body image. Perhaps for the first time in years, the body no longer serves as the primary channel through which emotions are expressed. The individual begins to challenge ideas about herself that have been tenaciously held, such as the need to be perfect or the belief that thinness equates with self-worth. For example, one AN patient who had achieved weight stabilization and normalized eating was astonished to receive a work promotion, believing for years that she would only succeed in her career if her weight remained below 100 pounds.

A surge in cohesion and universality is seen as the members identify common, previously split-off and conflicted aspects of themselves. Also evident are the working dimensions of self-disclosure, challenge, and cognitive mastery leading to a sense of meaningful psychological learning. Upcoming sessions are eagerly anticipated, and for the moment the group becomes the most significant and meaningful event in their lives.

The member does risk some loss of self-esteem as previously unacknowledged parts of self are uncovered. However, these risks are usually mitigated by collaboration with other members in the introspective process. What members more commonly experience is an enhancement in self-esteem as they start to accept those aspects of the self originally deemed bad or undesirable (MacKenzie and Livesley 1983). Members find others are more attracted to them as they share more of themselves. This directly challenges the protective social facade that has prevented them from accepting any positive regard or compliments from others. This distorted belief is directly challenged by the positive attention from other members accorded to their efforts at understanding themselves.

Case 5

For example, Elizabeth, a 27-year-old AN patient who complained of depression, loneliness, and a lack of direction in life, typically presented herself to the group in a passive, calculating, accommodating, and self-deprecatory fashion. Anything she vocalized was predictably preceded by her scanning the faces of therapists and members in hopes of receiving clues as to what they would want to hear. She eventually began to challenge this presentation, acknowledging it was often a defense, and to show the part of herself that was more uninhibited and opinionated. She noticed other group members began to show more interest in her opinions rather than the anticipated disinterest. She was able to gain insight into her fears of abandonment and rejection and her subsequent need to always play it "safe." The members told her that her former meekness was often boring and that the more she expressed her own desires and feelings, the more they were attracted to her. This member eventually became very popular and well-liked in the group, which helped bolster her self-esteem and provide her with the needed encouragement to begin taking more interpersonal risks in her personal life.

The major responsibility of the therapist is to help the group attain its task of introspective self-understanding by helping the members to integrate past, present, and future interpersonal experiences. The group members are now able to assume more responsibility for the content of the sessions, allowing the therapist to play a gatekeeping role that focuses on integrating content with process. A positive and active involvement in the group process can be maintained through genuine and empathic interactions with members and through the avoidance of impersonal and judgmental interventions. The group task of psychological exploration is further reinforced by recognizing and acknowledging when a member takes a risk and reflecting on the underlying affect of the self-revelations.

Because the identity of patients with eating disorders is often fragile, they are apt to take on and experience another group member's difficulties as their own. The therapist must be alert to this and help the patients to distinguish their own feelings from the feelings of the member speaking. This process helps to develop a more clearly defined sense of self.

Intimacy. The introspective process described previously pulls the members into closer relationships. The group task of the intimacy subphase is to experience, manage, and explore the implications of close interpersonal involvement. These interactions initially tend to be motivated more by the individual needs of the members, but this egocentricity is gradually replaced by more reciprocity. The members now have an opportunity to focus on the roles they assume in group, which often mirror those assumed in outside relationships. Considerable interpersonal learning takes place as members experiment with new and modified roles. The emergence of underlying feelings of guilt and inherent badness may be expected as defenses are modified. This experience stimulates members to examine and reformulate the nature of their contemporary and historic relationships.

Case 6

For example, Karen, a 32-year-old AN+BN patient, became aware of her tendency to adopt a very sociable, mediating, and cotherapy role within the group that paralleled the role she assumed in her family of origin and among her friends. She was very supportive of other members, attempting to ensure that everyone had an opportunity to participate. She filled lags in the discussion, endeavored to keep the group on a positive emotional tone, and assumed a peacekeeping position whenever she sensed friction between members. Although this role was very complementary to the group in its formative stage, Karen's rigidity with this role began to restrict the group's progression into the phase of differentiation. With the group's confrontation and encouragement to relinquish the excessive reliance on this role, Karen gradually began to experiment with new roles, despite her extreme anxiety and fears that the group would fall apart if she were not always "on hand to glue it back together."

Once she was able to demonstrate more role flexibility within the group, Karen seemed more receptive to exploring her role in the family and how she first assumed a sociable, peacekeeping, somewhat "parentified" position as a preteen in response to the distress of her parents and helplessness surrounding the rebelliousness and acting-out behavior of her older teenage sister. She recalled how her parents actively reinforced this role: how they constantly reminded her that she was the "tonic" in the family who was responsible for keeping them happy and together. Currently, Karen was still living at home. Any personal needs or problems of Karen's were historically withheld from her parents and solved by herself, frequently through the process of denial and suppression. Karen gained insight into how her development of AN helped her maintain some semblance of self-control and cope with her anxiety.

The dilemma experienced by Karen was her desire to make other members feel involved and needed, as she did for her parents, while at the same time not placing any personal demands on others or appearing to take anything from another member. The anger engendered toward her parents during these explorations was very anxiety-provoking for Karen, as was her open acknowledgment of personal needs to the group members. Initially she voiced feeling extremely guilty for talking negatively about her parents, particularly considering all the reassurance they had offered her surrounding her eating disorder. With time, Karen not only became better able to tolerate her ambivalence toward family members but also began to modify her role within the family and among her friends. A major step toward Karen's growing independence was her decision to attend graduate school in an out-of-province program scheduled to commence shortly after her termination from the group.

Some members describe families of origin that have unspoken rules forbidding the acknowledgment or expression of negative affect. These members may encounter negative resistance from family members when they attempt to deal with differences and anger within the family setting. They may need to accept that their family will not likely change and that they must be content to hold different beliefs. Working through these types of family issues and relinquishing long-standing family roles such as the "caregiver" or the "mediator" can be difficult and painful.

Patients with eating disorders often report difficulty with intimacy and commonly recount the superficial quality of their previous relationships. Many of these patients have experienced sexual abuse prior to the onset of their eating disorders (see Chapter 10), and it is during this stage that they are usually able to more adequately address and work through the complexity of this issue. The revelations of other members may permit the acknowledgment of the sexual abuse both to themselves and others. Body image concerns are also reactivated as members come to recognize the close link these issues have to their conflicts over intimacy. Working through the intense affect associated with these matters represents a major therapeutic triumph for patients with eating disorders. It is at this stage in the group development that the members are liberated from the belief that their acceptability is irrevocably connected to weight and appearance (MacKenzie et al. 1986). Self-esteem is further enhanced as the members experience that they are both capable of being involved with others as well as being acceptable to others. The following example looks at a segment of a group in its 42nd session that was addressing sexual abuse.

Case 7

Marilyn, a 27-year-old BN patient with borderline personality features, was exploring with the group her intense intolerance of loneliness and emptiness. Some months earlier she had acknowledged a prior history of sexual abuse but had not as yet engaged in any in-depth discussion of this. Since the recent breakup of her common-law relationship, Marilyn found it distressing to be spending so much time alone in her apartment and revealed how during these times her thoughts would be flooded with memories of being sexually abused by her stepfather from ages 10 to 12. Another member instantly related to her, adding that she went to great lengths to avoid being alone as it was at these times that she too was most apt to ruminate about her past sexual abuse from an older brother and his friends. With the group's support, these members then embarked on a very emotionally laden account of their sexual abuse and some of the current ramifications the experiences had on their well-being and interpersonal relationships. This was the first time either of them had revealed these issues with anyone, and they conveyed how strange it felt to have released their powerful secrets. Marilyn was able to explore her ambivalent feelings toward her stepfather with whom she still enjoyed a close, loyal relationship. She had been deemed his favorite child and this status in the family had been, and still was, very important to her. She was also able to address her fear of being criticized by group members for still loving her stepfather and also anticipated she would resent any criticism about him by the members.

For the next several weeks the group maintained a focus on sexual abuse, victimization, and exploitation. In this particular group, five of the seven members related a past history of sexual abuse, although only two had acknowledged this during the pregroup assessment process. As expected, body image conflicts inundated this group. One 30-year-old AN patient, who was struggling to accept a higher weight and curvaceous figure after 16 years of restrictive eating, was extremely uncomfortable with the compliments she was receiving from friends and family. During one session, she tearfully divulged that her father began to make sexual advances toward her during the start of her puberty. Her solution to his fondling was to regain her prepubescent figure through restrictive dieting. The solution to this problem seemed effective as her father seemed to lose sexual interest in her and stopped making advances. She had repressed all thoughts of these incidents until recently, when her father again became flirtatious with her.

A number of issues initially addressed during the stage of differentiation are now worked through at a deeper level. For instance, the realization that it is not always necessary to be perfect or accommodating is further integrated. Members can practice letting go of this stance during "here-and-now" group interactions, followed by experimentation in their external environment. Their belief that they would be rejected for such action is actively challenged as they experience being responded to with greater interest, acceptance, and closeness by their group peers and significant others.

It is at this stage that the sense of prevailing emptiness described by many patients with eating disorders begins to dissipate. As the members interact less on an intellectual, superficial level and more on an emotional, personal level, they begin to experience relationships as more fulfilling and meaningful. The realization develops that their previous social facades and perfectionistic tendencies contributed in part to both the onset and perpetuation of this internal emptiness.

Intermember interactions can be guided by the therapist through a variety of interventions such as interpersonal observation, reflection, clarification, summarizing, reframing, empathic understanding, and tentative interpretations. The therapist continues to focus on group process and to emphasize interpretations that encourage generalization to current outside difficulties. Highly abstract interpretations should be minimized; instead, pragmatic, uncomplicated interventions that provide ideas for how to understand behavior and interpersonal events within the session should be emphasized (Dies 1983). Feedback that is descriptive and behaviorally oriented should be modeled for the members and reinforced whenever it is exhibited. The members should be encouraged to experiment and practice interactional skills and new adaptive roles learned within the group to maximize interpersonal learning and change.

During this stage of the group's development, the group is receptive to a more open level of therapist transparency. Self-disclosures that reflect "normal" emotional experiences, feelings, thoughts, and reactions of the therapist, particularly as they pertain to interactions and events within the group, can be effective in reinforcing personal expression among members. The therapist should be mindful to avoid disclosures that are intrusive and overly revealing or critical.

Mutuality.   The substage of intimacy progresses gradually to one of mutuality. The tasks facing the individual member are to experience and acknowledge that they can be important to someone else, and to accept responsibility for their interactions with the other. This requires an exploration of the meaning of closeness. MacKenzie and Livesley (1983) emphasize that this does not imply an increased sense of intimacy, but rather an appreciation of the fundamental uniqueness of each member.

The opportunity now exists to establish more clearly a sense of personal autonomy. Problems surrounding interpersonal issues of dependency, exploitation, reciprocity, and responsibility can be explored and understood in greater detail. The interpersonal difficulties encountered by many patients with eating disorders can be attributed in part to the extreme control they have exercised in a variety of ways, often indirect, throughout their lifetimes. This control dimension, which is symbolized by struggles over food, becomes a central focus in psychotherapy. It can be conceptualized as a continuum, with total dependency versus uncaring exploitation representing the extreme ends. In this advanced group work, the members can experience and develop an understanding that relationships need not be determined in a polarized fashion through dominance or submission, but rather can be based on mutual agreement and cooperation.

Case 8

For example, during the 63rd session of a 6-member eating disorder group, one patient, Frances, raised concerns about the growing disharmony between her and her family, most notably her husband. This 41-year-mother of two with chronic AN had historically been very dependent on her husband, deriving her sense of worth largely through his personhood and her slight appearance. Over the past few months, Frances had begun to address a number of existential issues that appeared to coincide with her youngest son leaving home to attend a university. At the time of her son's departure, she had become very depressed and noted she had not felt this empty since her postpartum depression following the birth of this son. The onset of her AN coincided with this postpartum depression. For the first time, Frances was able to work through her grief and address issues surrounding her long-standing low self-esteem, ineffectiveness, and powerlessness. A notable shift occurred in Frances's affect and interaction style in the group as she began to work through her issues and empower herself with a sense of self-worth, independence, and autonomy and as she began to redirect her sense of purpose in life. With the group's encouragement and support, Frances began to take interpersonal risks outside of the group setting. Although she continued to equate a lot of her self-worth to her slimness, it no longer represented her total identity.

Other members could relate to the turbulence these major shifts were creating in Frances's home life. Although her family members were in part enthusiastic about her progress, they also felt threatened by the change and were experiencing some difficulty with Frances's changing role in the family.

This is a particularly challenging time for those patients with eating disorders who historically have experienced marked difficulty in trusting others. They commonly equate closeness within a relationship to engulfment and loss of individuality. Problems in heterosexual relationships offer a prime application of these difficulties. Many of these patients have previously fused issues pertaining to sexuality and control in a polarized and dichotomous manner. Working through the tasks of this substage represents a major developmental milestone for these patients.

It is common at this stage for members to begin to perceive themselves as worthy of being loved and as capable of loving others. This stands in sharp contrast to their self-perceptions at the start of group. It is also common to hear a member voice her astonishment over her ability to be more flexible with herself and others.

In order to facilitate the acceptance of personal responsibility in relationships, the therapist continues to encourage direct translation and application of here-and-now interactions to outside interpersonal relationships and vice versa. Modeling of genuine, positive interactions helps members understand the value of openness and support. With cotherapy arrangements, open communication between the therapists can be more overtly modeled to help members integrate the concept that what one person does has implications for someone else.

Termination

In the time-limited group format described, the groups typically last 12 to

18 months. The decision of whether to extend a group beyond 1 year is usually influenced by how well the group has advanced. The desired goal is for the group to spend several months in interpersonal work beyond the differentiation stage and to have sufficient time to work through termination issues. Should the group decide to extend beyond 1 year, a new ending point is then negotiated. Ideally, all members of a group will terminate together. Preparation for the termination process should commence 3 to 4 months in advance.

Termination is a critical stage in the group developmental process that can serve as an important force in promoting the continuance of therapeutic change. The group task entails the disengagement of members in such a manner that they can function without feeling a sense of demoralization and hopelessness (MacKenzie et al. 1986). The members now must give up the containing environment of the group. This was the first crucial development in the group, and its threatened loss will activate all the original self-definition issues.

At termination, as in the engagement stage, the focus of psychological attention is centered on events and issues external to the group. Future plans and ambitions are compared and contrasted with events that occurred in the group. This should be accompanied by a reflection on the history of the group and the progress of individual members. These various tasks all serve to assist the group members in assimilating the group as a personally significant and enduring experience. If this important group work is avoided or viewed negatively, the incorporation of the experience may be obstructed and earlier group progress may be undone. The members' task is to accept personal responsibility for their behavior without the presence or support of the group. During the early phase of termination, members will commonly express doubts over their ability to continue to assume responsibility for themselves.

In a longer term group, termination inevitably evokes feelings of loss and separation. It is common for all dynamic psychotherapy groups to witness a resurgence of presenting complaints, which in eating disorder groups tends to revolve around themes relating to eating behavior. This is a potent reminder of the previous centrality of these problems and the transformation the individuals underwent to break the secrecy and isolation surrounding these eating patterns (MacKenzie et. al. 1986). It is as if they must leave behind a major part of themselves. These reactions typically dissipate as the group resolves the task of termination.

Although some patients may have attained significant improvement in both their interpersonal functioning and in the intensity of their eating symptoms, they may not be totally free from restrictive episodes or periods of bingeing or purging. A state of disillusionment over not having accomplished total resolution may ensue. This usually results in members having the opportunity to once again work through the perfectionistic and dichotomous style through which they were apt to perceive themselves and their relationships. For the patient with an eating disorder, adequate resolution of termination issues consolidates the view that "I can effectively manage my life without an eating disorder."

A group may be prone to avoidance in dealing with the task of termination. It is the responsibility of the therapist to keep the task in focus for the group (Yalom 1985). The therapist must repeatedly direct the members' attention to the issues surrounding termination. All of the members should be provided with opportunities to participate actively and constructively in this process. The therapist does not encourage members to introduce new content material, as this impedes or blocks the group from achieving the task of disengagement. The therapist's interventions should be directed toward helping the group focus on comparing external circumstances, projected objectives, and future plans with group events and on reviewing the history of the group and its individual members. The therapist should also personally participate in the termination process. Some groups use a formal go-around in which each member says goodbye to all of the others. Often food is brought to symbolize the event.

Countertransference Considerations

Conducting intensive interpersonal groups for eating disorders is a challenging and emotionally taxing process. Countertransference reactions—a normal fact of life for the therapist—abound. Countertransference is used here in its broadest sense to mean the totality of the therapist's unconscious and conscious emotional reactions, attitudes, and behaviors toward the patient. The therapist must work not only with multiple patients, but with patients who exhibit a wide range of ego and self organizations. This heightens the emotional intensity of countertransference reactions. Given the prevalence of eating disorders in Western society today, there is a good chance that a member of the therapist's family, a friend, or a significant other may have an eating disorder. In such instances, there is an even greater need for heightened understanding of countertransferential and attitudinal derivatives stemming from the therapist's personal life.

Common countertransference issues include: 1) feeling and displaying irritation, anger, boredom, or anxiety at a group's or patient's resistance or defenses, 2) assuming the role of the caretaker or nurturer, the "good" therapist or parent, or the all-knowing, omnipotent leader, 3) identification with the patient, and 4) competition in the cotherapy relationship.

It is particularly important that the therapist has thoroughly thought through her or his own values or concerns regarding weight and body image issues. For example, a subtle attitudinal bias toward thinness may be "leaked" to the group through choice of language or through dress style. It is useful for the therapist about to begin an eating disorder group to systematically review the psychoeducational material. It contains statements about "set point" theory. Does the therapist accept this idea for self, or is there an internal blame attached to weight issues? Countertransference reactions in all psychotherapy groups often center around themes of control. This is particularly true in eating disorder groups, where the therapist must constantly be on the alert for making an intervention of an over- or undercontrolling nature. Can the therapist adopt a neutral position when challenged about passivity, or will there be a self-doubting reaction?

The key to effective management of countertransference is first to properly understand it. When correctly understood, the therapist's countertransference can be a considerable asset to therapeutic work. When not understood or identified, these countertransference reactions can deter or block the successful work of therapy for both the individual and the group as a whole. Continuous self-reflection and self-monitoring aid the therapist in understanding the patients' attitudes, beliefs, prejudices, preferences, fantasies, desires, feelings, behaviors, and personal difficulties. Supervision and the therapist's own personal therapy are two excellent avenues to attend to this extremely important facet of the therapist's clinical work. The following case examples illustrate some of the various ways countertransference reactions can manifest themselves in eating disorder groups.

Case 9

The therapist opened the 20th session of a 7-member group by asking what it was like for members coming to the session this day. In somewhat of a round-robin fashion, the members directed a brief synopsis of their week toward the therapist, interjecting flattering comments about the therapist's amazing ability to draw their secrets and concerns out in the open and about how they now couldn't imagine coping at all without the group. During an earlier session, the therapist's response to members' comments about how much they liked the group was to say that she too liked the group and, in fact, considered it to be one of her best experiences. From this point on, the group seemed very preoccupied with accommodating the therapist and ascertaining how the therapist ranked their group in comparison to others. This session followed in a similar vein. Most of the members addressed their remarks to the therapist and refrained from intermember participation unless strongly encouraged by the therapist. Any insights or progress were characteristically attributed to the therapist, regardless of the contributions of other members. The session deteriorated to a level where members sought advice and solutions to trivial day-to-day crises. One member suddenly dropped out of the group following this session, and attempts to contact the member were unsuccessful.

During a supervision session, the therapist commented that the group seemed stuck "in a sea of niceness" with one another. She was aware that the group was not progressing into the stage of differentiation, yet she was having difficulty helping them make this shift. Instead she felt continually pulled into rescuing members and engaging in problem-solving tactics. She reported feeling bored and increasingly impatient with members.

It is customary for patients with eating disorders to want to be the good patient and to overidealize the therapist. In the previous example, these transference situations persisted well beyond the usual time frame, largely because of the therapist's countertransference reactions. Unknowingly, the therapist's behavior began to be shaped by her need to receive repeated praise and admiration. Things that needed to be conveyed to the patients and group were not conveyed, and things that ought not to be said were said. The group's progress became blocked as the therapist and group engaged in an ongoing process of mutual admiration. The more superhuman powers the group attributed to the therapist, the more helpless and dependent they became. In fact, they even deskilled themselves to the point where they could not utilize their own interactional resources in the group and to where they could no longer imagine coping without the therapist. Unfortunately, the group lost one of its members before the transference and countertransference reactions were identified and addressed.

Case 10

Rachel, a 28-year-old single office worker, presented with a 10-year history of BN and a very turbulent family upbringing. Upon commencement of the group, she was immediately aggressive, negative, demanding of the group's time, and particularly critical of the therapist. Her pattern was to constantly interrupt members, minimize or oppose their concerns, and launch into detailed accounts of the various grievances and injustices she encountered at work and in relationships. She denounced and challenged the therapist's interventions and competence, constantly questioned the effectiveness of this type of group approach, and let it be known how she much preferred the type of therapy and expertise of her former individual therapist.

Although the group was both frightened and infuriated by Rachel, her behavior and vicious words immobilized them. They begrudgingly allowed her to continue to dominate the sessions in her victimizing fashion and became enraged at the therapist for allowing Rachel to join the group. The therapist, in reaction to Rachel's onslaughts, felt anxious and irritated by the interpersonal static her disruptive behavior was generating so early in the group's development. Initial attempts to manage Rachel's hostile and monopolistic behavior by encouraging her to acknowledge some similarities with other members were only met with heightened resistance, leaving the therapist feeling more helpless and incompetent. The therapist began to sense a growing negativity from all the group members and responded by unwittingly becoming more controlling. During one particularly tense session in which Rachel complained that she was starting to feel worse, the therapist recalled fantasizing about Rachel leaving the group and about vacation plans.

During a video playback supervision session, the countertransference issues plaguing the therapist and threatening the therapeutic work of the group were elucidated. A process of projective identification was occurring whereby the patient was projecting her unacceptable feelings of rage, inadequacy, and incompetence onto the group, particularly the therapist. The therapist received these projected feelings, resonated with them, and in turn began to experience feelings of incompetency and anger with this patient. The therapist not only began to question the suitability of the type of group modality for Rachel, but also worried that she was contributing to the patient's worsening state. In fact, some of the therapist's concerns about her own efficacy were enacted that, in turn, functioned to validate Rachel's projections and prophesies about the world. For instance, the therapist failed to try to understand Rachel's presentation from a historical perspective and allowed herself to react personally without adequate forethought. Moreover, inappropriate interventions were implemented in attempts to manage Rachel's dominating and critical behavior. Countertransference feelings to the group as a whole were also addressed. The therapist was aware of becoming overly controlling in the face of an increasingly angry and negative group and came to realize this was a defense against countertransference feelings of anxiety and frustration.

The supervisor helped the therapist develop more understanding for the patient when they began to review Rachel's past history. Rachel's mother, who suffered from a bipolar illness, had been involved in multiple marriages and common-law relationships necessitating frequent geographic moves and reconstituted family situations. Rachel had been physically and sexually abused by two of her mother's mates. On a number of occasions, Rachel's mother insinuated that the breakup of her relationships could have been prevented if she had been childless. Once the dynamics of Rachel's group presentation were assimilated with her past history, it became understandable that the therapist and the group were experiencing a very potent defense used by Rachel to shield herself from the intense anxiety about joining such a group. Rachel's method of coping with the experience of being shifted, rejected, and abused from one reconstituted family group to the next was to behave in the worst possible way in a new social or group situation. In this regard she was unconsciously attempting to test whether the group would reject and abandon or tolerate and accept her. Her bulimic behavior provided her with another powerful way to cope with her underlying feelings of ineffectiveness, rage, and lack of a cohesive sense of self.

Undoubtedly, the interpersonal sacrifice of Rachel's defense was great, denoting that the intensity of the pain was considerable. Understanding these dynamics enabled the therapist to adopt an empathic stance toward Rachel's behavior and adjust her interventions accordingly. Rachel responded to the therapist's invitation to hear more about her reservations and fears regarding joining the group and to hear more about what it was like to always feel different from others. The therapist also commented, "It must be hard to believe that you will not be kicked out of this group." These simple therapist interventions helped Rachel develop more understanding of herself and begin a therapeutic alliance with the group. The interventions also allowed the group members to develop an empathic stance with Rachel, which in turn made it possible for them to learn to tolerate and accept her behavior until such time as she was able to feel more comfortable and safe in the group.

Case 11

During a postgroup discussion of an eating disorder group that had been meeting for 5 months, the male therapist of a male-female cotherapy team voiced his feelings of irritation and growing impatience with a particular female patient, Sally. He was uncertain as to the source of his reaction. Was it stemming subjectively from his own past and his own personal idiosyncrasies, or was it coming from feelings that the patient induced that were pertinent to her core conflicts and issues? The female cotherapist did not appear to be experiencing this reaction. Over the next few sessions, the relationship of each therapist with Sally was monitored more closely. It became more apparent to both therapists that Sally's behavior was quite different with the male therapist, the only male in the group. It appeared Sally had been subtly derogating and provoking the male therapist.

This countertransference material was brought into the group when the interaction pattern arose again in the here and now. By examining both the therapist's and the patient's feelings, a new level of insight developed. Sally and the group began to understand her pattern of unconsciously needling men and how it was currently affecting her relationship with her fiance and had previously interfered with her maintaining jobs as well as relationships with men.

Summary

Longer term intensive group psychotherapy offers an important modality of treatment for patients with AN and BN. The holding environment and social microcosm created in the group provides an effective means to address the cognitive distortions and self-deficits that typify eating disorders. Resolution of these issues allows the individual to mature toward improved self-regulation and integration and experience greater autonomy and improved self-esteem. The peer interaction available in the group modality offers unique advantages in identifying and penetrating the resistant defensive style that characterizes patients with eating disorders.

References

Barth D, Wurman V: Group therapy with bulimic women: a self-psychological approach. International Journal of Eating Disorders 5(4):735–745, 1986

Beck AT, Rush AJ, Shaw BF, et al: Cognitive Therapy of Depression. New York, Guilford, 1979

Budman SH, Gurman AS: Theory and Practice of Brief Therapy. New York, Guilford, 1988

Dies RR: Clinical implications of research on leadership in short-term group psychotherapy, in Advances in Group Therapy. Edited by Dies R, MacKenzie KR. New York, International Universities Press, 1983

Fairburn CG: Cognitive-behavioral treatment for bulimia, in Handbook of Psychotherapy for Anorexia Nervosa and Bulimia. Edited by Garner DM, Garfinkel PE. New York, Guilford, 1985

Fulkerson C, Hawkins D, Alden A: Psychotherapy groups of insufficient size. Int J Group Psychother 31:73–81, 1981

Garfinkel PE, Garner DM (eds): Anorexia Nervosa: A Multidimensional Perspective. New York, Brunner/Mazel, 1982

Garner DM, Bemis KM: A cognitive-behavioral approach to anorexia nervosa. Cognitive Therapy and Research 6:123–150, 1982

Goodsitt A: Self psychology and the treatment of anorexia nervosa, in Handbook of Psychotherapy for Anorexia Nervosa and Bulimia. Edited by Garner DM, Garfinkel PE. New York, Guilford, 1985

Hall A: Group psychotherapy for anorexia nervosa, in Handbook of Psychotherapy for Anorexia Nervosa and Bulimia. Edited by Garner DM, Garfinkel PE. New York, Guilford, 1985

Hendren RL, Atkins DM, Sumner CR, et al: Model for the group treatment of eating disorders. Int J Group Psychother 37(4):589–602, 1987

Horwitz L: Group psychotherapy for borderline and narcissistic disorders. Bull Menninger Clin 44:181–200, 1980

Inbody DR, Ellis JJ: Group therapy with anorexic and bulimic patients: implications of therapeutic intervention. Am J Psychother 39:411–420, 1985

Laube JJ: Why group therapy for bulimia? Int J Group Psychother 40(2):169–187, 1990

Lieberman M, Yalom I, Miles M: Encounter Groups: First Facts. New York, Basic Books, 1972

Leibovich M: Why short-term psychotherapy for borderlines? Psychother Psychosom 39:1–9, 1983

Leszcz M: Group psychotherapy of the characterologically difficult patient. Int J Group Psychother 39(3):311–335, 1989

MacKenzie KR: Introduction to Time-Limited Group Psychotherapy. Washington, DC, American Psychiatric Press, 1990

MacKenzie KR, Livesley WJ: A developmental model for brief group therapy, in Advances in Group Psychotherapy. Edited by Dies RR, MacKenzie KR. New York, International Universities Press, 1983

MacKenzie KR, Coleman M, Harper H, et al: Group psychotherapy for bulimia: preliminary outcome figures. Paper presented at Psychiatric Research Day, Faculty of Medicine, University of Calgary, Alberta, 1985a

MacKenzie KR, Coleman M, Harper H, et al: Critical therapeutic events in the group treatment of bulimia nervosa. Paper presented at the annual conference of the Canadian Group Psychotherapy Association, Banff, Alberta, 1985b

MacKenzie KR, Livesley WJ, Coleman M, et al: Short-term group psychotherapy for bulimia nervosa. Psychiatric Annals 16(12):699–708, 1986

Neuman PA, Halvorson PA: Anorexia Nervosa and Bulimia: A Handbook for Counselors and Therapists. New York, Van Nostrand Reinhold, 1983

Oesterheld JR, McKenna MS, Gould NB: Group psychotherapy of bulimia: a critical review. Int J Group Psychother 37(2):163–184, 1987

Roth DM, Ross DR: Long-term cognitive-interpersonal group for eating disorders. Int J Group Psychother 38(4):491–510, 1988

Roy-Byrne P, Lee-Benner K, Yager J: Group therapy for bulimia. International Journal of Eating Disorders 3(2):97–116, 1984

Wong N: Combined group and individual treatment of borderline and narcissistic patients, heterogeneous vs. homogeneous groups. Int J Group Psychother 30:389–404, 1980

Wooley SC, Wooley OW: Intensive outpatient and residential treatment for bulimia, in Handbook of Psychotherapy for Anorexia Nervosa and Bulimia. Edited by Garner DM, Garfinkel PE. New York, Guilford, 1985

Yellowlees P: Group psychotherapy in anorexia nervosa. International Journal of Eating Disorders 7(5):649–655, 1988

Yalom ID: The Theory and Practice of Group Psychotherapy. New York, Basic Books, 1985

Specialized Group Treatment

♦ ♦ ♦ ♦ ♦ ♦ ♦ ♦ ♦

6

Inpatient Group Treatment

Jacqueline Duncan, M.B., M.R.C.Psych.
Sidney H. Kennedy, M.B., F.R.C.P.(C)

♦ ♦ ♦ ♦ ♦ ♦ ♦ ♦

The unit described here utilizes relatively brief periods of hospitalization. Its primary goal is the stabilization of eating behaviors that have reached a life-threatening point of decompensation. It may also alert the patient to other associated issues. Throughout the chapter, the authors emphasize the importance of not pushing the psychotherapeutic work too quickly and thus jeopardizing the fundamental task of stabilization. In the large Toronto system, patients may be referred at discharge to other intensive treatment programs, in particular the Day Hospital program described in the next chapter. In other clinical settings, longer inpatient hospitalization may be used to achieve a broader range of goals. By addressing these objectives in a day setting, considerable economic advantage is achieved.—The Editors

Group psychotherapy is an accepted, effective, and cost-efficient modality for the outpatient treatment of bulimia nervosa (Barth and Wurman 1986; Johnson et al. 1983; Lacey 1983; Mynors-Wallis 1989; Oesterheld et al. 1987; Roth and Ross 1988; Roy-Byrne et al. 1984; Stuber and Strober 1987). The effectiveness of group treatments for patients with anorexia nervosa has been less clearly described. The use of group psychotherapy as a component of intensive inpatient treatment for anorexia

---

* Molyn Leszcz, M.D., F.R.C.P.(C), provided helpful comments during the preparation of this manuscript.

nervosa (AN) and bulimia nervosa (BN) poses special challenges. This chapter illustrates the use of group psychotherapy as an effective component of the therapeutic program for this population. Inpatient groups may also facilitate participation in treatment following discharge from the hospital.

In the past, group therapy has been considered inappropriate for patients with AN. This opinion was based on the recognition that obsessive self-concern and a tendency for manipulation—both factors associated with an unfavorable outcome in group therapy—were prominent features of this patient population. More recently it has been argued that other needs of AN patients may make them appropriate for group psychotherapy (Polivy 1981; Polivy and Garfinkel 1984). Often these patients lack accurate information about nutrition, sexuality, and their bodies. They struggle with the demands and responsibilities of adolescence while experiencing the pressure to understand and accept the physical changes that propel them toward adulthood. In this patient population, such conflicts can produce a sense of estrangement accompanied by feelings of ineffectiveness and low self-esteem. Group psychotherapy has the potential to address these problems, by providing models of coping as well as offering consensual validation, instillation of hope, and interpersonal feedback from people who share the same difficulties. Membership in a group reduces feelings of isolation and entrapment. In addition to these advantages, increased self-esteem and a greater sense of self-control result from active participation in treatment.

Group psychotherapy for patients with AN has historically been approached with caution. In the Netherlands, Lafeber and colleagues (1967) developed an inpatient group for patients with AN. To overcome anticipated problems, they communicated initially with glove puppets, which eventually became unnecessary. Similarly, when our own inpatient group began, initial communication was begun with each participant drawing her family tree. After the first few sessions, the therapists were able to overcome their own anticipatory fears and dispense with these aids to communication. Piazza and colleagues (1983) began an inpatient group in their unit because of a persistent tendency among eating disorder inpatients to form "subgroups." These spontaneous gatherings had both helpful and harmful effects on the participants. The formal psychotherapy group sought to maximize the positive aspects of the informal group's socialization while reducing the negative effects.

Characteristics of Patients in the Inpatient Unit

Inpatients tend to have longer and more severe eating disorder histories.

In a comparison between inpatients and outpatients (Kennedy and Garfinkel 1989), inpatients had been ill for a longer time—approximately 8 years compared to 5 years. Patients with AN or AN+BN weighed significantly less at the time of presentation than their outpatient counterparts (70% compared to 75% of mean average weight). Measures of psychopathology revealed fewer differences between the outpatient and inpatient groups. However, on the Eating Disorders Inventory (Garner et al. 1983), inpatients with BN reported significantly higher self ratings of personal ineffectiveness, perfectionism, and interpersonal distrust than outpatients.

A recent study of personality characteristics of inpatients using the Millon Clinical Multiaxial Inventory (Millon 1985) indicates that as many as 93% exhibit psychopathology consistent with a diagnosis of personality disorder at the time of admission (Kennedy et al., in press). In particular, these self-report measures indicated borderline, dependent, passive-aggressive, avoidant, and schizoid features. When the same scales were repeated at discharge, the incidence of personality disorder diagnoses dropped only slightly to 79%. This suggests that the self-report measures were not simply reflecting acute states, though the initial level of distress may have been heightened by personal or family crises that precipitated the hospitalization. Admission to the hospital may in itself engender significant regression for these patients, making them appear very fragile.

The Inpatient Treatment Program

Three principal criteria can be used for admission to an inpatient eating disorder program:

1. Refeeding and weight restoration (mean length of stay 13 weeks);
2. Breaking the binge-purge cycle and promoting normal eating (mean length of stay 6 weeks); and
3. Time-limited weight correction for patients with a lengthy relapsing and remitting course of AN (mean length of stay 4 weeks).

Since 1982, approximately 30 people per year with AN and BN have been electively admitted to The Toronto Hospital after a preadmission assessment by the treatment team. Five beds are designated "eating disorder beds" within a 20-bed unit, where patients with mood disorders and other general psychiatric disorders are also treated. The program adheres strictly to a multidisciplinary team approach and utilizes cognitive-behavioral techniques and individual, family, and group therapies, as well as pharmacological treatments (Kennedy 1988; Kerr et al. 1987).

Approximately a week after admission, each patient meets with the treatment team to plan her treatment program. For the emaciated individual, nutritional treatment and weight gain to an agreed-upon target range are essential components of such a program. At the same time, individual and group psychotherapy programs are initiated. Family assessment and therapy are also key components.

Several essential components are included in every treatment program—for example, clarifying body image issues, challenging dietary myths about high- and low-calorie foods, and exploring alternatives to food and weight preoccupations. All of the patients on the unit are expected to attend educational group discussions as well as a weekly explorative psychotherapy group that lasts 1 hour. The principal goal of the latter group is to provide the patients with a forum to express and share common anxieties that arise from being in the program, while enabling them to benefit from the specific factors that are believed to be of therapeutic value in group psychotherapy.

Participation in all of the groups is considered to be a part of the treatment program and is not optional. Patients are expected to attend unless they are suffering from extreme emaciation or are actively suicidal. Thus, the participants at any one time can range from being extremely ill, self-absorbed, and totally lacking in motivation to being physically and mentally restored, insightful, optimistic, and planning actively for the future.

Rationale for Group Treatment Approaches

A number of factors have been cited as specifically beneficial for patients with an eating disorder in the inpatient setting. These include the promotion of safety and trust through universality, validation of self, alternating roles of helping and being helped, sense of participation in the treatment process, corrective interpersonal feedback, and instillation of hope (Polivy 1981; Yellowlees 1988). Interpersonal feedback from peers in the group setting has been noted regularly to be effective with patients for whom feedback in individual therapy has repeatedly failed to have an impact.

A patient was confronted by two of the other patients during a group session. The patient was nearing the end of the treatment program and was not assuming responsibility for her behavior as supervision was being gradually phased out. The group members accused her of being self-defeating and emphasized how depressing it was for them to see her doing so badly. They also felt unwilling to be honest with her in group when she was not being honest with them. Although distressed by the confrontation, the patient began to look at her behavior in the context of how it might affect others in the group. She was clearly astonished at discovering both how much the other patients were being affected by her behavior and how much they seemed to care about her progress. Over the next few weeks, she was able to adopt a more objective view and begin to modify her behavior.

The relatively rapid turnover of participants in the group inhibits the development of mature group functioning. Factors such as acquisition of insight through interpersonal learning are less likely to be achieved. Maxmen and Hanover (1973) found that inpatients particularly value the supportive factors that develop early in a group, such as instillation of hope, altruism, group cohesiveness, and universality. This is consistent with the idea that inpatient groups function as "brief" groups.

The group setting is frequently a venue for patients to share previously undisclosed secrets. Often, several members of the group have felt ashamed of the same behaviors involving food, or of previously unshared sexual experiences. This is of particular importance because approximately 40% of both AN and BN patients admitted to this unit reveal a history of previous sexual abuse. The process of self-disclosure entails a powerful universalization experience. In addition, it allows a distancing and desensitizing process that promotes mastery over the intrusive memories of adverse life experiences.

Benefits of Group Treatment Approaches in the Inpatient Setting

Inpatient group psychotherapy provides an opportunity to assess patients' interactional abilities and promotes increased staff interaction with patients (Davis and Dorman 1974). This promotes ward cohesion and diminishes tensions that might otherwise erupt into acting-out behaviors (Bailine et al. 1977). Group cohesion is further facilitated by the common experience of being in hospital and the high prevailing levels of distress. The therapy groups are helpful in diminishing an inpatient's sense of isolation and estrangement. Because patients are living together in the ward community, there is an opportunity to directly apply issues raised in the group, thus facilitating a process of interpersonal learning (Piazza et al. 1983). Leszcz (1986) has suggested that inpatients regard the short-term nature of the inpatient group as an impetus to engage in the group and not waste time. Patients are likely to continue in treatments with which they are familiar and comfortable following their discharge from the hospital (Mattes et al. 1977). A good experience with inpatient group therapy facilitates compliance with appropriate aftercare treatment.

Patients in the eating disorder program spend a minimum of 1 hour together after each meal, separated from the other patients on the ward. This magnifies the effect of interpersonal difficulties among group members following an interpersonal dispute. The next group session may begin with a distinct lack of cohesion. It is essential that these disputes be addressed promptly to facilitate the group process. This in itself can be very valuable, since patients with eating disorders traditionally avoid interpersonal confrontation and think only in terms of personal rejection when emotionally laden topics are addressed.

Being together for such a long time between group sessions may also allow the development of a separate "group identity" in which no therapists or "authority figures" are present. This has the potential to be a hindrance to therapeutic progress, as the patients may overidentify with having an eating disorder. The issue of subgroups has to be addressed. It is important that the therapists regularly reiterate the importance of following group rules and emphasize the responsibility individual members have for bringing material from outside exchanges back to the formal group setting.

Inpatient group therapy is most effective when it is valued as an intrinsic part of treatment by the staff on the ward (Astrachan et al. 1968; Leszcz 1986). The goals of the group must be synergistic with the goals of the overall program. Therapists should include other staff members in any discussions regarding the therapy and particularly in postgroup reviews. This is important because patients who suffer from an eating disorder have a recognized tendency to cause splitting among staff members (Yellowlees 1988). Leszcz (1986) describes the group as "a window onto the larger milieu" and cautions that unaddressed staff issues, such as struggles for leadership, may "produce a fertile nidus for both staff and patient splitting and acting-out" in the group (p. 735).

> One of the usual cotherapists was absent. Immediately preceding the group there was a tense discussion between staff members as to who should participate in the cotherapist's place. Although this was quickly decided, some previously unexpressed views as to the value of the group and who should lead it were brought to light. The ensuing group session was notably lacking in cohesion. Some members chose to sit outside of the group and the discussion was punctuated by long silences. The value of the group and the role of the group leaders were the main topics of discussion for the entire duration of the group. There are few secrets on an inpatient unit!

Practical Considerations for the Therapist

The prevailing level of distress in the inpatient setting is high and the involvement in the group by each individual is brief. Under these circumstances, the general principles of brief psychotherapy must be applied. The therapist should adopt a stance that is both active and supportive (Yalom 1983). The therapists should actively convey empathy and concern (Leszcz et al. 1985) as well as flexibility and eclecticism (Yellowlees 1988). The main roles of the therapists are to maintain the focus of the group on its task and to actively facilitate the pace and appropriate functioning of the group. In our experience, it is desirable to have two cotherapists—and if possible, one male and one female (Inbody and Ellis 1985). Ideally, one should have experience in the treatment of eating disorders, whereas the other should have a special expertise in group process (Yellowlees 1988).

Some strategies are particularly useful to the group therapist in this setting. Among them is clarification: a request for further elaboration on a topic, reexamination of a statement, summarizing or reflecting important material. This serves the purpose of highlighting the issue for the individual and for the group. It also provides reassurance for the group that the therapist is listening attentively and seeking to understand what is being expressed. Tentative confrontation by drawing attention to previously expressed, but currently unremembered, material may also facilitate group functioning.

The therapist can help members share with one another how each person's behavior on the ward and in the group is affecting the others. Group members themselves often have difficulty initiating this process in a constructive manner. The therapist may become alert to the existence of a problem with a particular member by sullen silence or an unwillingness to relate to that member. Patients with eating disorders tend to perceive their actions and attitudes in a self-centered manner. They may initially be resistant to the idea that their behavior affects others on the ward. Once the therapist has initiated the feedback process by breaking the silence, the group may be able to continue the process. The same feedback may need to be repeated by different members in different ways, until finally the member is able to see her behavior more objectively. This can be an enormously important learning experience for the individual in terms of future dealings with family and other involved persons outside of the group. The group members also gain in this process by having the experience of effecting change in one another through gentle but persistent effort.

The therapist should always be ready to offer praise and reinforcement when advances have been made, both within the group setting and in the ward program. This encourages motivation and provides the group with a useful model of how to express genuine concern and positive regard. Feelings that may underlie group statements or behavior should be tentatively reflected and explored by the therapist. Risk-taking should be encouraged and appropriately rewarded so that it becomes a positive learning experience for the individual and the group. Recapitulation of the family group can be facilitated by drawing attention to sibling-like rivalries as the therapists are cast in the role of parents. This regularly generates hostility and anger among new members. Invariably there is strong vocal resistance to interpreting the group as a family, and frequently a lively interactive session results.

A male therapist suggested that the group resembled a family. One member's response took the form of a vicious attack on the group, the therapists, and the unit. The patient had, for several years, engaged in a power struggle with her father and had left vomitus in his shoes on several occasions before she came to the hospital. Following her outburst, the therapists drew her attention to this previously expressed material. Initially she was unable to see any connection. But later in the group she spoke of her realization that she frequently would respond in an inappropriately hostile way to male authority figures. The thought of attempting to deal with unresolved emotions toward her father was so forbidding to her that she could not bear to think of the group as a family. From that point on her participation in the group was calm and constructive. She remained unwilling to explore her relationship with her father in any greater depth.

It can be helpful for the therapists to draw attention to the fact that the structure and formality of time and setting of the group has a resemblance to family mealtimes. This issue elicits initial distress followed by fruitful discussion, often providing the therapists with important insight into the experiences and fears of individual patients around food and family dynamics. Such a discussion provides an opportunity to deal with a prototypically stressful setting in a supportive environment.

This patient population can elicit powerful countertransference feelings from caregivers. It is important that group therapists in this setting recognize these feelings to forestall acting inappropriately on them. When there are cotherapists for a group, they can share their feelings during pre- and postgroup meetings. They can also mutually support each other during the group to ensure that such feelings do not hinder the group's psychological work. Failure to recognize countertransference reactions can result in the loss of valuable information about the effects a patient has on others. It can also have unfortunate consequences for the patient. For example, a therapist may act in a manner that is complementary to the patient's behavior and unwittingly produce a repetition of past traumatic experiences. Although it may happen that both therapists are experiencing the same countertransference feelings, it is more usual for one to be able to recognize what is happening and find a way to change the group focus. Such events need to be thoroughly explored after the group. Obviously, a good working relationship between the therapists is essential.

Occasionally the therapists may cautiously reflect countertransference feelings in the group. This is often helpful when the countertransference feelings are concordant and the patient is causing the therapists to feel trapped and ineffective just as she herself feels. Tentative exploration of these feelings in the group may bring a sense of relief to the individual by allowing her to feel that her current experience is being at least partially understood.

When groups are largely composed of patients with AN, therapists are aware of having to work harder and deal with higher levels of painful affect in the group. These patients have difficulty initiating psychotherapeutic work. They may be in hospital because of coercion from relatives or outpatient therapists and may initially be sullen and silent for most of the group time. Because inpatient groups are brief, there is an onus on both the therapists and participants to initiate psychological work quickly. This tension between resistance and time pressures may leave the therapists feeling drained. They may recognize that they have been rendered ineffective by the group. Groups are predictably more lively and confrontational when they include patients with BN, and this should be facilitated whenever possible.

Group therapists in inpatient units must ensure that adequate communication is maintained with other members of each patient's treatment network. This reduces the possibility of patients manipulating and splitting staff. It also helps the other staff to appreciate the role of group therapy as an integrated part of the program. If communication at a staff level breaks down, there is a clear potential for a split within the treatment system. The eclectic and explorative nature of the group can be seen as a threat to the wider program that utilizes mainly cognitive and behavioral approaches. When the program is working properly, this difference is complementary.

In order to maximize communication, the rehash meeting following each group session is attended by the therapists, the unit leader, and any nursing staff who are available. Staff can learn of affect-laden discussions that occurred in the group so that they can approach patients with appropriate sensitivity. This meeting also reduces the possibility of patients relating an inaccurate account of group events in attempts to split the treatment team. A biweekly meeting attended by all staff with a "hands-on" role on the unit provides a forum to share feelings and ideas about how the team is operating. Suggestions are encouraged about ways communication can be further improved between all the disciplines. This meeting also fosters mutual support among staff who are all dealing with difficult and often highly manipulative patients.

Certain themes recur regularly during the therapy groups. Therapists should be prepared to encourage these and explore in detail their implications for each member:

♦ Coming to terms with the diagnosis of an eating disorder
♦ Recognizing the need to give up the disorder
♦ Learning how to replace the function it has served
♦ Establishing a personal identity without the disorder
♦ Examining individual roles and alliances within families

♦ Examining personal attitudes toward perfectionism and control
♦ Acknowledging interpersonal relationship difficulties regarding trust and assertiveness
♦ Recognizing the pervasiveness of all-or-none thinking, particularly as this applies to body image and food
♦ Examining the pervasive preoccupation with one's physical appearance

A survey of opinions regarding therapy obtained 1 year following discharge indicates that the great majority of patients who have gone through the treatment program found group psychotherapy helpful: 40% of the patients rated group psychotherapy as "very helpful" and 80% rated it as at least "helpful." There is a tendency for older patients and patients with a diagnosis of BN to rate the group psychotherapy experience more highly.

We are currently measuring which therapist factors, setting factors, and group factors are most valued by the patients. This will assist us in maximizing the potential of this mode of treatment as part of the inpatient program. We are also interested in evaluating those dimensions of outcome functioning that are likely to be most influenced by group psychotherapy. This includes self-concept, the experiencing of emotional reactions, relationship problems, and communication skills. Inpatient groups have different characteristics than their outpatient counterparts. They take place within a setting where there are many additional therapeutic approaches. The patients are at a more severe point in their illness and the groups are open-ended and brief. Nevertheless, it is our belief that integrated group psychotherapy can significantly enhance inpatient treatment.

References

Astrachan BM, Harrow M, Flynn HR: Influence of the value system of a psychiatric setting on behavior in group therapy meetings. Social Psychiatry 3:165–172, 1968

Bailine SH, Katch M, Golden HK: Mini groups: maximizing the therapeutic milieu in an acute psychiatric unit. Hosp Community Psychiatry 28:445–447, 1977

Barth D, Wurman V: Group therapy with bulimic women: a self psychological approach. International Journal of Eating Disorders 5:735–745, 1986

Davis HK, Dorman KR: Group therapy versus ward rounds. Diseases of the Nervous System 35:316–319, 1974

Garner DM, Olmsted MP, Polivy J: Development and validation of a multidimensional eating disorder inventory for anorexia and bulimia. International Journal of Eating Disorders 2:15–34, 1983

Inbody AR, Ellis JJ: Group therapy with anorexic and bulimic patients: implications for therapeutic intervention. Am J Psychother 39:411–420, 1985

Johnson C, Connors M, Stuckey M: Short term group treatment of bulimia: a preliminary report. International Journal of Eating Disorders 2:199–208, 1983

Kennedy SH: Inpatient management of anorexia nervosa and bulimia nervosa, in Current Update: Anorexia Nervosa and Bulimia Nervosa. Edited by Garfinkel PE. Kalamazoo, MI, Upjohn, 1988

Kennedy SH, Garfinkel PE: Anorexia nervosa and bulimia nervosa—subjective and objective measures of outcome following inpatient treatment. International Journal of Eating Disorders 8:181–190, 1989

Kennedy SH, McVey G, Katz R: The effect of treatment on self report measures of personality disorder in anorexia nervosa and bulimia nervosa. J Psychiatr Res 24(3):259–269, 1990

Kerr A, Kennedy SH, Stern D: Inpatient treatment for anorexia nervosa and bulimia. British Review of Anorexia Nervosa and Bulimia 2:5–16, 1987

Lacey AH: Bulimia nervosa, binge eating and psychological vomiting. BMJ 286:1609–1610, 1983

Lafeber C, Lansen J, Jongerius PJ: Group therapy with anorexia nervosa patients. Voordrachtenreeks Van de Nederlandse Vereniging Van Psychiaters in Dienstuerband (May issue) 1967. Reprinted in Lansen J: Group therapy with anorexia nervosa patients. International Journal of Group Psychotherapy 36:321–322, 1986

Leszcz M: In-patient groups, in American Psychiatric Press Review of Psychiatry, Vol 5. Edited by Frances AJ, Hales RE. Washington, DC, American Psychiatric Press, 1986, pp 729–743

Leszcz M, Yalom ID, Norden MD: The value of inpatient group psychotherapy—patient's perceptions. Int J Group Psychother 35:411–433, 1985

Mattes JA, Rosen B, Klein DF: Comparison of the clinical effectiveness of "short" versus "long" stay psychiatric hospitalization, II: results of a 3 year post hospital follow up. J Nerv Ment Dis 165:387–394, 1977

Maxmen JS, Hanover NH: Group therapy as viewed by hospitalized patients. Arch Gen Psychiatry 28:404–408, 1973

Millon T: The MCMI provides a good assessment of DSM III disorders: the MCMI II will prove even better. J Pers Assess 49:379–391, 1985

Mynors-Wallis LM: The psychological treatment of eating disorders. Br J Hosp Med 41:470–475, 1989

Oesterheld JR, McKenna MS, Gould NB: Group psychotherapy of bulimia. A critical review. Int J Group Psychother 37:163–185, 1987

Piazza E, Carni JD, Kelly J, et al: Group psychotherapy for anorexia nervosa. J Am Acad Child Psychiatry 22:276–278, 1983

Polivy J: Group therapy as an adjunctive treatment for anorexia nervosa. Journal of Psychiatric Treatment and Evaluation 3:279–283, 1981

Polivy J, Garfinkel PE: Group therapies for anorexia nervosa, in Helping Patients and Their Families Cope With Medical Problems. Edited by Roback HB. San Francisco, CA, Jossey-Bass, 1984

Roth DM, Ross DR: Long term cognitive interpersonal group therapy for eating disorders. Int J Group Psychother 38:491–511, 1988

Roy-Byrne P, Lee-Benner K, Yager J: Group therapy for bulimia: a year's experience. International Journal of Eating Disorders 3:97–116, 1984

Stuber M, Strober M: Group therapy in the treatment of adolescents with bulimia—some preliminary observations. International Journal of Eating Disorders 6:125–131, 1987

Yalom ID: Inpatient Group Psychotherapy. New York, Basic Books, 1983

Yellowlees P: Group psychotherapy in anorexia nervosa. International Journal of Eating Disorders 7:649–655, 1988

7

Day Hospital Group Treatment

Allan S. Kaplan, M.D., F.R.C.P.(C)
Ann Kerr, B.Sc., O.T.
Sarah E. Maddocks, Ph.D., C.Psych.

♦ ♦ ♦ ♦ ♦ ♦ ♦ ♦

At first glance, this day hospital program may seem fragmented into a bewildering variety of special topic groups. It begins to make sense when seen from the perspective of its function to replace the need for inpatient care for all but a small number of extremely ill patients. The day program is time-limited and of a small size, and almost totally organized around group activities. The various small groups provide structure around which critical issues can be addressed. It is as if the core eating disorder themes have been dissected apart and focused on separately. Many of the groups deal with specific eating behaviors. This approach stands in contrast to the standard psychodynamic orientation, in which emphasis is placed on understanding issues more than changing specific behaviors. The particular components of the program have been selected with great care. For example, after a game of volleyball, a discussion might take place about how the activity stimulated issues related to competition, a common psychodynamic theme for patients with eating disorders. Indeed, a psychodynamic orientation flows throughout the program and underlies the behavioral and cognitive strategies employed. The authors' emphasis on the need for frequent and detailed staff discussions around management issues must be taken seriously as a means to integrate the various components. It is expected that many of the patients will move on to further outpatient treatment to consolidate and apply the gains begun in the day program itself.—The Editors

This chapter describes a treatment program developed as an innovative approach to the management of patients seriously ill with anorexia nervosa (AN) and bulimia nervosa (BN). The program provides integrated intensive outpatient care in a day hospital group psychotherapy setting. The rationale for this complex treatment package and a detailed description of the treatment components is presented. The advantages and problems associated with the program are discussed, and outcome data concerning the effectiveness of the treatment are reviewed.

Rationale for Program

Seriously ill, emaciated, anorexic patients need inpatient hospitalization. Such treatment traditionally focuses on nutritional stabilization utilizing a multimodel approach. This approach incorporates behavioral strategies; individual, family, and group therapies; and adjunctive pharmacotherapies. It is generally effective in the short term in inducing weight gain in anorexic patients but is accompanied by a high rate of relapse postdischarge.

Attempts to treat patients with severe AN as outpatients either in groups or individually have met with little success. Some investigators (Crisp 1965) have expressed concerns about the appropriateness of group treatment for anorexic patients, because so many of the characteristics associated with poor group therapy outcome are typical of patients with AN (Yalom 1975). Specific concerns relate to the intense competitiveness around weight related issues that develop between patients as well as the denial of psychological issues in the emaciated state, leading to an unsupportive and fragmented group experience. The outpatient treatment of severely ill anorexic patients has been hampered by the intense power struggle that typically develops around disturbed food- and weight-related behaviors in the absence of complete external control. All group therapeutic approaches are complicated by the inability of a patient who is in a starved and emaciated state to cognitively attend to psychological issues.

The management of seriously ill patients with BN is less clearly documented. As with anorexic patients, hospitalization of bulimic patients usually leads to a temporary reduction of symptoms with a return of symptoms when controls are lifted upon discharge. A variety of outpatient therapies including pharmacotherapy (Garfinkel and Garner 1987), cognitive behav-

The authors would like to acknowledge the following people for their conceptual contributions to the group therapies in the day hospital program: Niva Piran, Ph.D., C.Psych., D. Blake Woodside, M.D., F.R.C.P.(C), Lorie Shekter-Wolfson, M.S.W., C.S.W., Janis Winocur, M.Sc., R.P.Dt., Leslie Langdon, B.A., D.S.C., Maureen Mahan, R.N., B.A., Alison Patenaude, R.N., and Jan Lackstrom, M.S.W., R.S.W.

ioral individual therapy (Garner and Bemis 1985), group psychotherapy (Mitchell et al. 1985), and family therapy (Schwartz et al. 1985) have been recommended for specific populations of bulimic patients.

The in-hospital treatment of both anorexic and bulimic patients is fraught with difficulties for both patients and staff. During hospitalization, serious character pathology often becomes evident. Severe regression can occur with hostile dependency, unstable mood, and impulsive behavior with a tendency to self-harm. Efforts by staff to provide external controls in an empathic manner are interpreted by patients as sadistic and punitive efforts to control. As a result, patients feel compelled to oppose therapeutic efforts. Attempts are made to split staff, and outward compliance with treatment expectations are combined with covert engagement in illness related behaviors. Patients may talk in therapy of change while secretly adhering to distorted attitudes and beliefs about their situation. In-hospital treatment of such patients requires specialized units with a high staff/patient ratio of skilled and vigilant professionals. This may result in expensive and inefficient utilization of limited resources. Innovative approaches are needed that can maximize the application of intensive treatment while minimizing the problematic aspects of inpatient units. The day hospital program described in this chapter is an attempt to create such a combination.

Advantages of the Program

The clinical advantages of treating patients in an outpatient group psychotherapeutic format can be considered from two viewpoints: those attributable to the outpatient nature of the program and those related to the nature of the group treatment itself. Outpatient care limits regression and dependency, as patients have to maintain themselves outside of the hospital during intensive treatment. Such an approach promotes autonomy and provides an opportunity for generalization of eating regulation skills that patients acquire in the day hospital. The patients are, on a daily basis, forced to actively confront disturbed areas of functioning (e.g., relationships, vocational issues, impulsivity) while simultaneously attempting to normalize eating and weight. This facilitates the difficult yet crucial process of internal integration of external controls. As patients are not and cannot be totally externally controlled, they are less likely to oppose the treatment and more likely to experience it empathically rather than punitively. Day hospital treatment is much less psychosocially disruptive than in-hospital care and allows patients to continue contact with significant others while receiving treatment.

The group nature of the intensive treatment program has its own inherent advantages. The group treatment provides an atmosphere of mutual support while increasing the power of therapeutic interventions through group confrontation and pressure. The isolation that often develops as a result of patients secretly clinging to their disturbed eating patterns is relieved by the process of mutual sharing of what have been believed to be degrading and humiliating behaviors. Disclosure in a group forces patients to "own" their illness rather than to deny or dissociate it. Such ownership of behavior is an important first step in being able to take control of and eventually change behavior. Group process diffuses the intensity of interactions, helping to limit regression and dependency.

Financial advantages to outpatient group treatment are clearly evident. Resources can be allocated directly for providing treatment rather than 24-hour supervision of patients in beds. The group format allows for treating a larger number of patients with efficient use of facilities and staff.

Problems of the Program

The day hospital program may not provide enough containment for some patients. The program offers a holding environment provided by supportive group interaction, but has less direct control of behavior than an inpatient unit can provide. Some patients, because of underlying character disturbance, do not or cannot supportively engage in the group process. For them, the intensive group interaction can lead to being scapegoated—with subsequent deterioration.

The outpatient nature of the program requires continual monitoring of mental status, as patients can become emotionally unstable with increasing weight and changes in eating behavior. The ability to deal with an unstable population at risk for self-harm requires considerable clinical skills. Such skills are taxed by the intense and continuous staff-patient interaction required to provide an empathically controlling environment. Staff can feel at times that they are attempting to fill a bottomless pit, and this can lead directly to burnout. Contributing to this staff experience are pathologic group processes whereby angry and intolerable patient feelings are projected onto staff, who are then devalued and made to feel as if they are sadistically tormenting patients. Being unaware of such issues can lead to a sense of therapeutic nihilism. It is essential that staff function as a closely knit, mutually supportive unit with frequent communication, treatment goals decided by consensus, and clearly established models of intervention.

Description of the Day Hospital Program

The day hospital group therapy program integrates biological, psychological, and sociocultural interventions over a 2- to 4-month stay for a maximum of 12 patients at any time. Treatment goals are clearly established: 1) behavioral change with normalization of eating patterns, 2) nutritional rehabilitation through weight gain and adequate caloric intake, and 3) identification of underlying disturbed psychological and family processes. The program operates 5 days per week, approximately 7 ½ hours per day. It is staffed by a multidisciplinary team consisting of a psychiatrist-director, a full-time psychologist, an occupational therapist, a social worker–family therapist, a nutritionist, a psychometrist, and two nurses.

The biological treatment involves a thorough medical evaluation including a physical examination aimed at assessing and reversing the physical complications of starvation and/or bingeing and purging. This includes the difficult task of weaning patients off chronic high-dose laxative abuse. Pharmacotherapy is often utilized, most commonly to treat intense affective states, alleviate gastrointestinal symptomatology, reduce preprandial anxiety, and relieve the insomnia that often accompanies disordered eating and starvation. Nutritional rehabilitation is achieved through the introduction of a balanced meal plan of 2,000–3,000 calories that incorporates phobic foods divided into three meals and two snacks per day.

With the exception of medical and psychological assessment and family therapy, all treatment occurs in groups. Each group is led by a minimum of two staff members, and all patients are expected to attend all groups. The group treatments incorporate psychoeducational, behavioral, cognitive, interpersonal, and psychodynamic principles. Most groups are semistructured, in that they have an educational component with a specific focus and follow a general outline. The groups can be divided into those that deal directly with disturbed attitudes and behaviors around eating and weight, and those that focus on more general areas of disturbance and dysfunction. Sociocultural interventions provide vocational counseling and help in establishing community supports and in arranging alternate living accommodations.

The program is structured around lunch, afternoon snack, and dinner, with all patients eating meals together as a group. Patients eat 2,000–3,000 calories per day, chosen from the hospital menu. They are expected to consume foods about which they are phobic in this controlled setting. Table 7–1 shows the organization of a typical week. The specific treatment groups can best be described under the heading of eating and noneating groups. The separation of groups into these two categories is somewhat arbitrary as connections are made between behavioral, affective, and interpersonal issues in all groups.

The Assessment Process

Each patient is assessed in a multidisciplinary team interview that takes approximately 2 hours. The purpose of the assessment process is to determine the patient's appropriateness for an intensive and outpatient pro-

Table 7–1. Weekly schedule for day hospital program

Monday	Tuesday	Wednesday	Thursday	Friday
10:00 - 11:30 Leisure & Time Management	9:30 - 10:30 Food Shopping	10:00 - 11:00 Weighing Group		
11:30 - 12:00 Community Meeting	10:30 - 12:00 Body Image Group	11:00 - 12:00 Symptom Strategy Group	11:30 - 12:00 Cooking	11:00 - 12:00 Menus
12:00 - 1:00 Lunch 12:00 - 1:15 Lunch Outing	12:00 - 1:00 Lunch	12:00 - 1:00 Lunch	12:00 - 1:00 Lunch	12:00 - 1:00 Lunch
1:00 - 1:30 Free Time	1:00 - 1:30 Community Meeting	1:00 - 1:30 Community Meeting	1:00 - 1:30 Community Meeting	1:00 - 2:00 DEBQ Feedback
1:30 - 3:00 Symptom Strategy Group	1:30 - 1:50 Free Time 1:50 - 3:00 Gym	1:40 - 3:00 Family relations Group	1:35 - 2:40 Relationship Group	2:00 - 2:45 Goodbye Group/ Education Group
3:00 - 3:30 Snack	3:00 - 3:30 Snack	3:00 - 3:30 Snack	3:00 - 3:30 Snack	2:45 - 3:30 Snack Outing
3:30 - 5:00 Creative Art Group	3:30 - 4:45 Sexuality Group 4:45 - 5:00 Free Time	3:30 - 4:30 Assertion Group 4:30 - 5:00 Free Time/ Cooking	3:30 - 4:00 Free Time 4:00 - 5:00 Nutrition Group	3:30 - 5:00 Leisure & Time Management
5:00 - 6:15 Dinner DEBQ Evening Planning	5:00 - 6:15 Dinner DEBQ Evening Planning	5:00 - 6:15 Dinner DEBQ Evening Planning	5:00 - 6:15 Dinner DEBQ Evening Planning	5:00 - 6:15 Dinner DEBQ Evening Planning

Note. DEBQ = Daily Eating Behavior Questionnaire.

gram centered primarily on group psychotherapy. The attending psychiatrist or psychiatric resident begins the assessment with an interview conducted in the presence of all program staff. This focuses on the patient's present eating behaviors, including methods of weight control, physical and psychological complications of the eating disorder, presence of comorbidity including substance abuse and mood disorder, and the potential for self-harm behavior. During this interview, the quality of relationships, especially as these may pertain to group therapy, is considered. The patient's capacity for both receiving and accepting help are examined closely. All staff may ask specific questions related to family, occupational, and nutritional status.

The second part of the assessment consists of the family therapist interviewing the family members with the patient and other staff present. The focus of this interview is to understand how the eating disorder affects current family functioning and what attempts the family has made to deal with specific behavioral aspects of the problem. Following this, the family leaves and the staff have an opportunity to discuss the case.

For the final portion of the assessment, the family and the patient return to discuss concerns arising from the assessment and, if the patient is deemed an appropriate candidate, to set an admission date. Specific expectations regarding impulsive behaviors, especially drug taking and self-harm, are clearly established, and a verbal contract is agreed upon whereby the patient accepts the nonnegotiable aspects of the treatment program. These include attempting to give up disturbed eating behaviors and attempting to follow the meal plan as closely as possible.

There are specific indications for admission to the day hospital program. These include the presence of a severe eating disorder according to DSM-III-R criteria (American Psychiatric Association 1987) that has failed to respond to outpatient treatment or that has a high likelihood of failing because of the degree of chronicity, frequency of bingeing or purging, or emaciation. Both patient and family have to be motivated to become involved in an intensive treatment program with a mutually agreed upon expectation of symptomatic change (i.e., weight gain and decreased bingeing or purging). The patient has to demonstrate the ability, however limited, to tolerate a group setting and to relate to other members.

There are also specific contraindications to admission. These include acute suicidal risk, acute medical risk (e.g., hypokalemia with electrocardiographic changes or severe emaciation), and severe drug abuse that clearly interferes with the normalization of weight, appetite, and eating.

Eating Groups

The group experiences described in this section are directly focused on food and eating behavior. They include specific eating related tasks as well as educational material related to food and eating.

Eating experiences: Meals, cooking, outings. The most intense group experiences are the meals—lunch, snack, and dinner—that are served 5 days a week in the patient dining room. All staff share in the responsibility of supervising meals, thereby imparting the therapeutic importance of normal eating. Tremendous peer pressure is brought to bear on the individual members of the groups as they struggle to face phobic foods, abandon food rituals, normalize eating behaviors, and tolerate strong urges to restrict, binge, and purge. The intensity of the experience is contained by the very consistent application of norms and rules for eating. The supervisory function is served by two staff members who are present throughout the meals and for after-meal discussion. The staff occasionally eat here as well, serving as role models for normal eating behaviors.

The supportive function is primarily served by peer support following the meal as group members individually take turns commenting on the experience of eating, their emotional reaction to it, and practical issues related to strategies to prevent purging and restricting during nonprogram hours.

> For example, a new patient begins to cry when prompted by the staff to put butter on her vegetables. She eats the meal in silence, carefully watched by the staff person who then tries to take the focus away from food by discussing a recent movie. After the meal trays have been removed, the patient is asked to express how she feels about her upset. She says that she is humiliated at being prompted by staff to eat differently than she might choose. She is reassured in the open discussion by more senior patients that the first few days are always difficult and that patients often cry during meals. Other group members reveal that the rules seem endless and confusing but that the eating becomes easier with time. Copatients then ask about her plans for the evening, recommending she use the group for support by either going with them for coffee or phoning one of them should she feel upset or anxious, particularly when trying to eat her evening snack.

> An example of difficulties experienced by a more senior member demonstrates the greater sense of group cohesiveness that develops over time. A senior member orders a particularly phobic food for dinner. She shouts derisively that there is no way she is going "to eat a bloody steak" and proceeds to poke at the steak with her fork. The staff person comments quietly and reassuringly that this is how steak is cooked and for her to go on with her meal. The patient wolfs down her meat in an angry way, but later comments to the group that she is sorry she had commented on the meat as she knows this makes it more difficult for copatients to eat their meals. She then connects her angry feelings to an

earlier disappointment in the day. Copatients then comment on the effect her outburst has on them, but support her ability to finish eating her meal, despite her angry feelings.

Most learning at meal times is done by modeling. The rationale for rules around eating are given by both staff and patients. The responsibility for completing a meal in the given time rests clearly with the patients. Staff are present to create a holding environment necessary to facilitate adaptation to new eating behaviors. It is extremely important that staff are internally consistent with the rules and norms for all patients. The potential for splitting among staff is increased with the application of a multitude of rules, and staff spend many hours clarifying the details of normal eating for the patients.

Other behavioral strategies are also imparted at meals. A hierarchy of phobic foods is established for each patient. Initially food from the hospital menu is chosen, then food from a special list, which includes more phobic foods such as fried foods and fast foods. When eating is stabilized, snack and lunch outings are introduced to allow for eating in more social settings, often where binges have occurred. Response prevention takes the form of bathroom supervision. Before mealtime, bathrooms are unlocked; otherwise they remain locked. Self-monitoring of eating behavior, feelings, and significant events are carefully recorded following each mealtime in a Daily Eating Behavior Questionnaire (DEBQ).

Feedback groups.   Any program that expects behavioral change is required to provide as much immediate feedback as possible. Two groups are designed with this particular focus, the DEBQ Feedback Group and the Weigh Group. The incorporation of diary writing and weekly weighing into a group format helps to make these experiences interpersonal rather than solitary. The diaries are reviewed by staff weekly. A feedback sheet is prepared and returned to each patient containing comments from the team on the individual's eating behavior and emotional state that week. Each patient is required to read her DEBQ feedback aloud to the entire group. Information that was previously private now becomes the domain of the group. Patients thus hear an overview of their progress in the group setting. Group interpretation of the feedback gives the patient perspective on it and a direction for the group to take with each of its members. The feedback sheets are not signed and are seen to represent the entire staff's views to prevent splitting of the staff by the patients.

In the Weigh Group, patients discuss their concerns about weight, apprehension at being weighed, and eating behavior previous to being weighed. Patients are weighed individually by one staff member and return immediately to the group to divulge their weight, display a graphic depiction of the weight change since admission, and discuss their feelings about changes. Patients are often surprised at the inaccuracy of their self-estimation of weight change. When the goal of treatment is weight gain, no change or weight loss is a personal victory but may be perceived as a failure by the group members, who have worked hard to facilitate weight gain for a patient. Staff need to be very active in providing support when a number of patients gain dramatically at the same time. It may be difficult at such a time for staff to be supportive without responding to patients' requests to reduce calories.

Menu Group.　This group and the following two groups are primarily educational in nature. Hospital menus are filled out once weekly in an informal group setting supervised by the nutritionist. Each patient has an individualized meal plan, and changes in the meal plan, particularly calorie changes, are presented in the group setting. Several important group issues are addressed in this group. The notion that the patients will be treated equally, yet as individuals, is extremely important. Each patient is seen to have different needs, yet no one can be an exception to the basic rules of following a prescribed meal plan. The effect of this equalizing process contributes to a sense of safety and fairness in the group. Caloric changes are presented as a team decision; the nutritionist is not allowed to make changes on her own. This diffuses the power struggle that often develops around prescribed calories.

Nutrition Group.　The Nutrition Group is a didactic, behavioral group. Each week different educational aspects related to nutrition are presented by the nutritionist to the patient group. Misconceptions about how food is handled physiologically are corrected. In the second part of the group, each patient plans her meals for the upcoming weekend. Senior members are paired with newer members to help them apply the exchange system of the meal plan and to help anticipate difficulties associated with eating normally.

Eating Attitude Group.　The Eating Attitude Group utilizes a didactic format to present fundamental aspects of eating disorders. Group topics are presented by each staff member on a rotational basis. All staff are familiar with all of the educational material. Topics include the physiological effects of starvation, set point theory, effects of purging, medications for eating disorders, strategies for changing behavior, cultural influences and eating disorders, alcohol and drug abuse, budgeting, discharge planning, and cognitive beliefs associated with eating disorders.

Noneating Groups

These groups deal with more general issues that are associated with the eating disorder but do not specifically focus on food or eating. In keeping with the view that eating disorders arise out of deficit states (Goodsitt 1985; Kohut 1974), a number of the noneating groups attempt to build skills in different areas of performance, particularly those areas that relate to impulse control and expression of feelings. The first four groups are concerned with these adaptational skills, whereas the remaining five are theme centered.

Assertion Group. The Assertion Group meets weekly and uses role-playing, behavioral rehearsal, and scriptwriting to facilitate the "here-and-now" process of learning assertive behavior. The assertion paradigm functions as a new belief system that supports the patient's efforts to communicate interpersonally with a greater sense of self-control, personal responsibility, and empowerment. Difficulty in expressing negative affect and setting limits are two common deficits. The assertion group is open-ended, and each group session is complete within itself. Senior group members are often given the role of teaching newer members the background material necessary to understand the assertion issues presented each week. Situations that pertain to eating are the focus of group attention: for instance, refusing a second portion, or standing up to the pressure to drink alcohol. Assertion is viewed as a tangible skill or tool that is applied within the program and outside the program. The patients are encouraged to practice these skills. Requests for advice on how to solve a specific problem are saved for this group.

Leisure and Time Management Group. The Leisure and Time Management Group provides an avenue for the process of generalization. Individualized plans for the weekend are discussed by patients on Friday afternoon and reported on Monday morning. These plans help to maintain the program structure, norms, and goals during nonprogram hours. Each patient is assisted by the group to form plans that will maximize the possibility of eating normally. Very often, it is the commitment to and support from the group that allows individuals to make major behavioral changes despite few personal supports away from the program.

Gym Group. Physical activity in the gym is held weekly, or twice a week if there are no patient discharges. During this time two staff members take the patients to the hospital gym to play volleyball. This activity was chosen for several reasons. Volleyball is both competitive and cooperative, and it can be played with varying degrees of skill and physical fitness. It is a social sport that is commonly played in the community. Lastly, it is not a sport driven by calorie reduction. The volleyball game is another sensitive barometer of the group process and is handled as a therapeutic activity. The group is processed afterwards, and issues around competition, performance anxiety, body image disturbance, and group integration are explored with the guidance of staff.

Creative Arts Group.   Another forum for nonverbal expression is the Creative Arts Group. The goal of this group is not necessarily interpretative, but rather to provide patients with a forum for nonverbal expression that is innately valued. Different media are used to deal with various affective states or experiences. This group explores alternative means of self-expression. The leader offers instruction in visual arts techniques and encourages experimentation with the tools provided. Following an introduction to methods available for the group session, patients work independently for some time and then reconvene to discuss the experience of their creative work.

Body Image Group.   The goal of the Body Image Group is to reconstruct the development of the individual's body image, to correct body image distortion, and to create more positive body image experience. Guided imagery (whereby visual and kinesthetic images are induced during a state of deep muscle relaxation) is used to capture the experiencing of the body. This technique is described by Hutchinson (1985) and has been adapted to a group format, which is described in greater detail in Chapter 8.

Sexuality Group.   The Sexuality Group is the most recent of the groups to be offered in the program and is in response to the frequency of reports of adverse sexual experiences. Discomfort with physical intimacy often affects eating behavior and leads to the need to control one's body by pursuing thinness. As for most of the other groups, a psychoeducational approach is used. Much time is spent reviewing the norms of this group as they relate to confidentiality, voluntary participation, and respect for differences in sexual practice and experience among the members. Each week, different topics are presented to the group (e.g., menstruation, birth control, sexual responsiveness, sex play, sexual abuse, and self-protection). The disclosure of sexual abuse is common, and the leaders attempt to relate the sexual abuse experience to the development and perpetuation of the eating disorder. The connection to the eating disorder is the focus of all the discussions. Use is regularly made of community support programs for sexually abused women.

Relationship Group.   For the Relationship Group, patients are divided into two smaller groups of about six members each to facilitate interpersonal interaction. The format for this group is based on an adaptation of the "Higher Functioning Inpatient Group" described by Yalom (1983). Patients identify a personal problem they see occurring repeatedly in their lives. The problem or "agenda" is then made interpersonal by identifying a copatient or staff member with whom this problem occurs. Working through agendas often involves expressing feelings directly to the person who evokes them, getting feedback from that person, correcting distortions in the interpersonal experience, and finally linking the interpersonal difficulties with the eating disorder. Strong transferences within the patient group and toward staff are explored. This is frequently the group where sexual issues such as abuse, incest, or violence are disclosed. These issues are labeled and understood within the context of the eating disorder but are dealt with more specifically in family sessions or follow-up therapy.

Family Relations Group. The Family Relations Group provides a structured introduction to a series of family centered topics such as family roles, family life cycle, and family separation. This group is described in detail in Chapter 9.

Community Meetings. Community Meetings involve all patients and staff and occur 4 out of 5 days for half an hour. Patients view this time as an opportunity to attend to instrumental tasks such as requesting help with welfare, reviewing medication concerns, making requests to use the telephone, or arranging family meetings. Staff consider the Community Meeting from a broader perspective, including the containment of patients through the reiteration of rules and norms of the program, and the focusing of the group on eating issues and on group process. Issues such as subgrouping, scapegoating, leadership, and change of membership in the group and staff are all important aspects deserving comment in this forum. Eating goals for new patients based on the initial assessment may be presented in this group.

Goodbye Group. This group focuses on the process of saying goodbye, including issues of closure and separation. Each patient has her own Goodbye Group when she terminates the program. To facilitate the process of saying goodbye, the departing member uses the paradigm Kubler-Ross (1975) has described in understanding loss. The stages of denial, anger, bargaining, depression, and acceptance are all defined and explored in terms of accepting the illness, connecting to the program and group, and leaving behind both the illness and the group. For almost all members, the Goodbye Group represents the first time that they have said goodbye directly. The experience evokes the recollection of many unresolved losses and difficulties members have had in attachment and separation. These Goodbye Groups, occurring almost weekly, are also a preparation for discharge of all members. Every discharge means a shift in members' seniority and anticipation of one's own discharge. Roles within the group are explored openly in the context of the changing positions the members occupy. Depending on group cohesion and the departing member's connectedness to the group, the group may give a small gift to the departing member, exchange farewell cards, or have a group goodbye outside the program time.

Program Evaluation and Outcome

The primary aims of the group therapies in the day hospital program are to change aberrant eating habits, particularly bingeing and purging behaviors, and to produce weight gain in emaciated patients within the context of eating regular meals. The amelioration of associated cognitive distortions, such as excessive preoccupation with weight and shape, polarized "all-or-none" thinking, and chronic low self-esteem, is also considered an important goal of treatment. Successful shifts in these psychological dimensions generally occur once changes in eating behaviors are accomplished. Therefore, it is anticipated that follow-up treatment will be required of group members in order for them to deal with these aspects of the eating disorder in greater detail. The day hospital provides an opportunity to identify such issues and begin the process of addressing them.

The effectiveness of the program in achieving its goals of normalizing eating and ameliorating associated psychopathology has been evaluated in a series of studies that have looked at symptom change and at predictors that might identify patients who are likely to do well or not do well in the program. Several follow-up studies have been completed (Maddocks and Kaplan, in press; Maddocks et al. 1990, in press; Piran et al. 1989).

Symptomatic Change

All patients complete an extensive battery of change measures on admission, discharge, and follow-up. The following results are based on female patients who meet DSM-III-R criteria for BN or AN and who completed a minimum of 6 weeks of treatment. Overall mean attendance was 11.6 weeks.

Bulimic eating symptoms. The program is successful in helping patients significantly reduce the frequency of their bulimic behaviors. Overall, 83% of patients who completed the program experienced significant improvement in their bulimic behaviors (see Table 7–2). The 56% rate of total abstinence from bingeing and purging appears to be a robust finding, replicating an earlier finding on a smaller sample of 23 bulimic patients

Table 7–2. Eating behavior outcome results for bulimia nervosa patients

Outcome	Final 4 weeks before termination %	2-year follow-up %
Good		
No bingeing/purging	56	46
Moderate		
Bingeing/purging not more than once per week	27	28
Poor		
Bingeing/purging more than once per week	17	26

who received treatment in the program (Maddocks et al., in press; Piran et al. 1989). Seventeen percent of the patients with bulimic behaviors did poorly. They continued to be highly symptomatic at the end of treatment, bingeing and vomiting more than once a week.

Follow-up data are particularly important in this patient population, because virtually all patients had been severely symptomatic and treatment resistant for over a decade prior to beginning the program. A preliminary study (Piran et al. 1989) evaluated short-term outcome of 21 patients at 1, 3, and 6 months following termination and found that treatment gains were maintained. A more comprehensive 2-year follow-up study has recently been completed (Maddocks et al. 1990, in press). All female patients who had completed a minimum of 6 weeks of treatment were eligible. A contact rate of 86% was achieved. Patients were weighed and assessed by structured interview for specific eating disorder psychopathology and mood status. They also completed a battery of self-report measures. Some patients had relapsed, whereas others had gone into remission. As shown in Table 7–2, overall, 74% of the bulimic patients continued to report improvement on follow-up.

The information concerning long-term follow-up is still limited because of the cross-sectional nature of the data and the small sample size. Future studies are in progress to investigate the phenomenology of the long-term course of patients after they have received treatment in order to identify factors that predict or signal relapse as well as factors associated with prolonged treatment maintenance.

Weight gain. The program is also successful in helping patients gain weight. The anorexic restricting subgroup (ANR) and anorexic bulimic subgroup (ANB) gained an average of 5 kg (11 lb) and 6 kg (13 lb), respectively, over the course of treatment. No significant differences were found between the ANR and ANB patients in terms of absolute weight gain or rate of weight gain during the program. Interestingly, patients with normal weight BN also gained small but significant amounts of weight.

A simple outcome classification system is utilized for AN patients based on behavioral criteria of weight gain and purging behavior. A "good" outcome indicates a discharge weight of 90% or above matched population mean weight (MPMW) or a gain on average of at least 0.7 kg (1.5 lb) per week and abstinence from vomiting. The "moderate" group consists of patients whose weight was between "good" and "poor" criteria or who were vomiting not more than once per week. A "poor" outcome includes patients who weighed less than 85% of MPMW at discharge or who demonstrated an average weekly weight gain of less than 0.3 kg (0.67 lb) during treatment or who were vomiting more than once a week during the last 4 weeks of treatment.

Overall, patients diagnosed with AN appear to do less well in the program than do BN patients when assessed on the behavioral criteria. About a third of the AN patients demonstrated a "good" outcome, with approximately another third in the "moderate" category.

Anorexic patients who also meet criteria for BN do the least well. Several factors may be responsible for this. The briefness of the program—approximately 3 months—may not allow sufficient time for a patient to address both eating disorder syndromes. Binge eating and purging is generally experienced as ego-dystonic; patients tend to be disturbed by such behavior and want to give it up. However, the caloric restriction and relentless pursuit of thinness that is pathognomonic of anorexia nervosa is experienced as ego-syntonic; patients do not view such activity and beliefs as illness behavior and cling tenaciously to them. This would set up conflictual tension regarding the motivation for change. These patients may require additional kinds of treatment to make the necessary behavioral changes consistent with recovery.

Psychological symptoms.   Psychological symptoms also were significantly lower at the end of treatment. Both diagnostic groups (AN patients and BN patients) were found to display similar patterns of symptom reduction. The Eating Attitudes Test (EAT; Garner et al. 1982) and the Eating Disorder Inventory (EDI; Garner et al. 1983) were used to assess specific eating disorder psychopathology such as weight preoccupation, feelings of ineffectiveness, body image disturbance, interpersonal distrust, maturity fears, and interoceptive labeling. Prior to treatment, scores on these measures were found to be clinically elevated in the range expected for individuals with eating disorders. By the end of treatment, scores had decreased to ranges achieved for females without eating disorders, indicating that patients were not excessively invested in a drive for thinner body shape, had an improved sense of self-worth and interpersonal relatedness, and had an improved awareness of somatic cues of hunger and satiety as well as emotional states.

The exception to these findings were scores for the Body Dissatisfaction scale on the EDI. Although significantly reduced from intake, scores for both AN and BN patients remained clinically elevated. This finding is congruent with patient feedback received during groups, particularly the Body Image Group. Patients often recognize body image disturbance toward the end of the program after nutritional stabilization has occurred and when their cognitive functioning improves. Some ANR patients who achieve a successful weight gain during the program become aware of negative feelings associated with the weight gain—feelings that were earlier denied or inaccessible because of starvation effects. Frequently, patients identify body image disturbance as an area they need to work on after they leave the program. Associated psychopathology such as depression, self-esteem, and anxiety were also found to be significantly decreased at the end of treatment.

Social adjustment. Patients at discharge report significantly better social adjustment, although posttreatment scores on the Social Adjustment Scale (SAS; Weissman and Bothwell 1976) remained somewhat higher than norms achieved for a community sample (Weissman et al. 1978). These results also support our clinical impression that patients often have just begun the process of vocational and social rehabilitation as they leave the program and require more time before the effects of the lifestyle disruption and chronicity of the eating disorder settle.

Predicting Outcome in the Program

The overall findings of these studies indicate that both BN and AN patients demonstrate significant behavioral and psychological changes over the course of their attendance in the program. An examination of preadmission factors that can distinguish patients who demonstrate a favorable response to the program from those who do not has been reported (Maddocks and Kaplan, in press). To date, only patients with BN have been investigated with regard to the prediction of treatment response because of the sample size requirements for multivariate statistics. The "good" and "moderate" responders were combined into a "positive" response group who demonstrated significant reductions in bulimic behavior. This group was compared to those who remained highly symptomatic at the end of treatment, the "poor" response group.

Both the "positive" and "poor" BN response groups revealed clinically elevated symptoms of mood disturbance and eating disorder psychopathology at admission. However, the "poor" responders had markedly higher levels of symptoms on these measures. A discriminant function analysis revealed that measures of depression, self-esteem, and anxiety provided the best discrimination between the two groups. The frequency of bulimic behaviors was not significant in determining how well a patient did in the program. Poor responders were predicted by their psychological symptoms of severe depression and cognitive preoccupation with weight, shape, and body image.

This treatment resistant subgroup of highly symptomatic patients may need special considerations, even in a program as intensive as the day hospital. For example, the more depressed and cognitively preoccupied patients with BN may require concomitant pharmacotherapy before responding favorably to other aspects of the program. Perhaps a more focused cognitive behavioral approach to deal with depressive symptoms and faulty cognitions in addition to the existing group therapies in the program might be considered for these patients.

References

American Psychiatric Association: Diagnostic and Statistical Manual of Mental Disorders, 3rd Edition, Revised. Washington, DC, American Psychiatric Association, 1987

Crisp AH: Clinical and therapeutic aspects of anorexia nervosa: a study of thirty cases. J Psychosom Res 9:67–78, 1965

Garfinkel PE, Garner DM (eds): The Role of Drug Treatments for Eating Disorders. New York, Brunner/Mazel, 1987

Garner DM, Bemis KM: Cognitive therapy for anorexia nervosa, in Handbook of Psychotherapy for the Eating Disorders. Edited by Garner DM, Garfinkel PE. New York, Guilford, 1985

Garner D, Olmsted M, Bohr Y, et al: The Eating Attitudes Test: psychometric features and clinical correlates. Psychol Med 12:871–878, 1982

Garner DM, Olmsted M, Polivy J: Development and validation of a multidimensional eating disorder inventory for anorexia nervosa and bulimia. International Journal of Eating Disorders 2(2):15–34, 1983

Goodsitt A: Self-psychology and the treatment of anorexia nervosa, in Handbook of Psychotherapy for Anorexia Nervosa and Bulimia. Edited by Garner DM, Garfinkel PE. New York, Guilford, 1985

Hutchinson M: Transforming Body Image. New York, The Crossing Press, 1985

Kohut H: The Restoration of Self. New York, International Universities Press, 1974

Kubler-Ross E: Death, The Final Stage of Growth. Englewood Cliffs, NJ, Prentice-Hall, 1975

Maddocks SE, Kaplan AS: The prediction of treatment response in bulimia nervosa: a study of patient variables. Br J Psychiatry (in press)

Maddocks SE, Kaplan AS, Langdon L, et al: Group therapy for anorexia nervosa: short- and long-term outcome. Unpublished manuscript, 1990 (Copy available from Dr. Sarah Maddocks, Department of Psychology, Women's College Hospital, 76 Grenville Street, Toronto, Ontario M5S 1B2 Canada)

Maddocks SE, Kaplan AS, Langdon L, et al: Two year follow-up in bulimia nervosa: the importance of abstinence as the criterion of outcome. International Journal of Eating Disorders (in press)

Mitchell JE, Hatsukami D, Goff G, et al: Intensive outpatient group treatment for bulimia, in Handbook of Psychotherapy for the Eating Disorders. Edited by Garner DM, Garfinkel PE. New York, Guilford, 1985

Piran N, Langdon L, Kaplan A, et al: Evaluation of a day hospital program for eating disorders. International Journal of Eating Disorders 8(5):523–532, 1989

Schwartz RC, Barrett MJ, Saba G: Family therapy for bulimia, in Handbook of Psychotherapy for the Eating Disorders. Edited by Garner DM, Garfinkel PE. New York, Guilford, 1985

Weissman M, Bothwell S: Assessment of social adjustment by patient self-report. Arch Gen Psychiatry 33:1111–1115, 1976

Weissman MM, Prusoff BA, Thompson WD, et al: Social adjustment by self-report in a community sample and in psychiatric outpatients. J Nerv Ment Dis 66:317–326, 1978

Yalom ID: The Theory and Practice of Group Psychotherapy. New York, Basic Books, 1975

Yalom ID: Inpatient Group Psychotherapy. New York, Basic Books, 1983

8

Body Image Groups

Karin Jasper, Ph.D., M.Ed.
Sarah E. Maddocks, Ph.D., C.Psych.

◆ ◆ ◆ ◆ ◆ ◆ ◆ ◆

This is the first in a series of chapters on specialized groups that are designed to address a particular component of the eating disorder presentation. The body image incorporates core perceptions and evaluations of self that form a bridge between general psychological development and the selection of eating disorder symptoms. The authors have used evocative structured exercises to break through the veil of denial and repression commonly surrounding the severely disordered anorexia nervosa or bulimia nervosa patient. These techniques are not commonly used in group psychotherapy, perhaps to its detriment. The therapeutic challenge is to be able to manage the powerful affect that can be released through these techniques. The structure of the exercises helps in this regard, as well as the support of the surrounding therapeutic community in which they are taking place. Focused techniques such as those described here could be incorporated into general group psychotherapy procedures.—The Editors

Body image disturbances are probably the commonest problem among women today, and are all but universal in the increasing numbers of women affected by serious eating disorders.

—Wooley and Wooley (1985)

Body image disturbance is essentially a socioculturally generated problem. Contemporary Western culture has unfortunately managed to make most women feel uncomfortable with normal female body size, to find problems with their bodies where there are none. Great amounts of time and effort are consumed trying to solve these nonexistent problems. For example, a recent article in a major daily newspaper claimed that liposuction was useful for rectifying the "violin deformity," an indentation between hips and thighs. This "deformity" was stated to affect 75% of all women. Because this is the normal anatomic shape of most women's bodies, the article amounted to a claim that women's bodies are naturally deformed. Studies indicate that most women believe that there is something wrong with their bodies to the extent that they are motivated to do something about it (Rozin and Fallon 1988; Wooley and Wooley 1985). Despite the fact that more women than men are underweight, 80% of women are chronic dieters (Steiner-Adair 1989). Few men who describe themselves as overweight are bothered enough to actively diet (Rozin and Fallon 1988).

In short, large numbers of women feel the need to do something serious about a "pseudoproblem." Because most women are either average or underweight, there is no need to do anything about their body size. Many would benefit from gaining rather than losing weight—the exact opposite of their beliefs. The body image therapist is therefore required to do a kind of "metatherapy." The client must understand that the need for therapy arose out of attempts to correct something that did not need correcting. Once this is seen, therapy can either end, because there is nothing else wrong, or it can begin, because the real problems can surface. A good deal of therapy with women is of this nature.

In a misogynist society, women are socialized to think poorly of themselves, to find themselves inferior simply because they are not male. Helping women increase their self-esteem is often a process of empowering them to feel good about being female. Low self-esteem and body image disparagement among women—both significant factors in eating disorders—are primarily socioculturally generated problems.

Thus, an important component of body image therapy is to help the client reject the offensive yet ubiquitous sociocultural message that thinness equals happiness. She has to germinate this view in the midst of hundreds of messages to the contrary, including the magical notion perpetuated through advertising that by losing weight one can be problem-free. She must begin to believe that a larger body can be acceptable.

This chapter describes techniques for dealing with body image issues that can be used in therapy groups. Application of these methods is described in two different programs, an intensive day hospital and a private practice office.

What is Body Image?

Research and clinical results concerning body image are difficult to compare because there is no generally accepted definition for the term "body image." Consequently, researchers and clinicians are not always discussing the same thing. For the purposes of this chapter, "body image" will be considered a person's experience of her own body. Briefly put, body image is the way one sees one's body and how one feels about and in it. This includes the following components (Bruch 1973; Hutchinson 1981; Wooley and Wooley 1985):

♦ *Cognitive*—thoughts and beliefs about the body (e.g., "I am 5 feet 3 inches tall, and I am destined to be fat;" "My body size and shape determine my value as a person");
♦ *Perceptual*—internal feelings and sensations (e.g., feelings of vulnerability and tiredness, sensations of hunger and pain, perceived body size and shape, including over- or underestimation of actual size and shape);
♦ *Affective*—feelings about one's body (e.g., pride, anger, shame);
♦ *Evaluative*—judgments, including moral statements (e.g., "I am too fat;" "The fat on me is disgusting");
♦ *Social*—acute awareness of others' feelings, attitudes, and beliefs (e.g., criticalness, desire, disregard, "You've got Aunt Helen's big hips");
♦ *Kinesthetic*—sensed fluidity of movement (e.g., openness, heaviness, gracefulness); and
♦ *Tactile*—sense of permeability and solidity, as in feeling that others can move right through one, feeling vulnerable to the suggestions or expectations of others, feeling as though one does not occupy one's body.

The development of one's body image is affected by direct and indirect feedback from others (Kearney-Cooke 1988); actual occurrences to the body (i.e., surgery, accidents, illnesses, physical and sexual abuse; Kearney-Cooke 1988); general self-esteem (Butters and Cash 1987); and gender socialization.

The term "disturbance" is also vague. We need to know whether the disturbance is a perceptual or cognitive distortion, or a disparagement of one's body size, the latter being an affective or kinesthetic experience. In this chapter, the following terms will be used:

Body image "distortion" refers to a significant discrepancy between one's perception of, or beliefs about, the size or shape of one's body and its actual size or shape. An emaciated person who believes herself to be fat or who visually identifies herself as significantly larger than she is suffers from such a distortion. Similarly, the person who underestimates the size of her body perceptually or cognitively has a distorted body image.

Body image "dissatisfaction" refers to disparaging or disliking one's body—the way one experiences the body.

Both body image distortion and body image dissatisfaction can be expressed by the individual as "being too fat" or as "feeling fat." Body image distortion and dissatisfaction can exist separately or can occur together. A person can perceptually distort body size or shape but may not feel dissatisfied with it. Or a person can perceive body size and shape accurately, yet feel dissatisfied with it.

Most clinicians treating individuals with eating disorders emphasize the importance of treating body image distortion in order for recovery to occur. However, it is equally important, in order to prevent relapse, that body image dissatisfaction be a target of therapeutic intervention. In other words, treatment should aim both at rectifying distortions and at developing a positive attitude toward the body. There has been a considerable amount of research relating to body image over the last three decades. Most of this research is focused on measuring body image distortion, and little is related to body image dissatisfaction and its treatment. In addition, there is limited empirical evidence concerning how to repair body image distortion and dissatisfaction.

As Garner and Garfinkel (1981) have suggested, for many anorexic patients, it is likely that body image distortion will correct itself following the resolution of more fundamental psychological issues. However, Vandereycken and colleagues (1987) argued that the neglect of body image therapy may be one of the reasons why long-term outcome for eating disorder anorexic patients is generally poor. The researchers begin their program for treatment of anorexia patients with an intrusive body image videofeedback technique designed to break through patient denial regarding emaciation. Wooley and Wooley (1985) have suggested that body image therapy be used with eating disorder bulimic patients who no longer require close monitoring of eating but who are not making further progress because of unresolved distortions of body image. It is possible that different strategies may be useful with different categories of patients (i.e., what is beneficial for bulimic patients at a given stage of treatment may not be so for anorexic patients at a similar stage). Few body image therapies have been tested rigorously, and more research is certainly necessary to answer these questions. Because treating body image distortion does not necessarily affect body image dissatisfaction, and because the latter may be more relevant to relapse prevention, techniques related to both should be developed and studied.

The therapies that have been documented to treat body image problems include individual cognitive approaches (Butters and Cash 1987; Garner and Garfinkel 1981); an eclectic group approach including relaxation, movement, bioenergetics, and videofeedback (Vandereycken et al. 1987); a guided imagery, movement, and writing group approach (Hutchinson 1981); and eclectic group approaches using guided imagery, movement, art, psychodrama, and ritual (Kearney-Cooke 1989; Wooley 1986; Wooley and Kearney-Cooke 1986; Wooley and Wooley 1985). Only Hutchinson (1981) and Butters and Cash (1987) have reported formal testing of their programs; however, neither of these were used with subjects who had eating disorders. Both programs did find significant improvement in body image in subjects receiving their treatments.

Why a Group Approach?

A group approach offers a number of advantages over individual treatment. The opportunity for support and interpersonal learning in an environment where the role of the leader is less predominant fits the particular needs of the patient with an eating disorder. There are additional specific reasons to choose a group approach to body image difficulties. Women in our society rarely support one another in accepting natural body shape and weight. It is more common for them to foster maintenance of dieting behavior and "thin is best" attitudes. In the group, it is possible to develop an alternate experience where the support from other women is given for self-nurturing behavior and self-and-body acceptance. This has a powerful effect in terms of encouraging group members to risk the social and personal consequences of not being thin and in validating self-caring and self-accepting behavior. They create a small counterculture in which the value of thinness is questioned. In this context, it becomes safe for group members to give and receive feedback regarding body image distortions.

Treatment Techniques

Because body image is a multidimensional phenomenon, it requires the integration of a range of treatment modalities and a flexible approach. Although nearly all clients share the common background of our culture's negative messages about women's bodies, each client's personal history will have colored her experience of her own body.

In group, the therapist not only has to help each client identify various components of her body image but must also facilitate the verbalization of these nonverbal experiences. Nonverbal therapy techniques such as relaxation, guided imagery, videofeedback, role-playing, psychodrama, movement, art, massage, and bioenergetics are therefore important tools. They are used to access thoughts and feelings associated with body image disturbance that are difficult to put into words. Verbal techniques (e.g., cognitive or psychodynamic) help integrate these experiences in the group forum (Butters and Cash 1987; Fairburn 1985; Hutchinson 1985; Kearney-Cooke 1989; Vandereycken et al. 1987; Wooley and Wooley 1985).

Relaxation. Individuals with eating disorders typically do not allow time for relaxation. They frequently use ultimately ineffective behaviors such as extreme dietary restriction, bingeing, or purging to manage the tension and anxiety associated with feelings of fatness or fear of weight gain. The prospect of confronting previously avoided feelings and attitudes toward one's body can lead to intense anxiety.

Tension can be reduced to manageable levels by beginning a group session with a short relaxation exercise. Relaxation can also be utilized as an important adjunct for other techniques because of its usefulness in reducing anticipatory anxiety and for the "priming" effect on other techniques such as guided imagery. Breathing exercises, progressive muscle relaxation, self-hypnosis, and imagery are a few examples of the many available methods of relaxation (Davis et al. 1982). Different clients will favor different exercises, and each client may be encouraged to use the relaxation method that she has found most effective.

Guided imagery. Hutchinson (1985) and Kearney-Cooke (1988, 1989) have pioneered the use of guided imagery for exploring the symbolic nature of body image disturbance. Specific imaginary scenes are used with the aim of evoking unconscious sensory and affective material. Imagery exercises can range in potency from the elicitation of innocuous images of group room furniture, to the exploration of the evolution of one's body image, to highly sensitive images that address feelings related to sexuality. As faulty thoughts and beliefs become conscious through guided imagery exercises, the client can then work on changing attitudes and behaviors that serve to perpetuate body image distortion and dissatisfaction—and disordered eating.

Videofeedback. Videofeedback has been used in body image therapy as a method of providing objective information about physical appearance and verbal and nonverbal expression. Although valuable, this technique does have considerable risks in that it is quite anxiety provoking and can be very aversive if used inappropriately. This may result in an exacerbation rather than alleviation of negative feelings about one's body (Trower and Kiely 1983). Therefore, videofeedback must be used with caution and with sensitivity to a client's emotional state.

Vandereycken and colleagues (1987) have reported the use of videofeedback in a highly confrontational manner with hospitalized anorexic patients as part of a multimodal treatment plan. Each woman at admission poses in a bathing suit in front of the video camera and subsequently views the tape with other anorexic group members while listening to verbal feedback regarding her physical appearance. They describe this method as a means of breaking through the denial of body image distortion. We find this approach intrusive and degrading and suspect it may have long-term disadvantages. It encourages patients, who are almost always women and many of whom have been sexually abused, to see their bodies as objects to be manipulated for something or someone. Patients may respond to the verbal feedback by admitting a distortion, but perhaps only as a function of negative reinforcement.

In North America, Wooley and Wooley (1985) and Kearney-Cooke (1989) have used videofeedback in a much less intrusive way by employing a graded approach. Their clients view a tape of themselves sitting around a table; in later sessions, they watch tapes of the group in a movement exercise. A nonconfrontational approach employed with sensitivity can be very useful as a means of generating an awareness and understanding of body image distortion.

Movement therapy. Movement exercises including dance are useful for helping clients get in touch with their bodies as a source of information, to generate a sense of pleasure out of activity, for the development of spatial perception, and to explore the meanings of being fat or thin (Hutchinson 1985; Kearney-Cooke 1989; Wooley and Wooley 1985).

Art therapy. Drawing, painting, and clay modeling are also recognized methods of bringing into consciousness an awareness of spatial misperceptions of body size as well as the developmental aspects of body image distortion, dissatisfaction, and eating disorders. For example, Kearney-Cooke (1989) uses clay modeling after guided imagery in group therapy to assist clients' understanding and affective expression of material evoked by the exercise.

Other techniques. Many other structured and action oriented techniques have been described. Role-playing and psychodrama are useful techniques for helping clients develop an understanding of the context of their body image disturbance and for working toward alternative, healthier ways of coping. Massage and bioenergetics are less commonly employed but also are aimed at accessing feelings and sensations associated with body image and developing positive body experiences (Vandereycken et al. 1987).

Group Therapy in a Day Hospital Program

Body image therapy is utilized as one component of a multimodal group therapy program in an intensive treatment day hospital setting. The overall program is designed as a brief intervention of about 3 months' duration with a primary focus on normalizing maladaptive eating behaviors. Admission criteria ensure that all patients have chronic histories of severe eating disorders and concomitant body image disturbance. This manifests itself as a deeply entrenched negative influence that affects most aspects of daily living. The group members feel very threatened by the prospect of having to confront feelings associated with weight and shape. Even seeing the words "Body Image Group" on the program schedule has at times increased the anxiety of new members sufficiently to result in avoidance of the group.

At the beginning of treatment, group members tend to feel hopelessly locked in their negative cognitions and cannot envisage ever feeling differently. Behaviorally, this is observed as vehement expressions of hatred for their stomachs, thighs, and entire bodies and an avoidance of activities such as bathing, being touched, or exposing their bodies. Frequently group members talk about never allowing themselves to take a bath for fear of seeing their own flesh, preferring to take hurried showers, often in the dark. One group member described showering for several years dressed in a sweat suit so as to avoid seeing her body. The wearing of swimsuits, short sleeves, or shorts is also avoided by some group members. Histories of physical and sexual abuse are common among these patients, as are self-mutilating behaviors such as scratching, hitting, scrubbing, cutting, burning, and picking at various parts of the body.

Bruch's (1962) assumption that "a realistic body image concept is a precondition for recovery in anorexia nervosa" is central to the concept of body image therapy. The primary goal of the weekly body image group is to help clients begin the process of labeling and understanding their feelings and attitudes toward their bodies and to work toward developing a more realistic and positive body image. The emphasis is on generating an awareness of body image and fostering an understanding of how negative thoughts and emotions have served to perpetuate the eating disorder.

A multimodal approach is taken using guided imagery, drawing, role-playing, videofeedback, and relaxation. Most group members appear to make significant attitudinal shifts by the end of treatment and leave with some feeling of acceptance of their bodies. However, most report that many of the issues identified during the course of the body image therapy are only partially resolved and require continuing attention in follow-up therapy. Body image therapy is conducted at an early stage in the treatment process when clients are nutritionally unstable. Thus, it is not surprising that the group members feel the need for additional treatment after the day hospital experience to consolidate their gains.

A module approach was designed to accommodate the open-ended nature of the treatment program. Each group session is considered a complete entity, although as a client progresses through treatment, the content and process of the therapy will naturally build and overlap. A 10-week course is used so that each client is exposed to each module during her stay in the program. The evolution of the body image therapy led to structuring groups according to three broad themes: awareness, understanding, and acceptance. The groups are for the most part female but may include one or two males. The majority of the group members have BN, usually one to three members have AN, and one or two are classified as having an eating disorder not otherwise specified.

Exercises that address the spatial, perceptual, and cognitive distortions associated with body image disturbance form the core elements of the therapy. By questioning the beliefs and assumptions underlying negative body image, the body image groups begin the process of understanding body image problems and foster a readiness for change. Developing a contextual understanding of body image disturbance prepares the group members for a gradual acceptance of their bodies. For example, examining developmental aspects such as mother-daughter relationships, sociocultural issues, sexuality (including sexual abuse), and loss issues associated with giving up a negative body concept all serve to promote a psychological readiness that will enhance subsequent shifts in body image concept.

Two therapists colead the body image group and work to gently challenge the beliefs and attitudes of the group members. A general aim is to redress the sociocultural absurdity of making thin body size the cardinal marker of a woman's self-worth. The process of supportive and collaborative exploration allows group members to feel in control. The atmosphere of the group tends to be initially tense, with clients finding it hard to verbalize feelings and thoughts connected with their body image disturbance. The therapists must be active during this initial group phase. It is useful for the therapists to restate the purpose of the group each week. This affirms the fundamental goal of the group of beginning the process of developing a positive body image. This message is often not heard during the first week of the program because of apprehension and/or impaired concentration associated with nutritional instability.

The cotherapists attempt to maintain links with previous sessions, often giving homework tasks such as looking in the mirror, taking a bath rather than a shower, or reading relevant self-help material. Members are asked to provide feedback about these assignments. Care is taken to introduce the theme of the current group session and to explicitly describe a forthcoming exercise in an attempt to lessen the anxiety of group members and increase their participation during the group. Structured exercises are developed around the three central themes of awareness, understanding, and acceptance.

Developing an awareness of body image distortion. Two awareness-generating exercises are illustrative of the therapeutic process.

The first is a modification of Askevold's (1975) technique of addressing spatioperceptual distortions of body size called "image marking." Group members are asked to draw themselves as if they were looking at themselves in the mirror. After drawing their mirror images on large pieces of paper taped to the walls of the group room, the person standing to the right is asked to draw the actual body contour while the member stands in front of her own drawn "mirror" image. This brings many interpersonal as well as perceptual distortions directly into the here and now of the group. Interpersonal distrust and denial are consistent themes. Most clients find it difficult to accept that the tracing of their actual body size is accurate. The usual sentiment expressed is that other group members are only being "nice" and that they are actually much larger than is shown on the paper.

Reality testing with each other and exploring why it is so hard to trust others' opinions of their bodies during the group begins the process of fostering trust among group members and breaking through their denial. Aspects of social desirability are also prominent in this exercise, with emaciated patients often drawing accurate outlines of their body size despite severe body image disparagement, in an effort to please the group. When asked if the drawings are an accurate portrayal of the way they see themselves, these group members often admit that they feel much larger. As an emaciated woman once stated, "If I had drawn what I feel, there would be so much of me, there wouldn't be enough wall space."

"Image marking" is a potent method of helping group members appreciate their perceptual distortions through direct nonverbal evidence of body size and an awareness of split-off reviled body parts. An important task for the therapists is also to focus group members' attention on aspects of their bodies that they like, encouraging integration of what is liked and disliked and fostering awareness of their bodies as whole entities.

A second exercise incorporates videofeedback. This awareness-generating strategy was developed using a framework that would limit its potentially aversive qualities. Most of us become anxious at the prospect of being filmed or observed; for the person with an eating disorder, this anxiety is sharply increased. One strategy that has worked well has been to videotape a group session for feedback the following week. The goal is to provide direct feedback not only about physical size and shape but also to shed light on the cognitive distortions that limit the integration of the experience of the person as a whole. Before viewing the tape, we encourage the group members to talk about their apprehensions. Eliciting "worst fears" and reframing catastrophic thoughts usually helps to dispel discomfort once members realize most of their fears are shared with others in the group. Selected segments of the tape (approximately 10 minutes) are then shown.

Through experience we know that most group members will have strong urges to become transfixed on their own bodies while watching the tape and will tend to focus exclusively on their negative perceptions. In order to help the group widen its collective lens, we ask members to concentrate first on observing the group as a whole and to make notes on how they perceive the atmosphere of the group: is it tense, supportive, cohesive? Then we ask each group member to view the person sitting on her right and make notes of the verbal and nonverbal expressions and style of that person as she appears on the tape. Lastly, we ask each group member to view herself and note her positive qualities. The ensuing discussion usually reveals a dichotomous view of self and others. Group members find others acceptable, regardless of their size and shape, but see themselves as totally unacceptable. This is a powerful living group experience. The narrowness of self-evaluation is apparent, being exclusively linked with thinness, whereas evaluation of others extends to include the whole person. Having to focus on one's positive attributes forces an integration of other qualities such as tone of voice, physical gestures, and personality style that in turn helps to build a holistic sense of self. Group members almost always derive a sense of accomplishment at having "survived" videofeedback.

Understanding negative body image. The central process of understanding a negative body image involves questioning beliefs and attitudes that underscore an AN or BN patient's sense of self. This centers on the idea that feeling good about oneself is exclusively linked to being thin.

One strategy that is very useful for helping clients begin to make use of negative cognitions is an exercise designed by Hutchinson (1985) entitled "Body Talk." This is a guided imagery exercise in which group members are encouraged to bring to mind negative feelings and attributions they have toward their various body parts. They are then asked to write a letter to the body part(s) they most criticize. After this the group members are asked to turn the paper over and write a response from the body part addressed in the first letter. This request is usually greeted with looks of disbelief and resistance, but nevertheless is nearly always fulfilled by group members.

The material arising from the letters provides a wealth of information and brings into the group the reality of the abusiveness involved in adhering to the thin ideal. Negative affect and self-denigration are predominant themes of the group process. The content and style of the prose of the letters also illustrates the stage a group member has reached in her willingness to relinquish her fear of weight gain and reliance on the thin ideal. Readiness for psychological change is often signaled by the quality of the dialogue revealed in the letter.

The following transcripts are examples of "body talk" letters. The first was written by an anorexic woman in her second week of the program. She had been eating regular meals for the first time in a year.

> Dear stomach, hips, and thighs: This week I am less kind and less tolerant of you. Stomach, if you are hungry I don't intend to listen to you; hips, you feel less bony, something must be done. Thighs, you jiggle too much and I find you depressing. I have let all of you get out of control and now I feel bad, unhappy, and a failure. I'm giving in to the enemy.

Her response was:

> Dear A: What can we say. We know that we are a big disappointment to you. We have let you down. Betrayed you. We also feel like failures, not that that is any consolation. We guess we will all have to try harder.

This next transcript was written by a woman with BN in her eighth week of treatment:

> Dear Thighs: You'll be excited to know that last week I talked to my other archenemy (my stomach) about the ongoing hate relationship we have, and arrived at the awareness that "stomach" cringes in shame and fear whenever my attention becomes focused on her. As I got in tune with her and realized how horrid she feels when I so much as gaze at her, I shivered and cried (in fact sobbed) tears of shame and remorse. I vowed to try very hard to be kind to her, to tell her how wonderful it was that she had conceived two children in there and should be proud. Well, thighs, I can now much more readily befriend you and stop expecting you to look like a model. Maybe jiggly bumps can be okay.

This was the response:

> Dear Master: I almost feel like I've been adopted by another. You sound so gentle, warm, and forgiving. I lived and dreamed for this moment. I've felt so helpless. God made me this shape, cellulite and all, and you keep eating all the junk food and then scream at me for the extra jiggles. It would be lovely to be friends, maybe even stomach can be friends too.

The quality of these two dialogues illustrates differences in readiness for change. In the first letter, group member A indicates her desperate struggle with the physiological necessity of renourishment, which is extremely threatening to her. In her letter, her body parts only collude with the writer in her sense of failure and fight against weight gain. In contrast, the second letter is from someone who has already begun to question and change her values and is ready to accept her body, albeit on the shaky terms of "maybe jiggly bumps can be OK."

Acceptance of one's body. Acceptance of one's body is experienced in this treatment program mostly as fleeting moments of complex thoughts, feelings, and behaviors. Feelings of sadness and grief at the loss of so many years of self-abuse signals the beginnings of acceptance in some group members. A raised consciousness regarding the perniciousness of society's messages to women is important for others. Being able to look at oneself for a few minutes in the mirror, or losing the preoccupation with thoughts of body size, forms the basis of acceptance for others. The process of coming to terms with an altered view of one's body generally requires more time than the 3 months available in the day hospital.

A Private Practice Body Image Group

A weekly private practice group provides an opportunity for more advanced work on the resolution of body image distortion and dissatisfaction, taking up where the day hospital program ends. The group also supports normalized eating and maintenance of a realistic body weight for those whose eating behavior is under better control and no longer requires close monitoring. Typical comments from women applying for group membership include: "It's the thing I've been avoiding, but I think I'm ready for it now," "I can't stand my body now that I've gained weight," and "It's the icing on the cake—my eating is under control; now I want to feel better about my body."

The group is closed, for women only, and runs for 12 weeks, with each session lasting 2 hours. Group members are selected based on 1) not requiring monitoring of food intake or weight, 2) comfort and facility with a sample guided imagery exercise used in the assessment interview, and 3) not being actively suicidal, seriously depressed, or abusing drugs or alcohol. Women with a history of suicide attempts, major depression, or borderline traits are accepted only if they are concurrently in individual therapy. It is common for women to be referred by another mental health professional. Most women who have participated in the group have been between the ages of 20 and 40. The group is small, usually about five members, and run by a single therapist. Even though members have normalized basic eating patterns, entering the body image group is a difficult challenge. Very deliberate efforts need to be made in structuring the group, in developing cohesion and trust, and in making all expectations overt. It is a mistake to assume that, because a group member is highly motivated to maintain her normalized eating behaviors, she is not also highly anxious about the material to be confronted in the group.

It is useful to begin the group with a session in which ground rules regarding confidentiality, attendance, group participation, feedback to other group members, smoking, and fees payment are discussed. If the members are given suggested ground rules on paper, after which they can question, discuss, and alter the rules, they also get a sense of control over those rules. In particular, it has been found that a discussion of how to give feedback to other members helps generate a sense of safety in the group. Because the group is closed, group members cannot learn appropriate group conduct by watching more senior group members. An explicit discussion of whether advice, judgments, opinions, simple sharing, and questioning are appropriate forms of interaction brings out group members' fears about what might happen in the group and allows them to develop feedback guidelines that help them feel safe. The therapist provides input about what limitations or benefits might be expected with various guidelines. Knowing that a discussion will be held about 3 weeks later to revise ground rules, if necessary, allows members to see the rules they have set as experimental and to change them according to the results produced by using them.

Sessions are highly structured at the beginning of the series and become less so as the group progresses. Each session begins with a relaxation exercise and a "check-in" where each person has a few minutes to say how she did during the previous week. The first five to six sessions are centered around a topic that the therapist presents. Information is given and questions and discussion are invited. Topics include sociocultural pressure on women to be thin; set point theory and the effects of dieting; health risks and benefits of overweight; a nondieting approach to eating; and strategies for dealing with weight-prejudice in oneself, one's family, and the world. Because most members have already been exposed to the information presented, they are encouraged to discuss how they relate to it personally and how this may have changed since the first time they heard it. Members often comment that they began normalizing their eating as a final desperate attempt to avoid bingeing, but that they had fully expected to gain weight uncontrollably. Now they actually believe that the weight gain will stop and that they can begin to trust their bodies' indications of hunger and fullness.

The second part of each session is devoted to one of a series of exercises, including guided imagery, kinesthetic, tactile, and movement exercises. These draw largely from the book *Transforming Body Image* (Hutchinson 1985) and from *The Body Image Manual for Therapists* (Kearney-Cooke 1989). The exercises are sequenced to encourage participants to do the following:

♦ Refocus their attention on how they want to feel in their bodies rather than on how they want to look,
♦ Become aware of current feelings about and attitudes toward their bodies,

- ♦ Trace some of the history of these current feelings and attitudes,
- ♦ Explore letting go of negative feelings and attitudes,
- ♦ Try out more positive feelings and attitudes,
- ♦ Notice that "body image" is potentially under one's control, and
- ♦ Generate a positive attitude toward their bodies.

These exercises are followed by partner and/or group sharing and sometimes by drawing exercises.

The informational topics presented in the first part of the sessions are designed to promote acceptance of the idea of "natural" or "set point" weight range and rejection of dieting practices. At the same time, the imagery exercises work toward developing positive regard for current body size and shape. This sequenced structure as much as group interaction moves the group forward. Written summaries of the information presented is handed out, and a small library of relevant books, tapes, papers, and magazine articles is made available for home use. Homework around the group topics is given.

Compared with body image groups for women without a history of eating disorders, this type of group can present special challenges for the group leader. In groups whose members have not had eating disorders, it is more common for group members to spontaneously generate discussion and share personal feelings. In groups whose members have or have had eating disorders, the therapist must actively encourage discussion and sharing. For example, imagery arising from guided imagery exercises may be very painful or frightening, bringing to the surface past sexual or physical abuse. It is helpful to provide enough group structure that members are gently introduced to guarded material and feel safe about sharing at least some of it.

An early session in the series of 12 will focus on the sociocultural emphasis on thinness. The therapist gives a slide presentation including slides of advertisements directed at encouraging women to diet and exercise, and slides showing the fashion in women's size and shape. During the slide presentation, the therapist will cover the following points:

1. The enculturation process through which a female begins to see her body as the instrument through which she gets social status, power, and approval;
2. The pressure in developed countries on women to be thin, not just not fat;
3. The pressure on women to be nurturing relationship-oriented people, while at the same time successfully competing in the aggressive business environment; and
4. The identification in North American culture of thinness with control (MacKenzie 1985).

Critical evaluation of the sociocultural context is encouraged. Addressing sociocultural issues early in the group can be valuable in developing group cohesion, as these issues give members a common starting point and are easy to talk about. Thus, members get to know one another in a nonthreatening way. An additional benefit is related to the way each individual sees the sociocultural context. Individuals tend to minimize the role of such a context, focusing on themselves as not measuring up; or they have a well-developed intellectual understanding of these pressures without easing up the pressure on themselves to be thin. When the sociocultural context is introduced early, participants can be encouraged throughout the group to identify ways in which they have internalized the pressure to be thin.

Sometime after group members have become more comfortable with one another, a session is devoted to exploring the historical sources of individual body image distortion and dissatisfaction. The initial part of the session is used to introduce the concept of "automatic thoughts" or the "internal voice." Group members are encouraged to identify the typical critical messages they give themselves about themselves generally or about their bodies. In the second part of the session, an imagery exercise is used to elicit material relating to events or people who have affected the development of each member's own body image. For example, one member, whose inner voice admonished her for the repulsive fat on her body, realized that her father had stopped being physically demonstrative after she reached puberty. She was blaming her body for the inexplicable loss of his previously spontaneous hugs.

To prepare group members for the possibility that images relating to past sexual or physical abuse may arise, a didactic section has been designed to discuss a range of experiences that can make women uncomfortable with their bodies (Niva Piran, Ph.D., C.Psych., personal communication, September 1989). Nearly all women have experienced unwanted staring at or touching of their bodies. There is a continuum of such experiences ranging up to rape and incest. It is both helpful and accurate to place abuse on such a continuum, because women who have been abused need to know that this does not make them defective individuals, that the abuse was not their fault, and that such abuse is characteristic of a society in which women are oppressed. Properly contextualizing abuse is an important precondition to acceptance of their bodies. It is also important for members of the group who do not have a history of abuse to understand these principles so that an atmosphere of safety is maintained.

Physical abuse, early puberty, illness, surgery, embarrassment on first menstruation, and development of a homosexual orientation can also give rise to significant discomfort with the body. The therapist emphasizes that members will be at different stages in dealing with such personal history.

Group members are encouraged to connect their own histories to their feelings about their bodies, and emphasis is placed on dealing with these connections in the group. The nature of the group precludes dealing with sexual abuse or physical abuse in a more intense way.

It is not unusual for some group members to be struggling with issues related to sexual orientation. A woman who is beginning to accept that she is lesbian may find special difficulties toward liking her body. For example, one woman found that each time she began to have a close relationship with another woman, she had an urgent need to lose weight. She found that by losing weight she could control the fear she felt about what being lesbian might mean to her sense of self, to her relationships with family and friends, and to the culture at large.

One of the exercises that most graphically illustrates group process and, in particular, the difference between this type of group and a group comprised of women without eating disorders is a movement oriented exercise. A whole session is spent doing and discussing this exercise in the later, less structured weeks of the group. "Moving Attitudes," from the book *Transforming Body Image* (Hutchinson 1985), requires that group members walk around the room expressing different attitudes through their walk, including anger, shame, and pride, as well as different affirmations, including "I am a uniquely beautiful woman, inside and out, and I know it," "I like myself and feel easy in my body," and "I am open to life and to my world." In the body image groups where women do not have eating disorders, this exercise tends to be both illuminating and fun for group members. Group discussion following the exercise focuses on insights gained during various of the attitudes or confirmations. However, in groups composed of members who do have eating disorders, women tend to find it a very difficult exercise. They feel extremely self-conscious about displaying anything through their walking, especially anything related to sexuality. Group discussion focuses on the difficulties members have doing the exercise—on the barriers and fears they feel in trying to express pride, sexuality, or openness in a way that might be perceived by others. Group members are encouraged to discuss alternate ways of drawing personal boundaries than through a closed physical presentation. It can come as a surprise to some women that others draw these boundaries verbally. This exercise also brings out experientially the idea that how one feels in one's body is not dependent on how one's body looks. This can help group members extend their developing ability to invalidate the idea of appearance as the single measure of control, worth, and desirability.

Close to the end of the series of sessions, another exercise from *Transforming Body Image* is used. In "Imaginal Massage," group members imagine themselves being massaged first by a loved person (in a nonsexual way), then by their own hands. This has proved to be a most powerful exercise. One group member said after this exercise that she was shocked to realize that it was not her body she had hated all this time, but herself. Another said that she could allow someone else to massage her and feel good about it, but that she could not feel good accepting a loving touch from herself. She expressed great sadness about her inability to give to herself. At the same time, these group members expressed some relief at recognizing that their bodies were not the real problem. They could let go of the idea that changing their bodies would make them like themselves.

Summary

This chapter has described two programs designed to address body image disturbance. Disturbances in body image are conceptualized as a "pseudoproblem" resulting from sociocultural messages that influence women, and to a lesser extent men, to change their body shapes when in reality there is no reason to do so. The perniciousness of society's norms that at present equate a woman's acceptability and success to a thin body shape have led to a rapid increase in the incidence of women developing eating disorders as a way of attempting to conform to these social pressures.

The two programs are designed to address body image disturbance at different points on a treatment continuum. Body image therapy in a day hospital setting addresses the emergent awareness of clients' experiences of their bodies as they undergo nutritional stabilization. The outpatient body image therapy is conducted at the later maintenance stage in the nutritional rehabilitation process. It aims to deal with resolving longer term issues concerning full integration and acceptance of self and associated sexual or gender identity issues. Despite these differences, there are some common themes apparent in both groups. The group sessions are structured by specific exercises and anxiety reducing strategies, and the work proceeds slowly and sensitively. The therapist stimulates interaction in the group while providing safety and containment. Finally, both groups work to create a counterculture in which clients can begin to explore alternative ways of evaluating themselves, of giving and receiving support and, most important of all, of accepting their bodies.

References

Askevold F: Measuring body image. Psychother Psychosom 26:71–75, 1975

Bruch H: Perceptual and conceptual disturbances in anorexia nervosa. Psychosom Med 24:187–194, 1962

Bruch H: Eating Disorders: Obesity, Anorexia Nervosa, and the Person Within. New York, Basic Books, 1973

Butters JW, Cash TF: Cognitive-behavioral treatment of women's body-image dissatisfaction. J Consult Clin Psychol 55(6):889–897, 1987

Davis M, Eshelman ER, McKay M: The Relaxation and Stress Reduction Workbook. Oakland, CA, New Harbinger Publications, 1982

Fairburn CG: Cognitive-behavioral treatment for bulimia, in Handbook of Psychotherapy for Anorexia Nervosa and Bulimia. Edited by Garner DM, Garfinkel PE. New York, Guilford, 1985

Garner DM, Garfinkel PE: Body image in anorexia nervosa: measurement, theory and clinical implications. Int J Psychiatry Med 11(3):263–284, 1981

Hutchinson MG (nee Hoffman-Sankowsky): The effect of a treatment based on the use of guided imagery on the alteration of negative body-cathexis in women. Unpublished doctoral dissertation, Boston University School of Education, 1981

Hutchinson MG: Transforming Body Image. New York, Crossing Press, 1985

Kearney-Cooke A: Group treatment of sexual abuse among women with eating disorders. Women and Therapy 7(1):5–21, 1988

Kearney-Cooke A: Reclaiming the body: using guided imagery in the treatment of body image disturbances among bulimic women, in Experiential Therapies for Eating Disorders. Edited by Hornyak IM, Baker EK. New York, Guilford, 1989

MacKenzie M: The pursuit of slenderness and addiction to self-control: an anthropological interpretation of eating disorders. Nutrition Update 2:173–194, 1985

Rozin P, Fallon A: Body image, attitudes to weight and misperceptions of figure preferences of the opposite sex: a comparison of men and women in two generations. J Abnorm Psychol 97(3):342–345, 1988

Steiner-Adair C: The politics of prevention: weight preoccupation, weight prejudice, and eating disorders. Paper presented at the Public Forum, Nurturing the Hungry Self Conference, Toronto, Ontario, October 1989

Trower P, Kiely B: Videofeedback: help or hindrance? a review and analysis, in Using Video. Edited by Dorwick PW, Biggs SJ. London, John Wiley and Sons, 1983

Vandereycken W, Depreitere L, Probst M: Body-oriented therapy for anorexia nervosa patients. Am J Psychother 41(2):252–259, 1987

Wooley OW: Body dissatisfaction: studies using the color-a-person body image test. Unpublished manuscript, 1986 (Copy available from Dr. O. Wayne Wooley, Eating Disorders Clinic, Psychiatry Department, University of Cincinnati Medical School, M.L. #559, Cincinnati, Ohio 45267)

Wooley SC, Kearney-Cooke A: Intensive treatment of bulimia and body-image disturbance, in Handbook of Eating Disorders. Edited by Brownell KD, Foreyt JP. New York, Basic Books, 1986

Wooley SC, Wooley OW: Intensive outpatient and residential treatment for bulimia, in Handbook of Psychotherapy for Anorexia Nervosa and Bulimia. Edited by Garner DM, Garfinkel PE. New York, Guilford, 1985

9

Family Relations Groups

Lorie F. Shekter-Wolfson, M.S.W., C.S.W.
D. Blake Woodside, M.D., F.R.C.P.(C)
Jan Lackstrom, M.S.W., R.S.W.

♦ ♦ ♦ ♦ ♦ ♦ ♦ ♦

This chapter does not deal with family therapy per se. The groups described here expose the patients to ideas about family functioning that can be pursued further in actual family therapy or in other psychotherapy groups. The use of structured exercises makes the experience a powerful and arousing one. The authors stress the importance of the structure of the exercises and of leader responsibility in modulating the affect that is aroused. This work is going on at the same time as efforts to control the eating behavior itself are being undertaken. The Family Relations Group is in some sense a compromise solution to the need to introduce family-of-origin issues while at the same time not derailing the primary task of managing the eating behavior.—The Editors

Treatment of the patient with an eating disorder includes not only individual therapy but family and group therapy as well. Garfinkel and Garner (1982) suggest that the eating disorders, anorexia nervosa (AN) and bulimia nervosa (BN), are not only multidetermined in nature but also require a multidisciplinary approach in treatment. The literature indicates that there is greater therapeutic success with families of younger patients who have been ill for a shorter time than with older patients who have been ill longer (Russell et al. 1987). However, as the age of onset of eating disorders has increased over the past decade (Garfinkel and Garner 1982), attention has focused on creative ways of working with this older and very diverse population.

Many adult patients with eating disorders have not had recent contact with their families or are living away from home with very intermittent contact. Many patients remark that they initially did not see how "the family" could play an important role in their treatment. These same patients state following therapy that their families were indeed a major problem. Indeed, they had chosen to cut themselves off from their families as a way of dealing with the pain of problematic relationships. For some, these unresolved issues seem to get in the way of a full recovery. Although such patients may be able to behaviorally control their weight, the self-esteem issues that are so intrinsic to the treatment of eating disorders are often connected with their role within the family of origin. As a result, traditional family therapists have had to examine new ways of working with this population, dealing with issues that involve the patient's family without necessarily having the opportunity to engage in formal family therapy.

These concerns led to the development of a group focused on family relations to deal with family issues in the absence of family members. The objectives of the group include the following:

1. To help patients understand and begin to deal with family issues that might perpetuate the illness;
2. To help patients recognize that their feelings regarding their families are not "crazy" or "unique" (Weiner 1986);
3. To encourage patients to challenge others' beliefs about the perceptions of the family's involvement in the disorder; and
4. To help patients apply their learning from the group experience to concurrent family therapy sessions where applicable.

The literature on family groups has usually focused on understanding and treating the family as a group (Bell 1961, 1976; Dreikurs 1951) or the use of multiple family group therapies (Gritzer and Okun 1983; Strelnich 1977; Wooley and Lewis 1987). Our intention was to develop a group that helped patients deal systematically with issues that typically come up in family therapy. These include boundary diffusion, indirect communication styles, and methods of conflict resolution, as well as issues specific to eating disorders such as the family's involvement in the patient's eating patterns. The name "family relations" was given to emphasize the interpersonal aspects.

Group Structure and Composition

An initial decision was made to structure the process of the group around psychoeducational material and experiential exercises. This was based on the concern that because most of our patients reported problematic family relationships, an unstructured group would become caught up in endless "there-and-then" reminiscences without applying them to present circumstances. This could result in the patients feeling overwhelmed with past memories and guilty about having said hurtful things about their families. As the "family relations" group is only one component in a Day Hospital program for severely symptomatic patients, other therapeutic opportunities seemed more appropriate for dealing with such reactions.

The group focus is on normal family functioning, rather than on family dysfunction. This allows all members to participate whether they view their own family as normal or problematic. Attention is maintained on "here-and-now" issues that can be related to the primary goal of treatment—normalized eating. This focus on normality helps to concentrate the efforts of the group on proactive steps they can take to help themselves in each of their family situations.

Because the concepts of family functioning are not clearly understood by many people, it is essential to have methods to demonstrate these ideas. Psychoeducational handouts and experiential exercises are utilized to structure each session. The handouts serve both to focus the attention of the group on the specific topic and to provide a sense of organization and safety to topics that previously may have been experienced by the patients as confusing or dangerous. Experiential exercises provide a concrete forum for group members to experiment with strategies for changing their own behavior.

The group consists of patients with AN or BN attending an intensive Day Hospital. However, the group could be incorporated into any setting where group treatment is being used for these patients. This is true whether or not formal family therapy is offered. Some ideas about structuring the group differently for various treatment settings will be discussed later in the chapter.

Although the group is homogeneous in that the patients all have an eating disorder, family and socioeconomic backgrounds are quite diverse. Homogeneous groups are best for those persons who can accept and cooperate in treatment by viewing themselves as having problems in common with others and for whom identification provides the strongest medium for self-acceptance and for change (Weiner 1982). Homogeneity around the diagnosis of an eating disorder is quite helpful in the Day Hospital program generally. However, it has been less central in the family group because of the diversities and backgrounds and the differences in life cycle states. The following vignette illustrates this:

A married 56-year-old woman initially introduced her present nuclear family but did not discuss or mention her family of origin. Her mother was still alive and was sending care packages to the patient regularly and expected a phone call from her daughter every morning. Initially, the patient saw her family situation as very different from the younger patients and capitalized on her experience as a mother. However, as she progressed in the program, the younger patients indicated that it sounded like she was still struggling with some of the same parent-child issues that they were. As a result, the patient began to include her mother and sisters in the introduction of her family and in fact agreed to setting up family sessions with her mother as an adjunct to her treatment.

The inclusion of male patients in the group has not been a problem. In fact, these patients are helpful in diffusing some of the stereotypical ideas that patients with eating disorders have about gender influences on power relationships in their family.

The "family relations" group is open-ended. Whenever a new member is added, the session begins by having each member introduce herself and describe who is in the family. This family roster can be a useful marker of change in perception of the family situation. For example, one patient never included her sister who had died as a teenager until after it was clarified that her eating symptoms had begun shortly after the sister's death.

Structured Topic Areas

Sessions are organized around eight principal content areas, each with its own series of structured exercises (Table 9–1).

Topic 1: The Role of the Family

The goal of this session is to develop an appreciation that families function both to produce stability and to encourage growth and development. In addition, the session introduces the idea that families are governed by rules. Some of these rules are explicit and open (overt), whereas others are implicit and secret (covert). An exercise of family sculpting is used to demonstrate these issues.

The idea that families can be both stabilizing and growth inducing is often difficult for patients with eating disorders to accept. Some families believe that family structure must be very rigid, with stability at all costs and a tight control on the members. Others describe families where personal freedom is so highly valued that there is no parental guidance and the children become small adults not permitted to experience a normal developmental process. Still others come from families that have been struck by catastrophe, where the family's stability has been shattered by external forces and the children have been forced to assume adult or even parental roles at an early age. Some patients report an acceptable balance between stability and growth and can describe the experience of growing up in such a family and contrast it with the experience of other patients.

Discussions of this material leads naturally to a discussion of rules, whether through the experiences of patients from very stable (rigid rules) or very unstable (no rules) families. First, the group must understand the difference between the two types of rules and provide examples. The discussion quickly moves to a discovery of implicit rules, and it becomes evident that these rules are the ones that are causing the most trouble for the group members. With an adolescent group, explicit rules might also be troublesome.

After this general introductory discussion, the exercise of sculpting is

Table 9–1. Structure of family relations group

Topic	Major themes	Exercises
Role of family	◆ Stability and growth ◆ Implicit and explicit rules	Family sculpting
Family roles	◆ Traditional and idiosyncratic roles	Want Ads
Family life cycle	◆ Developmental stages of families ◆ Changes in relationships secondary to the life cycle	Strings
Communication styles	◆ Effective and ineffective communication styles	Role-playing of Satir's (1988) styles in a family
Disagreement and conflict resolution	◆ Normalizing disagreement ◆ Effective conflict resolution	None
Autonomy and separation	◆ Launching ◆ Strategies for developing more autonomy	None
Role of pets	◆ Function of pets in family	Pet photos
Role of food and appearance	◆ Family typologies	Role-play a meal

introduced. The exercise has a dual function: to demonstrate visually the concept of family structure, and to allow the group to experiment with "changing the rules" by changing the sculpture.

The exercise is conducted with one patient sculpting her family as described by Sherman and Fredman (1986). The patients who are participating as family members are encouraged to voice their feelings about the positions into which they have been placed, and to make suggestions about how they could be more comfortable. Common sculptures produced by our patients involve the patient sitting on the ground, or with one parent very close and protective and the other distant and detached.

Initially the position of family members is held static, and the outer group makes suggestions concerning changes the patient might make. This typically involves adopting a more commanding stance, such as moving from a sitting to standing position. Then we ask the sculptor (the patient) to suggest changes. These almost always involve attempts to move other family members. This is not permitted. By encouraging self-movement, we are emphasizing that the patient can only be in charge of her own actions, not those of others. However, after the patient has assumed a new position, the others are allowed to reposition themselves so as to feel more comfortable. This demonstrates how changes on the part of one family member may affect other family members. The session concludes with a brief discussion on the theme of the responsibility of the individual to clarify her own activities in the family.

Topic 2: Family Roles

This topic is completed in two sessions, with the exercise being prescribed as homework for the period between the two. The goal of this topic is to help the patients clarify their own role in the family, and to develop strategies for changing aspects of that role that they decide are not desirable.

The majority of the initial session is taken up with a discussion of traditional and idiosyncratic roles. Many patients experience difficulty in defining idiosyncratic roles, and considerable time is spent in clarifying the idea of "unspoken" or "covert" roles. Typical idiosyncratic roles identified by adult patients with eating disorders include: mediator, savior, black sheep, and scapegoat. Comparatively few patients identify the sick role as one they have adopted, although almost all will later include their illness in the exercise to follow.

At the conclusion of the first session, the process of changing inappropriate roles is discussed and an exercise prescribed. This involves composing a newspaper employment want ad to advertise for a replacement for the patient in her family. Patients who are married or in stable common-law relationships are asked to prepare two ads, one for their family of origin and one for their current family. The ads are then read at the next session. The typical response is a long, very detailed job description that quite completely describes the idiosyncratic roles of the patient in her family. The reading of these ads often starts out in a humorous vein, but the mood of the session quickly turns somber. It is not unusual for some patients to be unable to read what they have written or to read it in tears.

To avoid further regression, specific examples of parts of the roles that individuals would like to change are sought. The group is encouraged into a discussion of developing strategies to promote such change. A brief review of the process of the two sessions concludes the topic.

Topic 3: Family Life Cycle

This session focuses on the normal developmental stages of families and is well suited for a wide range of ages. Even in quite heterogeneous groups, members can fit their own experience into the stage they happen to be at presently. A choice was made not to focus directly on pathological family life cycles because of the difficulty many of our patients experience in their own life cycle. For most of our patients, the primary goal is to get "back on track" with life cycle issues.

This group starts off differently from many of our other topics in that there is only a very brief discussion. This is followed immediately by an exercise to visually demonstrate the stages of the life cycle. We use the "strings" exercise (Satir 1988). This exercise involves the use of pieces of string to represent relational patterns within families. The exercise starts off with two members of the group role-playing an engaged or newly married couple. Some time is spent allowing the pair to experiment with how they are going to manipulate the strings, and there is no interference with whatever method they choose to demonstrate closeness, distance, and so on. It is explained carefully that each individual controls only one end of the string representing her part of the relationship, and the other person controls the other end. The couple is then moved along in their life cycle by adding children (at least two), children's friends, boyfriends and girlfriends, marriage of children, the birth of grandchildren, and usually a sick grandparent coming to live with the couple. As each additional member is added, the growing group manipulates the strings in response to the change. A check is made regularly with each participant to see how things are different at each stage.

The number of strings in play rapidly grows, as does the complexity of the patterns. Not surprisingly, the effectiveness with which the initial couple were able to negotiate the strings of their relationship has a profound effect on the string patterns observed later on. For example, a common way for the patients to demonstrate "closeness" is to intricately braid the strings together, or attempt to loop them around the whole of the other person. When such awkward and intrusive methods are chosen, the introduction of new members into the family, even children, becomes difficult or impossible. In these cases, even quite uneventful family life cycles become overwhelmingly complex, as they degenerate into an incomprehensible mass of braided and twisted strings. Interestingly, it is common for one of the group members acting as an adult child in the family to choose a less enmeshed way of demonstrating closeness and produce a small subarea with less entanglement that can be used as a comparison. Because of the complexity of the exercise, major disruptions to the family life cycle such as deaths or marital breakdown are not introduced. However, patients participating in the exercise may spontaneously decide to pursue such a course. It is routine to introduce the sick parent of one of the original couple, who comes to live with them as their own children are growing older.

The exercise takes most of one session. As homework, group members are asked to consider where their families are in the life cycle. They are asked to consider whether this is appropriate, and what will need to change for their families to be able to "get back on track" if they are stuck. The following session comprises a discussion of this homework, which tends to center on a discussion of families having difficulty with launching adult children. In the discussion of strategies for change, it is emphasized that the group members are now entering a time in their lives when their own life cycle issues should become more prominent. Thus, an attempt is made to focus the discussion around strategies that will allow them to move ahead, rather than become stuck in fruitless and painful discussions of parental difficulties.

Topic 4: Communication Styles

This topic focuses on effective and ineffective patterns of communicating. Satir's (1988) archetypes of leveler, placater, blamer, computer, and distracter are used, to which we have added the concepts of directness and clarity. The session begins with an initial discussion regarding examples of direct/indirect and clear/masked communication, briefly examining which of the patterns work well and which do not. This might include ideas about how internal, personal fears and established family patterns perpetuate less effective styles.

The group members then role-play descriptions of Satir's archetypes of four ineffective styles. The first part of the exercise is left deliberately vague and is not attached to any particular person's family. Direct connections result in material that is too overwhelming for the patients. As homework, group members are asked to think about which styles their family members most commonly utilize. They are also asked to think about a particular situation they have encountered in their own family where they felt that they were not communicating.

In the second session, at least one group member's family is role-played, with the member directing the scenario. Suggestions are then solicited from the other group members as to how the group member who is role-playing the patient herself could communicate more effectively (i.e., generate a positive leveling response). It is critical to focus the comments on changes that the "patient" could make, rather than on changing the rest of the family. Once an appropriate leveling response is generated, the others in the role-playing are instructed to work as hard as they can to resume their originally assigned ineffective communication styles. The leveling response makes this more difficult, and the following discussion can focus not only on how much harder it was for the other members, but also on how much better the "patient" felt delivering the response, even if there was no change on the part of the other members.

As in the sculpting exercise, this communication exercise focuses the attention of the group on changes that they can make in their own patterns of relating to their families. It is vital to emphasize that although change in others' behavior may occur, this is not entirely predictable.

Topic 5: Disagreement and Conflict Resolution

This topic focuses on normalizing the existence of disagreement within families and demonstrates the many different methods that families use to resolve conflicts. This topic usually takes one session and does not contain an exercise.

The discussion is started by introducing the concept of disagreement as a normal part of family life and surveying the group as to how this has been viewed in their own families. Two major points of view generally emerge. For some, disagreement has never been an issue, as the patients report never having experienced any conflict. This first pattern of absence of disagreement is often the response to very real and threatening life events, such as death or prolonged illness. Occasional families may fit Selvini-Palazolli's (1974) description of a "facade of unity," hiding profound but unspoken parental marital unhappiness. The second major perspective is from the point of view of families where conflict has been more or less continuous. In both cases, group members are usually able to identify that the situation is a reflection of ineffective methods of resolving conflict. Members who feel their families have adequately dealt with conflict can use their experiences as a counterpoint to those of the rest of the group.

A stage method is presented for improving conflict resolution skills. The first stage is to recognize that a disagreement or conflict exists. The second is for the patient to decide what she wants to say about the situation. Then the patient must decide to whom it should be addressed, and how to approach it in an assertive manner. An unresolved current conflict in the life of one of the group members is used as a focus, using the discussion to generate ideas that may be of use to all of the group members. The targeted member is asked to report back to the group on how the ideas have affected her family conflict resolution.

Topic 6: Autonomy and Separation

This topic addresses issues that are particularly significant for a younger adult group and are often highly emotionally charged. One session is spent on this topic and there is no specific exercise. The initial part of the discussion is centered on autonomy, using decision making as the example. Examples of decisions that the group members feel have been more or less autonomous are elicited. The therapists are particularly alert to identify two extreme patterns: reactive, impulsive decision making, or decisions made in total isolation that are represented as autonomous.

An important part of the discussion is to review the issue of "age appropriate autonomy" within families. Many of our patients have family experiences where significant adverse life cycle events have caused parentification of children, leading to an illusion of autonomy at a very young age. These individuals tend to make decisions in a very enmeshed fashion, being highly vigilant of the needs of others in the family who are perceived to be fragile. Other families may have been perceived as very rigid, and not allowing for the development of appropriate autonomy.

These themes lead into the topic of launching, the life cycle stage of leaving one's original home and establishing an independent existence. This portion of the discussion is used to clarify what is meant by appropriate separation. Many of our patients can see only total isolation from their families as a route to separation. It is emphasized that achieving age-appropriate autonomy is a prerequisite for true launching.

The greatest affective response to this topic is derived from the discussion that relates to familial determinants of developing autonomy. This usually involves the recollection of painful memories of family interactions. Group members often become more aware of feelings of grief and sadness for lost opportunities in their own family, or of the inability of other family members to provide them with hoped-for nurturance and support. The latter is particularly true for those members who have experienced early and/or precipitous launches where there are often fantasies about a reunion with a magically transformed "perfect" family.

It is helpful to provide some structure to enable the group to feel a sense of mastery over the affect that is generated by these themes. The therapists may help to focus the later part of the group session on concrete suggestions for the development of more age-appropriate autonomous behavior. Typical suggestions include greater responsibility for financial or vocational matters.

Topic 7: Role of Pets

This topic was added to the list at the request of our patients. For many of them, pets are the only "people" available. This is especially true for those who have become very isolated due to the severity or chronicity of their illness. There is a small literature surrounding pets (Levenson 1972) suggesting beneficial therapeutic and life-enhancing effects of animal companionship. Although much of this literature has dealt with the special problems faced by the isolated and housebound elderly, many of our patients are in similar situations for different reasons.

Group members are asked to bring in a picture of their pet for the session. At the beginning of the session, each group member introduces her pet to the group in much the same way as we have previously asked them to introduce their family. Some group members are so isolated in their lives that they may not have even a pet. In such cases, they are asked to provide a description of some other object that has served the same function as a source of emotional support, such as a stuffed animal.

> A group member described abandoning her twin children to her husband 15 years previously as a consequence of feeling unable to care for them due to the severity of her illness. Once on her own, she purchased a group of three glass sculptures portraying an adult and two infant whales, which she placed on her mantel. It had never before occurred to her that these represented her lost family. One of the consequences of having had this identified was a strategy for re-contacting her children that she was eventually able to carry out.

Following the introduction of the pets, the discussion is focused on the purpose the pet has served for each member or for the families of the members. This has ranged from a replacement for a lost relationship, to facilitating either closeness or distance in relationships. For example, one patient introduced an entire family of stuffed animals that belonged to her and her fiance. She described a ritual they had developed whereby conflictual situations were resolved through role-playing with the stuffed animals. In another case, a married group member described purchasing a stuffed bear that slept between her and her husband; as she became more ill, and the couple postponed their plans for a family, the stuffed animal "married" and had "children" of its own.

Most of our patients enter this topic with considerable enthusiasm and lightheartedness. This almost inevitably changes early in the group as the members begin to talk about the experience of losing a pet and how they or their family have dealt with such losses. It is not uncommon for the members to be overwhelmed to the point of tears for much of the group session. This is especially true if there are numerous members who have not dealt with losses more generally. Another interesting observation is the eating habits of the pets vis-à-vis the eating habits of the patients. Patients may report either starving or overfeeding a pet depending on what they themselves weigh.

This topic is concluded by summarizing the purposes that pets have served for the group members. In particular, the issues that have been raised are related to general family issues, particularly those of distance, closeness, and loss.

Topic 8: Role of Food and Appearance

This is the only topic that deals directly with eating disorders. The topic is flexibly scheduled so that it can be done 2 to 3 weeks prior to major holidays where food will be an issue, such as Christmas, Easter, or Passover. The material is derived directly from the description given by Schwartz and colleagues (1985) of food and appearance related to three family typologies in BN.

1. In the "Americanized family," the emphasis is on appearance and achievement. Typically, the desired appearance is one of slim athleticism; fashionable and current mode of dress is also required.
2. By contrast, the "Ethnic family" emphasizes appearance much less, viewing loyalty to the family system as far more important. Although this loyalty may involve adhering to certain culturally-determined dress codes, it also involves accommodating a wide variety of cultural norms that may conflict with general North American norms. In such families, weight is rarely an issue; instead, an individual's worth will be partially determined by how much she eats. In such a family, food refusal or purging may be regarded as a significant rejection of the person who prepared or purchased the food.
3. The third type of family described is the "Mixed family," where one parent is from an Americanized family and the other from an Ethnic family. Children in such families may become caught between conflicting values around food and appearance, such as the mother feeling hurt if her children do not consume large portions of the food that she has prepared and the father insisting that the children maintain a slender shape.

The previous discussion serves to clarify some of the familial contributions to the patient's situation, not only from the perspective of predisposition but also in terms of perpetuating factors. This discussion often includes commentary about grandparents' views on weight, shape, and food. The impact of extended family members is frequently ignored in family assessments.

The session then moves on to more practical issues around coping with whichever holiday meal is about to occur. We ask patients to describe the family rituals around this meal, highlighting the aspects of the meal that they expect to be particularly difficult. Two main scenarios are usually described. The first involves well-meaning family members "pushing" food and encouraging the patient to eat more by subtle means such as controlling the serving of the food or, more blatantly, by loud public requests. The second common issue relates to family or relatives being hypervigilant, overly inquisitive, or insensitive in some way.

Each member's particular concerns are clarified by the end of the first session and planning begins for role-playing during a second session. One of the group is asked to volunteer their family, so that suggestions may be generated as to how the member could better cope with the situation. As in other exercises, the member volunteering directs the action with other group members playing the patient herself and her family members. The results of this role-playing are frequently dramatic. Overtly bizarre behaviors around eating are often directed into the exercise. The directing group member may be quite unaware of the unusual nature of the behavior.

> A patient role-played a scenario in which her mother was constantly on the move during the meal, getting up to serve others and bringing in new courses. Toward the end of the meal, one of the other members commented on the fact that the mother had eaten nothing, to which the directing patient replied that her mother never ate any of the food she prepared for such meals, but would sit down during dessert with a plate of leftovers from the previous day.

It is important to structure the role-playing so that some concrete suggestions can be made for the benefit of the group member. These suggestions must focus on strategies that involve change on the part of the group member—change that will make her feel more comfortable in the situation. In the example given above, the suggested change was for the patient to tell her mother that it made her uncomfortable when her mother did not eat with the rest of the family.

Evaluation of the Family Relations Group by Patients

The effectiveness of the Family Relations Group is not formally measured apart from the Day Hospital program as a whole. However, patients complete a program evaluation in which they rate each group in the program separately. These are reviewed regularly by the staff conducting each group. Comments are generally positive and reflect both the value and challenge presented by the topics: "Very interesting. I have a better understanding of how the family functions. This group upset me because it reminded me of how screwed up my family is and hit a sensitive spot!"; "Helped me identify issues that caused a lot of pain or confusion in the past and how to start small changes on my part;" "a difficult group but very helpful." Many comments are focused on specific issues that are salient to the individual—for example, autonomy and separation, pets, or communication styles. Other comments reflect the understanding patients appear to have developed concerning the interactional nature of the family system. For example, patients regularly comment on the value of the experiential components, such as strings, skits, and role-playing.

Critical or negative comments have included the opinion that the group is too intellectual. This may reflect the frustration individuals have experienced attempting to resolve family issues. Critical comments include the following: "I can see where it might be helpful, but I'm too confused right now about my family;" "I have had a lot of family therapy and I am tired of the topic;" or "Could have been more effective. Lots of big words in papers. Group interaction helpful."

It is the clinicians' opinion that the Family Relations Group has augmented the effectiveness of the family therapy component of the Day Hospital program. Patients use the information learned in the group to develop alternative understandings and beliefs about their family processes. These new belief systems often allow patients to take a new stance within their families, thus freeing themselves to develop new opportunities and relationships.

Group members also become supportive of the efforts for change within the family. Members willingly role-play conversations that an individual may wish to initiate within their family sessions. The group will provide guidance and support as their peers prepare for or react to family sessions. Peer pressure is exerted if members do not follow through on addressing issues. The group will not accept excuses for not inviting a family into therapy. The group also confronts blaming behavior. Peers are given an empathic ear only insofar as individuals do not avoid taking responsibility for their own actions. The group norm of being supportive in the face of difficult family dynamics and of being highly critical of those who blame their families or excuse themselves from responsibility or action provides an environment that makes family therapy a powerful and effective tool.

Summary

This chapter has described a unique method of addressing relevant family issues in a population where family involvement may not be possible. In our experience, the most important family issues among adult patients with eating disorders are those centering around autonomy and separation. These are issues that can, if necessary, be addressed by the individual herself. The use of a group format to address these issues has the advantage of harnessing peer pressure to address problems that may have been avoided for years. Adult patients often have moved away from home in an effort to "resolve" family issues, and the expense of arranging family meetings may be prohibitive. For older patients, important parental figures may be unavailable because of death or debilitating illness.

The limitations of this type of group relate to three factors. First, for younger adolescent patients where issues of identity formation and control are prominent, family therapy is more appropriate. Second, a subgroup of adult patients will have ongoing family conflict of such severity that some family therapy will be needed, if only to facilitate an appropriate disengagement. (In our own experience, this group totals less than 10% of our patients.) Finally, the Family Relations Group produces a degree of regression. There is some danger in integrating such a group into a less structured treatment setting. Family issues are potent generators of intense affects in these patients, especially in the early phases of treatment. In a setting with less control than a Day Hospital, therapists must carefully weigh the amount of highly charged, regressive affect they are willing to tolerate.

Experiential exercises mobilize considerable affect. Our exercises are used to demonstrate a nonpathologic family process, one step removed from the actual family experiences of the patients. Very specific assignments are made with the goal of obtaining greater mastery over a problematic family situation. We would caution against the use of such exercises without carefully determined goals. Keeping these cautions in mind, a family relations group can be a valuable adjunct to treatment programs for eating disorders.

References

Bell JE: Family Group Therapy Public Health Monograph, No. 64. Washington, DC, U.S. Government Printing Office, 1961

Bell JE: A theoretical framework for family group therapy, in Theory and Practice. Edited by Guerin PJ. New York, Gardner Press, 1976

Dreikurs R: Family group therapy in the Chicago Community Child Guidance Centre. Mental Hygiene 35:291–301, 1951

Garfinkel PE, Garner DM (eds): Anorexia Nervosa: A Multidimensional Perspective. New York, Brunner/Mazel, 1982

Gritzer PH, Okun HS: Multiple family group therapy: a model for all families, in Handbook of Family and Marital Therapy. New York, Plenum, 1983

Levenson B: Pets and Human Development. Springfield, IL, Charles C Thomas, 1972

Russell GFM, Szmukler GI, Dare C, et al: An evaluation of family therapy in anorexia nervosa and bulimia nervosa. Arch Gen Psychiatry 44:1047–1056, 1987

Satir V: The New Peoplemaking. Mountain View, CA, Science and Behavior Books, 1988

Schwartz RC, Barrett M, Saba G: Family therapy for bulimia, in Handbook of Psychotherapy for Anorexia Nervosa and Bulimia. Edited by Garner DM, Garfinkel PE. New York, Guilford, 1985

Selvini-Palazolli MP: Self-Starvation. London, Chaucer, 1974

Sherman R, Fredman N: Handbook of Structured Techniques in Marriage and Family Therapy. New York, Brunner/Mazel, 1986

Strelnich AH: Multiple family group therapy: a review of the literature. Family Process 16:307–325, 1977

Weiner MF: Identification in psychotherapy. Am J Psychother 36:109–116, 1982

Weiner MF: Homogeneous groups, in Psychiatry Update: American Psychiatric Association Annual Review, Vol 5. Edited by Frances AJ, Hales RE. Washington, DC, American Psychiatric Press, 1986

Wooley SC, Lewis KG: Multi-family therapy within an intensive treatment program for bulimia, in The Family Therapy Collections. Edited by Hansen JC, Harhaway JE. Rockville, MD, Aspen, 1987

10

Sexual Abuse Groups

Patricia J. Perry, R.N., M.Sc.N.

◆ ◆ ◆ ◆ ◆ ◆ ◆ ◆

Sexual abuse is so common in patients with eating disorders that it must be a central concern during the assessment process. It forms a subset of the general posttraumatic literature, with powerful gender-related social norm overtones. A first principle of treatment is directly retrieving and confronting memories of the events. Such memories may break through during the therapeutic process of treating eating disorders, and the therapist must be alert to their emergence so that a further experience of denial and repression is not triggered. Reactions to posttraumatic situations are often complexly determined. It is tempting for the therapist to become overly identified with the victim component and to lose a sense of neutrality toward the ambivalence often present regarding the perpetrator of the trauma. This may make it difficult to resolve the intensity of the intrusive memories.

Once the sexual abuse has been defused, it is not uncommon for further issues related to passivity or the role of victim to come to the fore—issues that have a significant impact on broader areas of interpersonal functioning. Often patients may be referred following or during an experience in a self-help group. Such programs offer an environment where the powerful topic of childhood sexual abuse can be raised. Not uncommonly, a professional approach has been unsuccessful in gaining access to the same material. There is some danger that the individual may become stuck in a persistent identity as a "survivor of . . . ," which may inhibit general psychological growth. The ideal would be a situation where there is a comfortable referral flow back and forth between self-help groups and professionally-led groups so that they can act in a complementary fashion.—The Editors

Experiences of sexual abuse appear to be widespread in the general population and are ruthlessly democratic, cutting across all social classes (Forward and Buck 1988). Formal research and informal interviews have identified an invisible population crying silently for acknowledgement, validation, and help. The first national U.S. survey of adults concerning a history of childhood sexual abuse found that 27% of women and 16% of men experienced victimization (Finkelhor et al. 1990). There is general agreement among clinicians who treat eating disorders that the frequency of sexual abuse in patients with eating disorders is significantly elevated. For example, Oppenheimer and colleagues (1985) found that approximately two-thirds of their sample had experienced adverse sexual events.

Sexual abuse can be envisioned as a "black hole," a zone of personal history actively avoided, frequently only dimly remembered, and certainly never actively explored. Individuals with eating disorders may go through a short- or even long-term treatment experience and never disclose that they have been abused. When the subject is tentatively disclosed, it may be minimized or normalized by either the patient or the therapist. For individuals who have eating disorders and were abused, group therapy can provide a safe environment for remembering, disclosing, and resolving issues related to sexual abuse.

Experiences of sexual abuse encompass sexual intercourse, sexual maltreatment, and sexual molestation, ranging from fondling to rape. Incest is defined as any sexually exploitive act or behavior that violates the special trust that exists between a child and a parent figure. Any sexual act that interferes with the child's rights, boundaries, and dignity should be considered abuse. Adults who were sexually traumatized as children have been termed psychological time bombs (Peters 1973), waiting to explode at any moment. Courtois (1988) has described how the aftereffects of sexual abuse intrude into many life spheres: social and vocational; psychological/emotional; physical; sexual; family; sense of self; relations with men; and relations with women. The ramifications of sexual abuse on personality development and general psychological functioning will influence the course and the treatment of individuals with eating disorders.

In this chapter, I discuss the impact of sexual abuse on individuals with eating disorders. The goals and the process of therapy are delineated, particularly as they pertain to the group modality. The chapter defines critical therapeutic issues that must be addressed when the sexual abuse comes to light. It describes clinical interventions to facilitate recovery and healing. Finally, it identifies special concerns and priorities that must be addressed if the abuse is to be dealt with in a group context.

Relationship of Sexual Abuse to Eating Disorders

The basis for the association between sexual abuse and eating disorders is not clear. There are several theoretical concepts relevant to the development of eating disorders that psychodynamically "fit" for sexual abuse. Traumatic sexualization (Finkelhor and Browne 1986) refers to a process of development whereby the child's attitudes, feelings, and sexuality are shaped by inappropriate sexual and interpersonal experiences. Being forced or enticed into sexual experiences that are too advanced for her developmental stage leaves the child feeling confused and frightened. She remains haunted by painful memories associated with sexual relations.

A sense of stigmatization and powerlessness is a long-term effect of childhood sexual exploitation. The child incorporates negative connotations associated with the abusive experience into her developing self-concept. The perpetrator insists on secrecy, coercing the child into maintaining silence while blaming and denigrating her. Powerlessness occurs when a child's sense of control and rights to privacy are violated against her wishes and her attempts to end the activity thwarted. As anxiety and fear mount, the sense of competence and mastery over self diminishes. This may result in depression and somatic complaints. The outcome of such experiences are pervasive feelings of guilt, shame, anger, fear, and shattered self-esteem. There may be a quality of personal humiliation and associated self-revulsion amounting to a sense of evilness.

As the child matures, suppression of these feelings serves to reinforce the sense of being different from peers and results in isolation. Early body image disturbance is one of the risk factors in the development of bulimia nervosa (Wooley and Kearney-Cooke 1986). A child with a history of negative body image approaches adolescence with insecurity and feelings of physical inadequacy. In the face of biological pressures to achieve an optimal body weight, bingeing and purging may emerge as a strategy for resolution of the tension over emerging evidence of sexuality. The bulimic woman has been described as the "missing woman," the facade behind which all affect is hidden and numbed by the binge-purge ritual. The bulimic episode can be understood as an attempt at purification from hateful and repulsive feelings associated with earlier sexual abuse. Drug and alcohol abuse, self-mutilation, or suicide may develop along with the eating disorder (Finkelhor and Browne 1986).

Crisp (1970) observed that the combination of a premature demand for sexual interest and an immature personality can precipitate anorexia nervosa. Bruch (1973) described anorexic individuals as having deficits in personality structure resulting in difficulty seeing themselves as self-directed and having an identity of their own. They feel confused about their bodily sensations and are disturbed by new sexual impulses that represent a challenge for which they are unprepared and that threaten the little control they have. Preoccupation with weight and rigid dieting may be understood as attempts at recouping the lost control. Basic ego deficits related to this sense of ineffectiveness are reflected in body image distortion and misperception of affective and visceral sensations. Selvini-Palazzoli (1974) describes this interoceptive mistrust as "intrapsychic paranoia," in which the anorexic patient not only mistrusts her body, but is afraid of it.

> I feel very confused and there are so many things I don't understand, so many contradictions. When I'm with Louis [first boyfriend], I feel calm and warm inside and safe. I like it when he holds my hand. I don't feel like no one sees me or knows I'm there. I don't feel invisible. But then I get scared. A light goes off in my head and this tells me the hurt is coming. I'm going to get trapped and I won't be able to get away. And I will get all dirty. I'm scared and I want to run away. But he hasn't hurt me. Louis makes me feel good, but so did my brother and he hurt me, he hurt me in so many ways that inside I still feel hurt and I'm still confused and I still don't understand. All I know is that I am terrified.

The Recovery Process of Sexual Abuse

The treatment literature is primarily descriptive and anecdotal. There is little empirical data on the treatment of sexual abuse, let alone the combination of sexual abuse and eating disorders. Most clinicians have developed their own strategies and techniques based on the treatment reports and theoretical proposals found in the clinical literature. Although these may not have been systematically evaluated to determine their effectiveness, they do fit a broader psychotherapeutic outcome literature that supports the effectiveness of most of the techniques utilized. As with any intervention model, the choice of treatment technique must be based on the specific needs of the individual, including personality structure, psychodynamic issues, and social/family context. The basic concepts of addressing posttraumatic stress reactions, of which sexual abuse is one example, can be applied in individual or group psychotherapy. Often a combination of individual and group therapy, either concurrently or sequentially, provides the most effective treatment.

There are some specific advantages to a group approach. Many of the clinical features found in sexual abuse victims are rooted in belief systems concerning what others will think. The code of secrecy is not just fear of punishment, but of shame about the behavior and fear of rejection if it is disclosed. The group setting offers a specific arena in which these faulty concepts can be tested. Seeing others talk of their experiences gives the new member permission to do the same. Other survivors look normal; the individual, perhaps for the first time, is therefore able to identify with others. The universalization experience involved in "breaking the silence" provides a powerful sense of support and hope (Leehan and Wilson 1985). This act of public disclosure triggers the possibility of reframing the self-blame and shame that is characteristic of the sexually abused person.

The environment of a cohesive group is a powerful catalyst for exploring the beliefs, rules, and messages that maintain powerlessness and helplessness. An active working group is able to empathically confront the denial, minimization, or distortion that perpetuates negative self-esteem. The individual is able to compare her own standards of self-judgment with how others see her and reduce the sense of stigmatization. Opportunities are provided for members to help each other develop trust and to practice new skills and behaviors.

All of these processes may go on in individual therapy, but the group accelerates the work and encourages rapid generalization. In conjunction with group therapy, individual therapy may allow initial disclosure of the trauma and safe expression of feelings and reactions to it. It also provides an opportunity for more detailed examination of the memories and their ramifications in present relationships. Individual therapy allows the establishment of a close relationship with a single valued person in a way that is somewhat different from the peer relationships developed in a group. Because sexual abuse often involves a parental figure, the opportunity for such an experience may have specific advantages.

If the abuse was chronic and repetitive, it is likely that longer term treatment will be required. Such experiences generally have a major impact on the personal development, character, and interpersonal style of the victim. Time is required to work with the strong defenses and to establish a therapeutic alliance. This is particularly true for those individuals who have survived by engaging in self-destructive behaviors such as substance abuse and suicide attempts. In the more severe case, it is anticipated that the therapeutic process will be erratic, with surprising breakthroughs alternating with periods of resistance.

Intake Assessment

The majority of individuals with eating disorders do not enter treatment with the express goal of disclosing or confronting the sexual abuse and its attendant symptoms. They are often unaware of the significance of the abuse and intend to withhold the memories of the experiences. They certainly may not be aware of any connection between earlier abuse and their eating disorder. Intake interviews for patients with eating disorders therefore must include questions about sexual abuse. By doing so, the groundwork is laid for openness in addressing the role of sexual abuse and its impact. It also gives the clinician an opportunity to inform and educate the individual that intrusive or vague symptoms such as crying spells, nightmares, flashbacks, trouble concentrating, or detachment and a sense of unreality might be related to the underlying trauma.

It is helpful for the assessment interviewer to use assumptive questioning such as: "Many individuals with eating disorders have had some experience with abuse, either emotional, physical, or even sexual, from parents, relatives, boyfriends, or strangers. What was your experience?" Some individuals will hesitatingly acknowledge the abusive experience; others directly admit to having been abused. Many will pause, visibly ponder the question, and say "I don't think so." The clinician must accept this response as a significant piece of information to be considered as therapy progresses. Those who do acknowledge the abusive experience need to know that specific problem areas will not likely improve until the underlying trauma issues are discussed.

Suitability for group psychotherapy is assessed to ensure that the patient is able to deal with group process and not be overly disruptive for the group. This will include the criteria and contraindications discussed in Chapters 2 and 5. Group members must possess a sufficient level of tolerance to deal with both the painful feelings that may surface and the intimacy of the group. Some individuals cannot discuss their own abuse experience without intense, uncontrollable anxiety or dissociative, depressive reactions. They may require individual therapy to begin this process. Group process is impeded when some members need constant monitoring and attention. For a patient in acute crisis, the group experience can be disorganizing and can exacerbate other destabilizing life events. Other contraindications to a process group involvement include acute suicidal tendencies, severe self-mutilation, life-threatening eating disorder, intense paranoia, an inability to control strong aggressive and impulsive tendencies, and alcohol or drug abuse. Because sexually abused women already feel isolated and different, there are advantages to forming the group with the maximum degree of homogeneity possible.

Critical Group Processes

Dealing with the central issue.   Memories of earlier sexual trauma often go underground for long periods of time, only to surface during periods of developmental stress or times of major psychological events. Disordered eating behavior may serve to stave off the painful memories of sexual abuse, providing a false sense of control (Goldfarb 1987). Within the group treatment process, the central issues that must be addressed with a sexually abused individual who has an eating disorder are both the reality and impact of the sexual abuse. The abuse was neither a fantasy nor a wish. As self-evident as this may seem, an integral part of the therapeutic process is to convey this belief to these patients: to validate their experience and not blame them. Individuals who think and feel they were abused but don't seem to have any memories most often were abused and should be approached with this assumption until proven otherwise.

The therapeutic process requires the reworking of the traumatic experience itself and integration of the self through the development of a therapeutic alliance with the therapist and group. The abuse must be addressed directly along with its original and compounded effects and symptoms. Models of traumatic stress, feminist theory, and family systems provide the theoretical framework for this work. Some members may divulge the abuse in the early stage of the group development. This must be accepted and acknowledged, although it is unlikely that the material can be dealt with in depth until the group is well engaged.

Memories are often accompanied by physical symptoms of sweating, trembling, and extreme anxiety. Panic attacks are not uncommon. Nightmares or flashbacks may herald the emergence of new memories. Visions that were vague and intangible take on a clear, distinct quality. Reliving and reexperiencing is raw terror: the re-creation of the scene of a child being abused and in its terror keeping the abuse secret. By reliving these scenes, the patient is gradually able to develop an adult perspective on these experiences and thus to become desensitized to them.

The therapist plays an instrumental role in helping the individual to recall the abuse and maintaining a safe and controlled atmosphere to provide the anchor for restoring accurate meanings and feelings attached to the experience. The healing process begins when the rage, despair, pain, and grief can be expressed and experienced. Dismantling the defenses that break the silence results in gradual learning of new skills. The goal of treatment at this time is to repeatedly validate her reality through being able to talk about the abuse and its effect on her. Herman and van der Kolk (1987) underscore the centrality of the validation of the victim's experience and stress that "the integration of trauma is a precondition for defensive organization; the validation of the trauma is a precondition for restoration of an integrated self-identity and the capacity for appropriate relations with others" (p. 119).

I'm feeling obsessed with abuse. That's all I think about. I think about him and I want to scratch his eyes out. I used to want to scratch my eyes out. Now I want to kill him. I think everybody can tell I've been talking about it. I feel like it's written on my forehead, "I've been abused." But it's getting different. I don't know how, it still hurts and I still have memories, but it's getting different.

Denial, repression, and minimalization have allowed the individual to survive the abuse. At the same time, these reactions serve to make her feelings inaccessible except when they break through in flashbacks and nightmares. Emotions have been sealed off, and an attempt is made to operate strictly on a rational basis. Therapy challenges this split and helps the individual to recognize and label these feelings. As therapy progresses, she can better articulate her emotions and use them for understanding and self-determination (Courtois 1988). Breaking the old patterns of silence and secrecy challenges the conditions under which the abuse took place. Acknowledgment and acceptance counters the denial and facilitates working through the emotional repercussions for each member of the group. Recounting the experience by one member elicits reactions and expanded reworking of their own experience by other members. Sharing their secret among the group members may free up the individual to go on to disclose the abusive experience to significant others. Members will often role-play these disclosures in the group and anticipate possible reactions and counterreactions.

Dealing with the perpetrator. The rage directed at the perpetrator is a necessary phase of recovery, a rage shared by the group as a whole. At the same time, there is usually a need to make sense of why it happened. Analyzing the perpetrator's distorted reasons is important for the individual because so much time over the years has been spent trying to understand the events. Working through this issue is central because the perpetrator's ideas have often been core ideas internalized and applied to the self. The consequences of sexual abuse are further compounded if it occurred within a family under the guise or in the context of love and affection. In these circumstances, the victim may hold a powerful mixture of both loving and rageful feelings toward the perpetrator and experience considerable self-doubt because of the ambivalence (Courtois 1988).

It is helpful for the therapist to discuss with the group some general facts regarding perpetrators. Someone who sexually abuses has often been abused, though that does not mean that everyone who has been abused will be an abuser. Perpetrators rarely are conscience stricken about the event. Indeed, they are usually incredulous about why such a big deal is being made out of it. Often they express sorrow when they are caught and made to face the consequences of the behavior. When they do express remorse, it is typically only in terms of themselves. The perpetrator views the victim as merely an object, allowing the victim's feelings to be unaddressed—thus minimizing the impact of the event itself. As the individual moves through the healing process, she will have less interest in understanding the event and may develop a rationale for the behavior of the perpetrator that does not involve her personal responsibility.

The healing process. Just as each individual has uniquely experienced the abusive trauma, so therapy must be tailored to respond to the specific needs of the individual. The process of therapy encourages expression of repressed memories and remembrance of internalized shame and guilt.

Expressing and sharing feelings of loss in the group process is an essential component to healing. In order to grieve for past opportunities and missed pleasures, it is necessary for group members to relive their childhood experiences. Acknowledgment that the sexual abuse has stolen innocence, trust, and capacity for joy and spontaneity is important. Grieving brings to the surface feelings of sadness, depression, and anger. Group therapy provides an occasion to grieve with the support of caring people and of the adult self. Often the survivor can acknowledge and accept her own losses only after she has identified and empathized with the losses suffered by others.

Anger is a natural response to abuse. It is pervasive in the group atmosphere right from the start of therapy. Feelings of rage are accompanied by feelings of loss and sorrow. The acceptance by the group of the anger is a positive healing force. Anger must be kept directed accurately and appropriately at the abuser. Shifting the accountability and responsibility helps the survivor understand her powerlessness in a compromised situation. It serves to heighten the potential for self-empathy and self-esteem. For some abused individuals, violence has been an enduring part of their lives, but the anger has been expressed in disguised forms of self-destructive and self-abusive behaviors. The process of beginning to address the anger directly can result in a breakthrough of explosive rage and intense anxiety.

> I was reading and my mind started racing. I felt panicky and then I had a flashback. I was on the floor on my back and he was rubbing his penis in my face and pressing it in my mouth. I felt trapped and angry. I felt like I was going to burst. I wanted to scream and kick him and beat him. I get so panicky, I have to stay put. I want to cut or burn myself. God, I hate myself when I think like that. I don't know why I'm so split, part of me is so out of control. It feels like the walls are closing in and I want to run, but I have to stay here. It will pass.

Learning the difference between the emotion of anger and the expression of angry violence may be difficult for the abused person. It is helpful to learn to identify the cues to anger. The group can assist by accepting and legitimizing the anger and developing ways to discharge it in constructive, safe, and nonharmful ways. Ground rules regarding the acting out of anger in the group must be clear. Physical action or hurting oneself is not allowed. The therapist must be prepared to intervene if it appears that anger will escalate to the point of physical interaction between members.

A group member may experience intrusive symptoms to such a degree that a time-out period is required. Time-outs are basic tools for controlling violence. They provide structure that allows the individual to break abusive patterns. Ground rules concerning this issue are required to prepare members and create a sense of safety in dealing with such matters. The individual should be instructed to tell the group of her reaction and communicate directly. She should take responsibility for her feelings and assure the group she is committed to avoiding violence. She should not leave the vicinity of the group. She can choose to be alone or be accompanied by a group member. When she is more settled, she should rejoin the group. Time-outs and emotions should be fully discussed in the group for both closure and reassurance. Members can share similar experiences and suggest coping strategies.

Panic attacks.   Group therapy is a good place to get in touch with deeply buried feelings that are extremely frightening. This process may result in the development of panic attacks as hidden material comes to the surface. These may appear during group sessions or outside, particularly when a group member is not occupied with a specific task (e.g., before sleep). Part of a panic reaction is the feeling that something catastrophic is about to happen. This reinforces the level of anxiety. The group can help to contain a panic reaction from spiraling out of control. A group atmosphere of patience, support, encouragement, and empathy assists the desperate individual to regain control. It also facilitates the more withdrawn and scared members to interact. Simple relaxation exercises can be taught that will help members control panic reactions if they occur outside the group.

Forgiveness.   The issue of forgiveness inevitably arises during the group process. Forgiveness implies that the patient ceases to feel resentment and no longer seeks revenge or compensation from the abuser. Developing compassion or forgiveness for the abuser or for the family members who did not protect or support the abused individual is not a required part of therapy (Bass and Davis 1988). It is wrong to suggest that the survivor must forgive the person who abused her; it minimizes and denies the validity of the patient's feelings. The process of forgiving can short-circuit the healing process. It is essential to encourage the survivors to forgive themselves for having been caught in a vulnerable situation and for being unable to protect themselves from the sexual abuse. This allows them to direct their compassion and understanding to themselves so that they can heal.

Trying to get something from the abuser can be a trap to successful recovery. This might take the form of seeking financial compensation or a statement of guilt, apology, or respect. The survivor must focus concern on herself, her current life, and her future—not on changing the perpetrator.

Tasks of the Therapist

The group therapist must have a working knowledge of traumatic stress and sexual abuse. Effective group leadership demands that the leaders be knowledgeable of how the dynamics of abuse and family dynamics affect the group process. It is particularly important that the group leaders not re-create the childhood scenario through ignorance or by playing the role of an uninvolved or passive authority figure. This places the responsibility on the survivor for the caretaking role. A major goal of therapy is the identification and modification of this very role. The therapist must be an active, knowledgeable leader, struggling to understand the complexities of the abusive experience (Kearney-Cooke 1988). Stability of group membership, regular attendance, and individual reliability are important to the development of group cohesion and trust.

The issue of confidentiality is of special importance in group therapy. The issues of secrecy, shame, and trust are of very high significance for each group member. Clear, mutual understanding of the bounds of confidentiality to ensure privacy and comfort are mandatory for trust to develop. The subject of extra-group socializing must be addressed by the group and a policy regarding contact outside the group decided on by the group as a whole. The group policy must be sensitive to the needs of all the members. Members are asked not to discuss other members or group issues on the outside. They are asked to be open about contacts. Group members are encouraged to negotiate their needs and to share whatever amount of contact feels comfortable.

The group therapist who works with individuals who have been sexually abused must actively convey openness and acceptance. A position of passivity will be perceived as being judgmental and unavailable—often a recapitulation of the family picture. Unresponsiveness duplicates the dynamics of the past, inhibiting self-disclosure and exploration. The therapist needs to convey respect and understanding and the belief that what happened was not the member's fault. The therapist who tries to be the authority and control the therapeutic environment re-creates abuse dynamics. The basic group therapeutic stance should be one of openness and sharing. Intimacy and closeness are suspect for the abused individual. Thus, the reality of the relationship in the here and now must be stressed. Armstrong (1989) has suggested that, through the process of experiencing empathic understanding from the therapist, "the survivor may eventually introject the experiences as her own damaged self is repaired and develop the capacity to self-soothe, allowing her to view her own past with compassion" (p. 556).

Throughout the course of treatment, information about sexual abuse and the stress response syndrome should be continually offered by the therapist and discussion of it encouraged. The therapist may have to correct previous misinformation. This educative component helps the patient to restructure her understanding of the past and validates the nature of the patient's emotional reactions. Similarly, it is helpful to discuss the course of recovery. This might emphasize the fact that the process will be upsetting and painful before things get better.

Dealing with abusive experiences requires tremendous energy from the therapist and group members. First experiences of remembering and flashbacks are overwhelming and emotionally draining. This is the time for the therapist to encourage group members to "simplify" their lives by eliminating anything that is not "essential" and not adding extra pressure or responsibility to daily living. Time is needed for these individuals to dwell on the therapeutic issues. Discouraging major life decisions stabilizes confusion about the changes group members feel they should make at this time.

Patients often feel that they should be coping better, a holdover of an attitude that their emotional reactions need to be suppressed.

Keeping a daily journal can be useful. This creates a reality to the abuse and assists in breaking the silence. It provides an intermediate environment that is safe enough to face the pain so that healing can begin. Many clinicians treating sexual abuse think that writing, reading, and talking are the crucial steps in beginning to heal.

> I took your suggestion and did some writing. I don't know if it makes any sense to you but I would like you to read it. It helps to write. It didn't solve any of the confusion but it organized it. Now my head doesn't feel so crowded this morning.

Because of the intensity of the group process and the great demands the emotional content places on the therapist, much of the literature on abuse suggests that groups have coleaders. Cotherapy provides mutual support and shared observation and processing of group interaction patterns and issues. It can decrease the intensity of the transference, particularly the idealization of the therapist. Most abuse survivors perceive female leaders as being safer, more trustworthy, and more understanding of the victimization issues. Female group therapists can provide group members with positive role models of strong, competent, and responsive women.

It has been suggested that a female therapist might be more effective if she herself had a history of sexual abuse. Unquestionably, the therapist must be able to work objectively without her own issues constantly getting in the way. Her past provides a powerful aid to understanding; however, she needs to be able to separate it from client issues. Survivors may feel that a "nonabused therapist" could not possibly understand or empathize. Sometimes this therapist is idealized as having a "normal" life or as having greater insight and fewer problems. Over time, however, these issues of abuse versus nonabuse lessen. It is useful for them to be openly discussed in the group.

Ten Rules for the Therapy of Sexually Abused Women

These rules need to be repeatedly reinforced in the group process.

1. If an individual thinks she was abused and her life shows the symptoms, then she was abused.
2. Healing is possible; recovery is never as painful as the abusive experience.
3. One hundred percent of the responsibility for the abusive experience lies with the perpetrator. It was not her fault; she did not want it, cause it, enjoy it, or bring it on herself.
4. The individual has the right to consistent support and encouragement to face the terrifying emotions and memories.
5. The pace of the therapy is set by the individual.
6. Trust is the basis of the relationship; the individual is believed unconditionally.
7. The therapeutic hour is a safe place; the individual will never be taken advantage of.
8. The individual experiences a wide range of strong emotions; she has the right to feel them and the responsibility to allow herself to express them.
9. The survivor does not have to forgive the perpetrator in order to recover.
10. Being compassionate and self-forgiving is essential for resolution.

Summary

This chapter has focused on the management of the sexually abused woman. The general principles can be integrated into the group management of patients with eating disorders. Although the issues may not apply to all members, it is likely that a sizable number will find the material of benefit. The thrust toward taking responsibility for self and mastering intrusive ideas about the perpetrator is a good general process of autonomy building. Thus, it nicely complements similar themes relating to eating behaviors. Common issues of damaged self-esteem are usually found. The therapist dealing with individuals with eating disorders must be familiar with this sexual abuse literature in order to comprehensively respond to the needs of group members.

References

Armstrong MW: Therapy of incest survivors: abuse or support? Child Abuse Negl 13:549–562, 1989

Bass E, Davis L: Courage to Heal: A Guide for Women Survivors of Child Sexual Abuse. New York, Harper & Row, 1988

Bruch H: Eating Disorders: Obesity, Anorexia Nervosa, and the Person Within. New York, Basic Books, 1973

Courtois CA: Healing the Incest Wound: Adult Survivors in Therapy. New York, WW Norton, 1988

Crisp A: Reported birth weights and growth rates in a group of patients with anorexia nervosa (weight phobia). J Psychosom Res 14:23–50, 1970

Finkelhor D, Browne A: Initial and long term effects: a conceptual framework, in A Source Book on Child Sexual Abuse. Edited by Finkelhor D. Beverly Hills, CA, Sage, 1986

Finkelhor D, Hotaling G, Lewis IA, et al: Sexual abuse in a national survey of adult men and women: prevalence, characteristics, and risk factors. Child Abuse Negl 14(1):19–28, 1990

Forward S, Buck C: Betrayal of Innocence: Incest and Its Devastation. Markham, Ontario, Penguin, 1988

Goldfarb L: Sexual abuse antecedent to anorexia nervosa, bulimia, and compulsive overeating: three case reports. International Journal of Eating Disorders 6(5):675–680, 1987

Herman F, van der Kolk BA: Traumatic antecedents of borderline personality disorder, in Psychological Trauma. Edited by van der Kolk BS. Washington, DC, American Psychiatric Press, 1987

Kearney-Cooke A: Group treatment of sexual abuse among women with eating disorders. Women in Therapy 7(1):5–20, 1988

Leehan J, Wilson L: Grown-up Abused Children. Springfield, IL, Charles C Thomas, 1985

Oppenheimer R, Howells K, Palmer RL, et al: Adverse sexual experience in childhood and clinical eating disorders: a preliminary description. J Psychiatr Res 19:357–361, 1985

Peters JJ: Child rape: defusing a psychological time bomb. Hospital Physician 9:46–49, 1973

Selvini-Palazzoli MP: Self-Starvation. London, Chaucer, 1974

Wooley SC, Kearney-Cooke A: Intensive treatment of bulimia and body-image disturbance, in Handbook of Eating Disorders. Edited by Brownell KD, Foreyt JP. New York, Basic Books, 1986

11

Adolescent Group Treatment

Fern J. Cramer-Azima, Ph.D.

♦ ♦ ♦ ♦ ♦ ♦ ♦ ♦

The treatment of adolescents with eating disorders must be modified to take into account the powerful developmental issues that coincide with the eating symptoms. These include the very strong effects of peer pressure on self-esteem and the connection between these and the vulnerability to developing an eating disorder. The author concludes that groups should be formed on the basis of homogeneity for age, not for the eating disorder, including treating those under age 15 separately from those in later adolescence. A peer group approach offers an opportunity for greater definition of the emerging adult self. With adolescents, a careful assessment of the impact of family dynamics on the eating symptoms is mandatory. Often—perhaps usually—the group approach will need to be augmented with family therapy either simultaneously or sequentially.—The Editors

I t is curious that there are relatively few articles dealing specifically with group psychotherapy for adolescents suffering from eating disorders, especially when one considers that this is the developmental stage of onset for anorexia nervosa (AN) and bulimia nervosa (BN). An overview of the literature reveals that adolescents have often been part of the population under investigation but not isolated for special study. Group techniques for their treatment include psychoeducation (Connors et al. 1984), cognitive/behavioral (Schneider and Agras 1985), family (Minuchin et al. 1978), and adjunctive treatments combined with psychosocial, nutritional, and pharmacotherapies. Stuber and Strober (1987) have reported on the positive adjunctive use of group psychotherapy for bulimic adolescent females, analyzing the clinical results over the initial, middle, and termination phases of the 6-month treatment. In an 8-month cotherapy treatment of girls and young women ranging from ages 13 to 21, Inbody and Ellis-Jones (1985) reported a lowering of depression and improvement in self-confidence and improved self-image. These authors attempted to correlate the specific conflicts of the patients to appropriate psychotherapeutic interventions.

The inpatient treatment of patients with eating disorders usually involves a multimodal model with some integration of group therapy. Piran and colleagues (1989) have reported on a day hospital program that utilizes a combination of several groups in the areas of nutrition, socialization, recreation, family, and psychotherapy.

General Treatment Considerations

Homogeneous and Heterogeneous Groups

Patients with eating disorders are treated primarily in homogeneous groups, either with AN or BN patients. Patients who are bulimic seem to be most prevalently treated in group. This may be because anorexic patients are particularly intransigent and difficult to sway from their rigid controls. However, comparative data are not available to contrast differential treatment outcomes for these two different subgroups. In inpatient settings designed specifically for patients with eating disorders, common eating symptoms and behavior patterns may provide an initial bonding link between patients with BN and those with AN. Differences between the two subgroups may lead to difficulty in effectively managing them in the same group as more advanced psychotherapy is undertaken.

In most psychiatric inpatient or outpatient facilities, there are insufficient numbers of patients with adolescent eating disorders to form a separate group, and they are most often included in existing groups. In some ways, this can be advantageous. The therapist without special expertise in treating eating disorders may be less likely to initially focus on the eating disorder. Instead, the focus will be on the conflicts that contribute to the symptoms in every group member. Additionally, the substrate of orality, body image, and gender identity can be addressed to everyone in the group. The presence of both sexes increases interpersonal learning and coping strategies in this highly conflictual area.

Short- Versus Long-Term Groups

Short-term modalities of 6 or 8 months or 1 year are increasingly being advocated. For acute hospitalized adolescent patients, intensive daily groups are indicated to focus on the eating disorder. Long-term groups

(Cramer-Azima 1989) are advisable for adolescents with significant pathology and concomitant motivation that warrants in-depth treatment for 2 or 3 years. Adolescents 16 and over who are motivated and self-reflective are capable of pursuing long-term goals. Roth and Ross (1988) similarly have advocated long-term cognitive interpersonal groups for adults.

Often the psychotherapists, both in individual and group format, utilize an eclectic integrated approach combining psychodynamic, behavioral, cognitive, and educational techniques (Steiger 1989). An important question that needs to be addressed is whether the group psychotherapist should be the one to deal with eating habits, diet, and nutrition within the group. Many teenagers may rebel against what they consider to be a parental intrusion and control over their eating. Stuber and Strober (1987) have also called attention to this factor. Where possible, it would seem advisable to separate out the idea of the eating behavior instructor or teacher from the role of the psychotherapist.

Sequential and Combined Therapies

Conjoint or sequential individual, group, and family therapies are often indicated where the eating disorder is acute, especially with the younger adolescent. After a brief hospitalization, continuance in a longer term outpatient or day hospital program is likely to maximize better treatment outcome for these patients. Older adolescents dealing with issues of individuation and separation often are highly ambivalent about family involvement. The latter may be necessary where the life of the patient is endangered because of the degree of self-starvation. An innovative group for parents of adolescents with AN or BN has been suggested by Eliot (1990). In this group, two of the additional cotherapists are parents of an adolescent with an eating disorder.

Group Psychotherapy Principles for Adolescents

Evaluation of group psychotherapy for adolescents (Cramer-Azima 1989) strongly suggests that the greatest benefit is derived from an active leadership style combining empathic confrontation with gradual interpretation of defenses. Most clinicians working with adolescents utilize a combined developmental interactive model and stress that the process of the group over time is a major therapeutic factor.

The group modality is especially advantageous for adolescents because of their specific need for relationships with their peers. Reciprocal exchange of thoughts and feelings permits a level of self-disclosure in the group that is often not possible in dyadic therapies, where rebellious silences pervade the transference to parental authority figures. In the group, the adolescents place special importance on what their peers deem acceptable. Learning that their problems, including the eating disorder, are not unique promotes faster sharing of information with less resistance and denial. Adolescents will frequently find it shameful and embarrassing to acknowledge their aberrant eating behaviors and underlying psychological conflicts, perhaps for the first time. As this process unfolds, it becomes increasingly clear that the problems facing them as adolescents and young adults are linked to their eating disorders. This includes their ambivalent and rebellious attitudes toward parents and their concern with body image, sexuality, and dependency.

The group context provides a safe, supportive, and empathic setting where the boundaries and rules are defined by the therapist(s). The gradually growing trust, loyalties, and support allow the formation of a group climate that facilitates self-disclosure and problem solving. The essential value of the group for adolescents is the meaningful interchange of their innermost thoughts and feelings and the reflection of their own self-worth by the acceptance by their peers.

Most group therapists working with adolescents are active in their leadership and utilize a developmental framework accentuating psychoanalytically-oriented and cognitive-behavioral approaches emphasizing here-and-now interactions. There is frequently a variety of blends and integrations of theory as well as technique. The interactional psychodynamic framework is readily combined with elements of the cognitive framework.

As in all therapies, the essential ingredient is the analysis of content and process that over time allows the unfolding and reactivation of past memories in the present ongoing group context. The group affords an increased expression of thoughts and feelings that allows each member to be understood from many more points of view than could be hypothesized by a single therapist. Additionally, these projections open a window into the speaker's own pathology. The allies and dissidents deviate in their perceptions and responses, as if the group were a system of revolving mirrors, reflecting intrapsychic and interpersonal coordinates for every member. These differing responses to a particular speaker promote both the working-through process and provide a corrective monitoring system for the group therapist.

There are several important features of multiperson therapy. It provides a social context in which the rebuilding of more accurate interpersonal relationships can occur. The development of an "esprit de corps" motivates and energizes the loyalty and cohesion of the membership. The development of a group composition that permits better functioning members to interact therapeutically with ego-weak and more conflicted members is helpful. The mediation between dominant and submissive, independent and dependent roles assists in clarifying relationship issues (Cramer-Azima, in press).

The psychotherapist working with adolescents with eating disorders must facilitate the formation of a meaningful, trusting relationship combined with the task of identifying and undoing long-held emotional disorders supporting the gorging and/or fasting rituals. Elsewhere (Cramer-Azima 1989) I have proposed that central to the therapeutic working-through is the correct blend, timing, and sequencing of the therapeutic triad of confrontation, empathy, and interpretation. Confrontation accentuates the verbal enunciation of thoughts and feelings, whereas empathy involves the experiential process incorporating the other person's feelings and thought. Each member displays a stronger or weaker confronting or empathic communication style. Some members are in need of more active confrontation; others benefit from a longer period of support and silent understanding. Interpretation takes place at a point in the therapeutic process after sufficient empathic confrontation and clarification have allowed unmasking of defenses and recognition of underlying unconscious conflicts, and it occurs in synchrony with the individual and the group process.

Psychodynamic Correlates of Adolescents With Eating Disorders

Group therapists dealing with adolescents must be aware of the specific subset of dynamics that are associated with BN and AN in order to tailor the accuracy and timing of their interventions. At the same time, it is clear that the group process and the interactional dynamics provide self-disclosure and problem sharing with peers that is not available in dyadic or family therapies.

A vast literature has accumulated in the field of eating disorders. This chapter will focus on the group and psychosocial characteristics of the adolescent. Yates's overview (1989, 1990) of the historical course, psychology, biology, treatment, and research reveals the complexity and lack of agreement in many areas of understanding or treatment of these disorders. An integrated biological, psychological, and psychosocial model is once again recommended.

Clinicians appear to choose the theory and technical intervention from their academic repertoire that are compatible with their own personalities. The best of all worlds would be the choice of an experienced group therapist well versed in an understanding of the eating disorders. To put it bluntly, a specialist in eating disorders is not necessarily a trained group therapist, nor is the latter often sufficiently knowledgeable about the biology and psychology of the eating disorders. Some of the reported inferior results may be due to these difficulties. Such problems are particularly likely when students or residents are assigned to run such groups without proper preparation for the complexity of the task.

It is important to remember that if a patient begins to decompensate, pharmacotherapy and/or hospitalization are to be considered. Frequently, patients may need pharmacotherapeutic intervention to render them amenable to psychotherapeutic approaches.

Psychodynamic Issues

Contributions from the fields of psychoanalysis, cognitive therapy and behavior therapy, and family and general systems have each broadened and helped our understanding of these disorders. Bruch (1973), Beck (1979), Crisp (1980), Fairburn (1985), Garfinkel and Garner (1982), Minuchin and colleagues (1978), and Selvini-Palazzoli (1974) are a selected few of the pioneers in this area.

Because of the nature of eating disorders and the adolescent developmental stage, theoretical perspectives dealing with deficits in interpersonal relationships and the development of the self are particularly relevant. These include object relations (Winnicott 1958), attachment-separation (Bowlby 1969), and self psychology (Kohut 1977). Why some emotionally disturbed teenagers develop the symptoms of AN or BN while others do not seems to be related to a complex combination of genetic, metabolic, and constitutional deficits, as well as familial and environmental factors. The histories of many adolescents with eating disorders show an overly ambivalent or symbiotic attachment to mothers, with marked difficulty in separation. Mahler and colleagues (1975) have referred to this as the "rapprochement" phase, and Winnicott (1958) uses the term "transitional" phase. The concept of the group itself as a transitional object (Levin 1982) may provide an understanding of how group therapy can promote a shift in object attachment concerning both past and present relationships. Frequently, patients refer to these "internal objects" that they can feel and have to get rid of or avoid in order to manipulate their body image and weight. The fear of giving up on developmental challenges and becoming a sexual person, and in the future a parent, is terrifying to these teenagers.

A review of the existing classification of the subtypes of eating disorders and their diagnoses and defense mechanisms is of importance in deciding upon the specificity and planning of the psychotherapeutic intervention (Steiger 1989). The restricting subtype disorders of AN are linked to early enmeshed, overprotective, and overinvolved parenting. Defenses include introjection, denial, and withdrawal. There is a predominance of avoidance strategies, including food and people. Associated diagnoses include obsessive-compulsive disorder and schizoid personality. By contrast, the symptoms of the bulimic subtype of AN appear to result from parental neglect and enforcement of too early separation. These children need to maintain some connection with the neglecting parent and try to become high attainers with images of perfection—to hide, as it were, the possibility of anybody detecting their early neglect and loneliness. Personality disorders and borderline pathology are frequent among patients in the bingeing group, and psychotic intervals may occur. Defenses for patients with the bulimic subtype of AN, in contrast to the introjective style of patients with the restricting subtype, rely more on externalizing defenses of projection. A third group of patients, and possibly the most difficult to treat, combines the restricting and bingeing subtypes, often with an alternation of symptoms and diagnoses.

Inbody and Ellis (1985) have listed the following unique cluster of dynamics of the patient with an eating disorder: distortion of body image, fear of weight gain, perfectionism, encouragement of risk-taking, fear of emerging sexuality, isolation and alienation, magical thinking, double-bind conflicts, mistrust of males, and rigid sexual stereotypes. In addition to these conflictual areas, therapy is made even more difficult when combined with stubborn resistance to change, severe cognitive distortions, and counterdependency. It is interesting that, with the exception of compulsive preoccupation with eating and weight loss, most adolescents seen in psychotherapy groups show many or all of these problems. Preoccupation with body image and slimness are prevalent among teens in general, especially in North American culture (Chernin 1985).

Younger adolescents (13 to 15 years of age) function better in homogeneous short-term groups with a task oriented, cognitive behavioral framework that is psychoeducational, stressing coping strategies. For older adolescents (16 to 19 years of age), a framework that combines psychodynamic and cognitive approaches is indicated. Short-term modalities stress problem solving in the here and now and setting of future goals, and deal less with the past. Emphasis is on ego support, not uncovering or interpretation. The aim is restructuring the belief system, expression of feelings, modifying aberrant eating patterns, and improving coping skills.

The longer term, more intense modalities are indicated for the more severe pathologies, often with accompanying diagnoses of obsessive-compulsive, depressive, and borderline features. In some units, the nutritional disorder is handled separately, and in others the group therapist combines the active symptom management with the psychotherapy. The danger of the latter is the encouragement of resistances and dependency on the "parental" rules.

The goals of the longer term group favor the psychodynamic framework and the working-through of basic issues of attachment-separation, body image, management of interpersonal control, gender identity, and promotion of autonomy. The generalized goals are the comprehension of the relationship between intrapsychic and interpersonal conflicts, and the ability to analyze the early clues that lead to a reoccurrence of the emotional problems and eating symptoms. Symptom alleviation is not identified as equivalent to treatment termination—an important factor to be shared with the group.

Therapeutic Alliance

In the initial selection of the adolescents for an intensive group psychotherapy, there should be a careful assessment of their ability to self-reflect, analyze their present predicament, and describe their eating disorder. Motivation and frustration tolerance are important predictors of the type of therapeutic alliance they can form in the group process.

The concept of the therapeutic alliance (Cramer-Azima 1973, 1989; Glatzer 1978; Greenson 1965) refers to the construction of a positive collaborative, realistic endeavor that must be established between the patient and the therapist. In group therapy, this also develops between the patients themselves as they genuinely search for solutions of their emotional disorders, and in this context, their eating problems. With adolescents, the therapist must adopt a genuine, outgoing, active working relationship punctuated with empathic warmth and a sense of humor. The eating disorder must be adequately confronted, with attention to proper timing, and not avoided. It must be made explicit to the patients that a working alliance is necessary to describe and explore all the facets of their problems and symptoms. If the therapist colludes from the beginning in an attempt to deny or evade the real purpose of the therapy, the patients will receive a message to delay their own self-expression. Each time a confrontation is made by the therapist or another group member, the patient's own awareness is heightened and its impact is felt by the entire group in a vicarious resonance.

In the selection stage, expectations regarding self-reflection and the importance of speaking about inner thoughts and feelings should be reinforced by the therapist. Then and later in the group, the therapist models how to listen, relate empathically, and self-reflect, and mirrors back to the group what has been seen, heard, and comprehended from the verbal and nonverbal communications.

The therapeutic alliance is elaborated at greater depth in the ongoing group process by statements made by the therapist, such as the following: "Our therapeutic goal is to say what we feel and think, to gradually admit more of our thoughts that are presently unclear, and to search for clarification of our hidden internal worlds. Working together, we will mutually explore, clarify, and understand the nature of our problems as we search for better solutions." Enlisting the membership to become active copartners in this contract strengthens the motivation and purpose of the therapy.

The Alliance With the Symptom

As a general principle, my approach is to build a firm, cooperative, trusting relationship—to confront the nature of the problems, but not to delve into the symptoms. The therapist becomes an understanding ally of the symptom and shows a readiness to accept it, befriend it, contain it, with no immediate goal to change. The word symptom is clarified to mean not just physical aspects such as anorexia, purging, headaches, or stomach pain, but also psychological repetitive ideas, acting out, defiance, and so on. Similarly, in the cases of drug taking, phobias, or psychosomatic symptoms, the therapist does not disqualify their existence. Rather, the strategy is one of empathic acceptance and confrontation, with clarification that the distorted behavior is a reflection of underlying problems, through remarks such as "I am sure that there is no immediate solution to your eating problems, and until you have a more meaningful rewarding life, it is not likely you will be able to surrender this habit."

The therapist's early alliance with the symptom—and in a heterogeneous group there may be a wide array of symptoms—demonstrates empathic acceptance of the deviant patterns, for the present, and enforces a nonjudgmental tone. "In a way both defense and underlying conflict are confronted in a supportive tolerant way that does not threaten the individual or the group with the expected ridicule and chastisement. The stage is then set for collaborative interpretive working-through, which if successful leads to the surrender of entrenched defective personality patterns" (Cramer-Azima 1989, p. 14).

The development of the working alliance and the acceptance of the symptom addresses all group members and stresses the commonality of emotional pain. As the group process gains momentum, the recapitulation of the developmental steps of the adolescent also takes place. The acceptance of the symptom promotes for the most part an easier way for all members to talk of their symptoms, defenses, and gradually the details of their actual eating practices. The horror of many of these rituals are best understood by the peers themselves.

Case Illustrations

Case 1

Jane was an obese 16-year-old who showed a history of BN and borderline features. In the first 3 months of the group she was almost totally silent, did not remove her coat, and kept her books on her lap most of the time. Occasionally she made eye contact with the therapist, usually at a point in the dialogue when she became disturbed. Following the example of the therapist, the group members greeted her each session but did not ask her questions. One day the therapy room was warmer than usual, and either because of this or because she was becoming more relaxed, Jane took off her coat, spilling her books and parcels all over the floor. She became startled and fearful, grabbed her coat, and folded it over her lap. Someone remarked that it was really very hot in the room and the therapist asked if she were getting ready to open up and talk. The patient burst into tears and said "Well you see I have made a mess; what a slob, I've vomited over everything." Louise tenderly said: "No, you only spilled your books, but I know how you feel. You keep everything inside until you think you will burst, but maybe it is time you tell us about yourself because you are our mystery lady."

Jane over time revealed her hoarding of food and her bingeing rituals in the dark of night. She pretended to her parents that she had to get to school at 8 A.M. each day, and this meant she had to leave home at 6:30 A.M. Her routine was to walk through a nearby cemetery and find a tombstone behind which she would vomit up her night's bingeing intake. She then felt a sense of peace and quiet, and slowly would make her way to school.

Jane was a very intelligent adolescent whose depression lowered her concentration in school. In the group she often said "What will I vomit up today?" She told us of her love of animals and that she had a menagerie of 5 cats, most of whom she found in the cemetery. They were her only friends. She had no rapport with her parents, who were constantly quarreling. Her father was alcoholic and she hid from his violence. As the group therapy progressed, confrontation was gradually upgraded to help her divulge the "pockets of pain." She kept all types of food in the pockets of the many garments that she wore.

Gradually Jane normalized her eating, gave up bingeing, and began to lose weight. Her school grades increased dramatically, and she gained a lot of praise from her teachers and her therapy group. Toward the end of the first year, Jane told us that she wanted to move into a group home, because, she said, "I will never get better at home." She visited the social worker and by the end of the summer she had left her home, on the best terms she could manage. In the following year she began to make plans to go to nursing school, saying that she wanted to look after people better than she had been. She was able to speak of her neglect as a child, her sense of abandonment, and how she was forced to create a fantasy world with the food and cats she collected.

Today Jane is a competent nurse. She has regulated her eating and to date, 4 years later, she is symptom-free.

Case 2

There are few male anorexic patients reported in the literature. For this reason, this short case report has been chosen.

John was a very thin 16-year-old with obsessive-compulsive disorder who did not readily admit his eating problem. Rather, he chose to say that he liked to sleep in the mornings and would therefore miss his breakfast, and had no time to eat lunch. He was a resident of a group home, being placed by his mother at age 2. He told the group that he was in a foster family and called the mental health professionals his mother and father. He spoke quite freely of his loneliness, his inability to make friends, and his difficulties studying. This group was held in a room with a one-way screen, as it was part of a research project, and John would continually look at himself in the mirror, pat his hair, and smile. His pattern in the group was to give helpful advice to others and only start to talk about his difficulties in the last 5 minutes. As one member remarked: "You don't give us much to chew on."

Gradually the compulsive nature of his eating and personality disorder began to unfold. He did not let anybody touch things in his room, and he was fastidious in cleaning. He often would not wear his own clothes, and borrowed or stole from others in the foster home. He was extremely conscious of his body image and fluctuated between voyeurism and exhibitionist self-display. He wanted to remain small, young, and dependent, and never have to leave his newly found "parents."

The progression in this case was very uneven and marred by reality conflicts that each time submerged him into regression, panic, and fasting. Feeling helpless that he could not live on his own, he contacted his biological mother. She sent him a card but did not actually phone or come to see him. He plunged into apathy and lost weight. During the group summer break, he was seen individually, reentered the group in the fall, but showed little motivation to continue.

The approach with John has involved networking with social services and the school that is continuing. The fragility of the early mother/child bond suggests a very difficult prognosis. The outcome for John has been only fair, but this is the reality of the treatment of eating disorders associated with severe pathology.

Summary

The predominance of reports on the eating disorders are focused on AN and BN, with little written on the psychological treatment of patients who are obese or who are finicky eaters. Identification of aberrant eating patterns in childhood may lead to earlier detection and treatment, which may give more rewarding results (Jaffe and Singer 1989). Questions as to selection, composition, and matching with different types of group treatments are also in need of further research. The use of therapeutic alliance and interpersonal measures would offer an important way to evaluate and predict differential outcomes regarding both psychological issues and eating disorder diagnoses.

Currently, the combination of cognitive and psychodynamic themes seems most suitable for adolescents, who need changes in deviant eating attitudes and behaviors as well as a deeper exploration of the underlying conflicts maintaining these disorders. In most instances, the active physical symptom management is better separated from the group psychotherapy and (if possible) should proceed it. Follow-up groups after hospital discharge are particularly recommended, for relapse occurs quickly if treatment is terminated at the point of symptom alleviation without attending to related family and personal issues.

Regardless of the theoretical model of group treatment, development of an adequate therapeutic alliance appears essential. It is always hard to lift the defensive veils and recognize the major underlying issues. Although general dynamics have been detailed for the eating disorders, each case has its unique history. The rigidity, denial, and manipulation in these cases "eats into" the resilience of the group therapist. The language of devouring, vomiting, starving, and biting are constantly felt by the therapist. These pressures may provoke a countertransferential response. In some cases, it may be of greater value to place one or two patients with eating disorders in a heterogeneous group where more of the members have normal eating patterns.

The complexity and intransigence of many of these disorders suggest a networking of services shared by a team of specialists in the areas of nutrition, physiology, recreation, and individual, family, and group therapies at different stages of the treatment continuum. Peer group therapy for adolescents appears to offer considerable value in the treatment of eating disorders, for it provides the psychosocial context, par excellence, for the rebuilding of self-esteem and interpersonal competence.

References

Beck AT, Rush AJ, Shaw BF, et al: Cognitive Therapy of Depression. New York, Guilford, 1979

Bowlby J: Attachment and Loss, Vol 1. New York, Basic Books, 1969

Bruch H: Eating Disorders: Obesity, Anorexia Nervosa and the Person Within. New York, Basic Books, 1973

Chernin K: The Hungry Self: Women, Eating and Identity. New York, Harper & Row, 1985

Connors ME, Johnson CL, Stuckey MK: Treatment of bulimia with brief psychoeducational group therapy. Am J Psychiatry 141:1512–1516, 1984

Cramer-Azima FJ: Transference-countertransference issues in adolescent group psychotherapy, in Group Psychotherapy for the Adolescent. Edited by Brandes NS, Gardner ML. New York, Jason Aronson, 1973

Cramer-Azima FJ: Confrontation, empathy and interpretation, in Adolescent Group Psychotherapy (AGPA Monograph No 4). Edited by Cramer-Azima FJ, Richmond LH. Madison, CT, International Universities Press, 1989

Cramer-Azima FJ: Group psychotherapy for children and adolescents, in Child and Adolescent Psychiatry: A Comprehensive Textbook. Edited by Lewis M. Baltimore, MD, Williams & Wilkins, 1991

Crisp AH: Anorexia Nervosa: Let Me Be Me. New York, Grune & Stratton, 1980

Eliot AD: Group coleadership: A new role for parents of adolescents with anorexia and bulimia nervosa. Int J Group Psychother 40:339–351, 1990

Fairburn CG: Cognitive-behavioral treatment for bulimia, in Handbook of Psychotherapy for Anorexia Nervosa and Bulimia. Edited by Garner D, Garfinkel P. New York, Guilford, 1985

Garfinkel PE, Garner DM (eds): Anorexia Nervosa: A Multidimensional Perspective. New York, Brunner/Mazel, 1982

Glatzer HT: The working alliance in psychoanalytic group psychotherapy. Int J Group Psychother 28:147–161, 1978

Greenson RR: The working alliance and the transference neurosis. Psychoanal Q 34:155–181, 1965

Inbody DR, Ellis-Jones J: Group therapy with anorexic and bulimic patients: implications for therapeutic intervention. Am J Psychother 39:411–420, 1985

Jaffe A, Singer LT: Atypical eating disorders in young children. International Journal of Eating Disorders 8:575–582, 1989

Kohut H: The Restoration of Self. New York, International Universities Press, 1977

Levin S: The adolescent group as transitional object. Int J Group Psychother 32:217–222, 1982

Mahler G, Pines F, Bergman A: The Psychological Birth of the Human Infant. New York, Basic Books, 1975

Minuchin S, Rosman BR, Baker L: Psychosomatic Families: Anorexia Nervosa in Context. Cambridge, MA, Harvard University Press, 1978

Piran N, Kaplan A, Kerr A, et al: A day hospital program for anorexia nervosa and bulimia. Int J Eating Disorders 8:511–521, 1989

Roth DM, Ross DR: Long-term cognitive interpersonal group therapy for eating disorders. Int J Group Psychother 38:491–510, 1988

Schneider JA, Agras WS: A cognitive-behavioral group treatment of bulimia. Br J Psychiatry 146:66–69, 1985

Selvini-Palazzoli MP: Self-Starvation. London, Chaucer, 1974

Steiger H: An integrated psychotherapy for eating-disorder patients. Am J Psychother 43:229–237, 1989

Stuber M, Strober M: Group therapy in the treatment of adolescents with bulimia: some preliminary observations. International Journal of Eating Disorders 6:125–131, 1987

Winnicott DW: Transitional objects and transitional phenomena, in Collected Papers. London, Tavistock Press, 1958

Yates A: Current perspectives on the eating disorders: history, psychological and biological aspects. J Am Acad Child Adolesc Psychiatry 28:813–828, 1989

Yates A: Current perspectives on the eating disorders, II: treatment outcome and research directions. J Am Acad Child Adolesc Psychiatry 29:1–9, 1990

12

Support and Self-Help Groups

Carla Rice, B.A.
Joan Faulkner, M.S.W.

♦ ♦ ♦ ♦ ♦ ♦ ♦ ♦ ♦

This chapter describes a professionally led support group for patients with eating disorders. It exists in the context of a network of services and has strong connections with specialized backup resources, including regular supervision for the therapists. This allows the support group to avoid some of the liabilities of such programs. For example, in less integrated programs, patients may get into medical difficulty with their disorder and not have access to appropriate treatment, perhaps being actively discouraged from seeking it. Without experienced leadership, it is possible for a contagion effect to develop between the members regarding pathological eating practices. The support group provides a powerful validating ethos that helps the individual to contain and address the symptoms. The authors carefully point out the complementary nature of the support group to formal treatment approaches. They manage the group so as to maintain the positive supportive environment that in many cases serves as a sustaining resource for patients engaged in more intrusive therapy programs.—The Editors

Self-help groups and support groups have become increasingly popular for addressing a variety of problems including eating disorders. It has been suggested that this might be in response to a shortage of knowledgeable professionals as well as the prohibitive cost of more traditional forms of treatment (Enright et al. 1985). This chapter will address some of the questions that have been raised by clinicians regarding the role and function of self-help and support groups for patients with eating disorders. What are the philosophical differences and similarities between self-help and support approaches? How effective are these groups? Are their treatment philosophies and strategies free of harmful effects?

Our discussion in this chapter has grown out of a literature review, debates with individuals from varied theoretical perspectives, clinical experience, and, most importantly, from the feedback of individuals attending the groups. Our purpose is to explore the philosophies underlying various types of support and self-help groups, address theoretical and practical problems inherent in each, and develop an alternative model for interpreting the role and function of support groups in the treatment of eating disorders. Moreover, because little attention has been paid to concrete clinical issues in the literature, we believe it is important to address practical considerations for planning and running support groups. Although we have attempted to place eating disorder support groups in a theoretical context, we are also concerned with providing practical information for clinicians, the kind of information we would have greatly appreciated when planning our first group.

Self-Help Versus
the Support Group Experience

The self-help and support group movement in North America originated from the belief that individuals who have struggled with a particular issue are experts in their own experience and because of this can provide valuable support, information, and insight to others faced with similar problems. Such groups grew out of the therapy movement as an alternative to medical approaches to treatment. Many were also predicated on the notion that sharing and support can empower individuals to change their life circumstances. Although the self-help/support group movement may have evolved in response to a lack of professional knowledge and frustration with traditional treatment approaches, larger systemic problems such as rapid social change may have contributed to the breakdown of traditional social networks and created the need for new systems of support (Silverman 1978).

Gartner and Riessman (1982) have identified fundamental factors distinguishing self-help and support groups from other therapeutic interventions. They argue that both types of groups can create a unique environment wherein participants sharing a common focus or problem can work for social and personal change through mutual support. Thus, these groups may have similar underlying goals and objectives that involve self-improvement through sharing and peer support.

Self-help and support groups have many similarities and commonalities that differentiate them from more traditional therapy groups. However, they also differ from each other. Self-help groups are usually leaderless; facilitation is shared, and each participant is considered an equal member in the group. Support groups, on the other hand, have at least one identified leader or facilitator, often with professional training. It is the leader's role to facilitate the sharing between members, to identify commonalities in experience, and to protect the safety and continuity of the group (Enright et al. 1985). The leader is not considered a full participant and is expected to use self-disclosure only when it is in the interest of group members.

There is some dissension in the literature regarding the effectiveness and appropriateness of the self-help group's philosophy and structure. Enright and Tootell (1986) have argued that eating disorder self-help groups can be potentially destructive to participants because of a lack of knowledge on the part of lay individuals of the physiological and psychological issues that may interfere with a person's ability to effectively use the group. Alternatively, Rubel (1984) suggests that self-help groups having an affiliation with a professional can provide a valuable first step in the process of resolving weight and shape issues, particularly for individuals unwilling to commit themselves to psychotherapy. Similarly, Larocca (1983) has argued that self-help groups can provide a fundamental component of an eclectic program by offering a support system that engages the individual in addressing change.

Anecdotal evidence from our experience suggests that self-help groups are less stable and may be less effective than support groups for individuals with eating disorders. Evidence from university-based peer educator programs suggests that peers can provide a vital link in treatment between individuals with weight/shape concerns and professionals. Peer counselors are successful in diminishing shame and guilt by being able to empathize with their clients' lifestyle and needs. This may be particularly true in regard to minority groups (Sesan 1989).

We have observed a number of self-help groups start up and fold within relatively short periods of time. Key members assume leadership positions, become overwhelmed by the needs of others, take on helper roles, cease to be helped themselves, and finally experience burnout. We believe these problems could be resolved with increased professional support for such groups as well as more opportunity for training and supervision of peer leaders.

Support groups avoid many of the problems with which self-help groups struggle and, for this reason, can play an important role in the treatment of eating disorders. The presence of professionally trained leaders provides continuity, consistency, and stability of the group. Leaders are able to guide group discussion, prevent conflicts from developing among group members, and intervene in the case of a crisis. Professional involvement helps to ensure that emotionally needy members do not dominate group discussion and that all members have an opportunity to disclose and have their needs met. Trained leaders can provide members with information about treatment resources and advocate on behalf of clients needing more intensive treatment. There is probably a role for both self-help and support programs in the treatment of eating disorders. The type of group best suited to a particular community or population will depend on local resources and the needs of the participants.

Support As Therapy

Most of the literature addressing the role of support groups in the treatment of eating disorders emphasizes the support group as an adjunct to therapy (Enright and Tootell 1986; Enright et al. 1985). Although we do not question the necessity of using standard therapeutic interventions such as nutritional counseling and psychotherapy in treating eating disorders, we do have some concerns regarding the conceptualization of the support group only as an adjunct rather than as a potentially powerful therapeutic tool with its own unique goals and objectives.

The functions of support groups vary from community to community and member to member. However, one common and crucial function of a support group is that it provides support systems for individuals who have lost their social networks or whose systems of support are unable to meet their needs (Pearson 1982). In addition, support and self-help groups enable individuals to begin taking responsibility for their own therapeutic change by learning to take an active role in the support group process (Larocca 1983). We believe these are extremely important and unique functions of the self-help/support group structure that can have empowering effects on individuals by giving them the confidence to make positive changes in their lives. In our own clinical experience, support groups have a number of additional functions.

1. Members report that groups with a support focus help break the patterns of isolation that often accompany eating disorders.
2. Support groups provide members with a safe, nonjudgmental environment where individuals can disclose behaviors and feelings they may feel guilty or ashamed about.
3. Group members learn about the underlying causes of eating disorders, what the various metabolic and biological effects of starvation are, and the processes through which their food and weight issues can be resolved.
4. Support groups may provide an environment where participants can

begin to identify some of the issues that may underlie the eating problems by assisting members in making connections between their life experiences and their struggle with food and weight.

5. Support groups often educate members about the process and goals of therapy and help them make informed decisions about treatment options.

6. They may create an emotional "container" when other treatment facilities are not available or accessible.

7. Members report that they use the support group setting to identify and validate important issues and feelings. Many members take these "validated" feelings to individual psychotherapy for more intensive processing.

8. The therapeutic support group offers hope to members who may question whether overcoming food and weight issues is possible. Observing or learning of the emotional and intrapsychic work of others serves a very important therapeutic function.

9. Many participants describe the importance of the support group setting in helping them place their struggles with weight and shape in the context of larger life struggles. Here, the weight and shape issues are not interpreted as illness but as coping strategies that are logical and rational given the individual's personal history.

Support groups have a number of unique functions that extend from providing an individual with the confidence and support to take responsibility for making changes in her life situation, to validating her feelings and contextualizing her experiences. However, it is important to realize that these functions differ in some fundamental ways from the role and functions of process-oriented therapy groups. Enright and colleagues (1985) identified four primary factors that distinguish supportive from process-oriented therapy groups. First, process-oriented groups stress stability of membership as a crucial factor in therapeutic change. Support groups, by their very nature, have a highly unstable membership; attendance is not required, and the format is usually open. Second, members of process groups are chosen carefully to maintain a balance that will ensure group cohesiveness. Support groups, on the other hand, are composed of participants having a wide variety of issues and needs as well as of life circumstances and histories. Third, process groups stress current relationships and interactions among group members, whereas support groups focus more on the participant's personal history and life circumstances. And finally, the goal of process-oriented groups is the resolution of issues identified by individual group members, whereas the goal of support groups is, in simplest terms, to provide members with support, validation, and information.

Although there is no question that more traditional interventions such as psychotherapy are necessary in treating individuals with food and weight issues, professionally-led support groups may provide a dynamic environment in which therapeutic change can occur. In fact, these support groups may function uniquely in creating an environment where an individual's experience is contextualized and validated by peers. Moreover, support groups may provide an introduction and "first link" to treatment programs and more intensive therapeutic interventions. Thus, these groups provide a crucial service that, in our experience, is often seen by an individual as a fundamental part of her therapeutic process. In summary, professionally-led support groups are neither an alternative to other therapies nor an adjunct to treatment; rather, they are a unique and dynamic part of the treatment process.

Philosophy of Treatment

The philosophy of treatment for our support group developed out of our work in a nonprofit, government-funded information service. The mandate of this program is to provide individuals, families, and professionals with information on the prevention and treatment of eating disorders and weight preoccupation. This is accomplished through 1) developing and distributing educational materials; 2) maintaining an in-house directory of treatment programs, organizations, and therapists; 3) providing a telephone support line; 4) running a nondieting, self-acceptance program for large women; 5) engaging in public education through public speaking engagements and providing the media with interviews and information; 6) sponsoring an Eating Disorder Awareness Week; and 7) offering a weekly 2-hour support group.

The support group is seen as an extension of the program's mandate because of its psychoeducational and supportive function. The group was originally set up to accommodate individuals who did not have financial resources for private therapy, who were unsure about the benefits of psychotherapy and needed an introduction to the processes of therapeutic change, or whose therapists were unable or reluctant to address weight and shape issues. The group is considered a "support" rather than a "self-help" group because it is professionally led and supervised.

The philosophy of treatment is a direct extension of the ideas of the self-help movement. We interpret an individual's weight and shape issues as real issues that not only have a profound effect on the person's physical and psychological well-being (Garner and Garfinkel 1982, 1985) but that have meaning in themselves (Steiner-Adair 1989). They therefore must be addressed in the context of her familial and cultural experiences. Related to the weight and shape issues are a whole host of issues around identity, autonomy, connection, and power that must be explored in order to ensure the person does not return to using dieting and weight control behaviors at some future period in her life.

We interpret the weight loss behavior as a coping strategy that is both rational and understandable given the individual's past experiences. It is only logical, for example, that a large-bodied woman would develop issues around food and weight in a culture where her value as a woman is equated with her appearance and where her fatness is interpreted as one of the worse possible sins against womanhood she could possibly commit (Schoenfielder and Wieser 1983). Alternately, it makes sense that a woman who has been sexually abused or raped would develop issues around her body as the hated and shameful site of her violation and powerlessness (Fallon 1988; Wooley 1990a, 1990b).

The theoretical stance taken in the support group is a modified approach to the multidetermined or biopsychosocial model (Anderson 1985). We utilize a concentric and interconnected understanding of eating disorders: familial and psychological issues are lodged within a larger social context, and psychological, familial, and social issues are conceived of as intersecting forces. These interweaving forces give rise to a unique individual with unique struggles.

The approach to treatment taken in the support group is a two-track approach. "Track one" involves addressing issues around eating, weight, and physical condition. "Track two" deals with the issues that have contributed to the development of the eating disorder and its perpetuation. Treatment focuses on track one psychoeducational issues with individuals who are new to the support group and to eating disorder therapies in general (Garner et al. 1985). More attention is paid to the track two issues with members who have been attending the group for a longer period of time. Both tracks need to be kept in balance in order to avoid trivializing an individual's struggle.

One of the most important philosophical stances taken in the group is the belief that individuals can fully resolve their food and weight issues and that an eating disorder is not an addiction. This perspective is in contrast to the philosophical approach of some self-help groups, such as Overeaters Anonymous, which incorporates a 12-step abstinence model for understanding BN. Such groups interpret preoccupation with food and binge eating as symptoms of an addiction to food (Garner 1985) and argue that individuals with eating disorders are always "in recovery." The abstinence model implies BN can only be controlled through abstaining from certain foods (usually calorie-dense and fattening ones), rather than overcome by learning to integrate all foods into a regular meal plan. Because it promotes restrictive eating, such an abstinence model may perpetuate the bingeing and purging behavior and prevent the individual from fully resolving food issues. The addictive approach is not congruent with the re-establishment of normal healthy eating patterns reported by many clients with eating disorders (Rubel 1984).

Implementing the Professionally-Led Support Group Model

The primary aims of the group are to provide participants with relevant information on eating disorders, to promote the development of positive feelings toward one's own body and self, and to provide a context in which related issues and experiences can be contextualized and validated. Significant emphasis is placed on food, weight, and shape issues. In addition, facilitators assist participants in recognizing and acknowledging the myriad underlying psychological issues that must be addressed by each individual in order for her to resolve the eating problem. These issues may be explored in the context of psychotherapy or discussed by the group if appropriate and relevant to members. Facilitators do not take a psychodynamic approach in discussing these issues, but instead, maintain a supportive posture to facilitate change.

Referral Screening

Our program receives many calls daily from people who have heard about its services from therapists, the media, speaking engagements, or by word of mouth. When an individual expresses interest in the group, a telephone interview is conducted to determine that the individual is not actively suicidal or highly unstable. This is not an ideal screening process, but time and personnel constraints do not allow for personal screening interviews. Further screening is conducted once the individual commences the group. If a facilitator determines that an individual is so emotionally unstable that she is a deterrent to other members, she may be referred to a more intensive program. At all times, the well-being of the whole group and its underlying objectives must be considered.

Group Structure

The group meets on a weekly basis for 2 hours. It is open-ended, and members may attend as often or as little as they wish. This open-ended structure dictates that each group session must be treated as a separate, distinct experience. Content will differ and interactions vary depending on the mix of members in attendance. At times, the group has grown to 15 individuals, forcing the program to establish a waiting list. A support group of more than 10 participants becomes less conducive to meaningful interaction.

Group members must be over the age of 18. Adolescents with eating disorders have their own unique issues that are best explored in an age-appropriate group. The support group is primarily composed of female participants, but at times males have constituted up to one-quarter of the membership. The fact that men have been present in the group is discussed explicitly in the terms of similarities and differences in their eating behavior, body image issues, and socialization as it pertains to the expression of affect. We have been careful to ensure that male participants have the opportunity to express their needs while not monopolizing group discussion. Additionally, facilitators must be aware that the current literature suggests a high percentage of those with eating disorders have been sexually abused (Fallon 1988; Goldfarb 1988; Wooley 1990a, 1990b). Feelings related to this issue may arise as a result of discussions within the group and may be intensified by the presence of men.

The group comprises individuals with both anorexia nervosa (AN) and bulimia nervosa (BN). This mix is justified by the fact that many members engage in both anorexic and bulimic behavior or move from one constellation of behaviors to the other. Although this mix evokes feelings in some members, particularly around differences in weight and body image, addressing the issue directly can diffuse the problem and lead to constructive interactions. For example, individuals with BN sometimes express their desire to be as thin as those with AN. A participant with AN will reply that maintaining a low weight has not resulted in the fulfillment and happiness she previously thought attainable through weight loss. This interaction may lead to a discussion of the relationship between body image and self-esteem.

No fee is charged to attend the support group. We have found that this has not interfered with a sense of commitment to the group. All participants are required to have a consent form filled out by a family doctor to ensure that a physician is monitoring the individual's physical health. This is a requirement of the institution where our group meetings are held and helps to ensure members are not in immediate medical danger.

Members may place their names and phone numbers on a list that is distributed to group members. This list is used when an individual feels she needs the support of other group members between meetings. We also advocate using the telephone if an individual wants help in delaying or avoiding a binge episode.

Group Rules

For members to speak openly, they must feel assured that their revelations will stay within the group (Yalom 1985). Hence, confidentiality is an essential requirement. Members are also requested to abstain from the use of alcohol or other substances prior to the group meetings.

Group Facilitators

The support group is professionally led by two trained counselors. Often one of these counselors is a peer who has herself experienced eating problems. Hartman (1987) has described the facilitator as assuming many different roles, including those of supporter, consultant, protector, liaison, advocate, and model. As support persons, the facilitators encourage peer interaction, nurture the progression of the group, and empower group members to set the agenda. As consultants, the facilitators impart pertinent information on eating disorders, provide resource material, and assume responsibility for membership screening. As protectors, the facilitators intervene in the case of a crisis, assume responsibility for ending the group on time, and intervene in disruptive interactions of group process. In their liaison role, the facilitators serve as a link to other organizations, publicize the various therapies available, and provide information about treatment resources. As advocates, the facilitators engage in public education such as Eating Disorder Awareness Week and advocate on behalf of clients in need of more intensive treatment. Finally, facilitators act as models through their respectfulness, genuineness, and ability to express themselves openly and assertively.

It is crucial that group facilitators be supported by some form of supervision. The facilitators meet briefly after each group to review the session and their personal reactions to it. They also meet with a clinical supervisor on a weekly basis to discuss group issues and the feelings arising from them. Problems the group is struggling with and issues affecting its functioning are reviewed.

Self-Harm

The issue of self-harm is occasionally raised by group members. Facilitators must be prepared and willing to address the issue if it arises. Access to a local emergency crisis center or hospital emergency department is essential.

Attendance of Families

From its inception, the group has been closed to family members. We feel strongly that the objectives of our support group are not well served by mixing family members and individuals with AN or BN. Many individuals struggling with eating disorders would not use the support group context to identify and validate various feelings if their mothers, fathers, siblings, or partners were present. Mixing family members and their relatives with eating disorders may also create a potentially explosive situation wherein feelings of guilt and anger could dominate and allow neither side to benefit. Furthermore, the mutually supportive and validating function of the group would be threatened by the power dynamics between parents and children and by the lack of commonality in perspectives, experiences, and feelings about the eating problems. Although family members are not allowed to attend the eating disorder support group, we do encourage them to attend family support groups. Like those with eating disorders, family members can benefit from sharing and mutual support.

Clinical Themes and Issues

The support group is a self-directed group. Individuals raise issues they are working on or concerned about, and leaders facilitate a discussion between the participants. Although new participants are likely to focus on food and weight issues, experienced members may address the eating disorder as it relates to other issues in their lives. In addition, with time members often assume increasingly active and responsible roles in the group by educating newer members, setting group norms, and acting as role models.

A fundamental function of the support group is an educational one. For new participants, this may consist of discussing the facts and fallacies of eating disorders. For members attending the group for a longer period of time, education will focus on using therapy effectively as well as coping with the eating disorder behavior and related problems. The complexities of eating disorders are always acknowledged and often examined. More than once, for example, a new member will say, "If only I could lose weight, I would be able to overcome my eating disorder." When this occurs, the groups members and facilitators spend a considerable amount of time discussing how dieting and the effects of starvation are related to the symptoms of eating disorders and how dieting behavior exacerbates the underlying problems. In addition, they will facilitate a discussion of why it is so important to the individual with the eating disorder to lose weight, how the weight loss is reinforced, and why an individual may feel unable to accept herself at a higher weight.

For those group members who are in transition or currently unable to afford therapy, the support group becomes an "emotional container" where the individual is encouraged to begin addressing and resolving immediate issues. The individual might bring up a particular problem she is confronting, such as applying for a job. This is often a stressful situation, particularly for someone who is feeling out of control in many aspects of her life and trying to regain a sense of effectiveness. Facilitators encourage group members to provide suggestions from their own life experiences and support the individual in her struggle.

The facilitator must be aware of potential differences in interactional styles and degrees of self-knowledge. It is an oversimplification to say that an individual with BN is more likely to interact and be willing to explore her feelings than a person with AN. However, those with AN more often need encouragement to participate. Sometimes it is necessary to gently indicate to a woman with BN that she has to allow time for contributions by other members.

There are a number of common themes that emerge in the eating disorder support group. They are central issues for patients with eating disorders and need to be systematically explored when they arise. These themes have been divided into issues related to weight and shape, issues related to the therapeutic process, and issues related to the development of an eating disorder.

Issues Related to Weight and Shape

◆ Understanding the relationship between starvation and bingeing
◆ Identifying weight prejudice
◆ Discerning body image distortion and disparagement
◆ Understanding how food and weight preoccupation interferes with academic, career, social, and familial pursuits
◆ Learning the mechanics of normalized eating
◆ Using distraction and delaying tactics to avoid bingeing
◆ Relieving stress
◆ Coping with eating and weight gain
◆ Learning how to handle friends and family when food and weight are discussed

Issues Related to the Therapeutic Process

◆ Understanding the positive nature of the therapeutic process
◆ Learning that one's problems, feelings, fears are similar to those of others
◆ Trusting others
◆ Checking out feelings and ideas to be discussed in therapy
◆ Understanding the differences between lapses and relapses in the recovery process
◆ Being supported and valued by the group

Issues Related to the Development of Eating Disorders

◆ Understanding the relationship between self-esteem, self-concept, and body image
◆ Recognizing how perfectionism can be damaging by discussing the impossibility and harmful effects of the "superwoman" image
◆ Understanding how women learn to negate and repress their needs and how individuals in the group can begin to recognize and meet their own needs
◆ Recognizing how early childhood traumas such as sexual and physical abuse relate to eating disorders
◆ Understanding the relationship between alcoholism in the family and eating disorders
◆ Recognizing how the issue of control relates to the eating disorders
◆ Identifying cognitive thinking patterns such as all-or-nothing thinking and magical thinking

Every effort is made to ensure that all members of the group are referred to therapists who have an understanding of and willingness to address the complex issues related to an eating disorder. Week after week, the message delivered to the group is that individuals with eating disorders have issues they must confront and that weight preoccupation is often a means of coping with these issues.

Many members attending the support group are involved in intensive psychotherapy but find they can benefit from additional discussions and interactions with peers. They value the nonspecific help of group membership. For some, it is the sharing with understanding others that they find particularly beneficial. For others, it is the nonjudgmental acceptance and active support of group members that helps to facilitate change. They may find it useful to hear that others have difficulty with the same sort of problems and to understand the solutions others have found for them. It is enhancing to self-esteem to have the experience of helping others.

References

Anderson AE: Practical Comprehensive Treatment of Anorexia Nervosa and Bulimia. Baltimore, MD, Johns Hopkins University Press, 1985

Enright AB, Tootell C: The role of support groups in the treatment of eating disorders. American Mental Health Counsellors Association Journal 237–245, October 1986

Enright AB, Butterfield P, Berkowitz B: Self-help and support groups in the management of eating disorders, in Handbook for Psychotherapy for Anorexia Nervosa and Bulimia. Edited by Garner DM, Garfinkel PE. New York, Guilford, 1985, pp 491–512

Fallon P: A feminist systems approach to the treatment of bulimia. Paper presented at the Third International Conference on Eating Disorders, New York, April 1988

Garner DM: Iatrogenesis in anorexia nervosa and bulimia nervosa. International Journal of Eating Disorders 4:701–726, 1985

Garner DM, Garfinkel PE: Anorexia Nervosa: A Multi-Dimensional Perspective. New York, Brunner/Mazel, 1982

Garner DM, Garfinkel PE (eds): Handbook of Psychotherapy for Anorexia Nervosa and Bulimia. New York, Guilford, 1985

Garner DM, Rockert W, Olmsted MP, et al: Psychoeducational principles in the treatment of eating disorders, in Handbook of Psychotherapy for Anorexia Nervosa and Bulimia. Edited by Garner DM, Garfinkel PE. New York, Guilford, 1985, pp 513–572

Gartner AJ, Riessman F: Self-help and mental health. Hosp Community Psychiatry 33:631–635, 1982

Goldfarb L: Sexual abuse antecedent to anorexia nervosa, bulimia, and compulsive overeating: three case reports. International Journal of Eating Disorders 6:675–680, 1988

Hartman S: Therapeutic self-help groups: a process of empowerment for women, in Women's Therapy Groups: Paradigms of Feminist Treatment. Edited by Brody CM. New York, Springer, 1987, pp 67–81

Larocca FEF: The relevance of self-help in the management of anorexia and bulimia. St. Louis, MO, Res Medica (St. John's Mercy Medical Center), June 1983

Pearson RE: Support: exploration of a basic concept in counselling and informal help. Personnel and Guidance Journal 61:83–87, 1982

Rubel J: The function of self-help groups in recovery from anorexia nervosa and bulimia. Psychiatr Clin North Am 7:381–393, 1984

Sesan R: Peer educators: a creative resource for the eating disordered college student, in The Bulimic College Student. Edited by Whitaker LC, Davis WN. New York, The Haworth Press, 1989

Schoenfielder L, Wieser B (eds): Shadow on a Tight Rope: Writing by Women on Fat Oppression. Iowa City, IA, Aunt Lute Book Company, 1983

Silverman PR: Mutual Help Groups: A Guide for Mental Health Workers. Rockville, MD, National Institutes of Health, 1978

Steiner-Adair D: Developing the voice of the wise woman: college students and bulimia, in The Bulimic College Student: Evaluation, Treatment and Prevention. Edited by Whitaker LC, Davis WN. New York, The Haworth Press, 1989, pp 151–165

Wooley S: The psychology of women. Paper presented at the Fourth International Conference on Eating Disorders, New York, April 1990a

Wooley S: Childhood trauma, eating disorders and the psychology of women. Paper presented at the Making Connections Conference, Toronto, Ontario, October 1990b

Yalom ID: The Theory and Practice of Group Psychotherapy. New York, Basic Books, 1985

13

Continuing Care Groups for Chronic Anorexia Nervosa

Ann Kerr, B.Sc., O.T.
Molyn Leszcz, M.D., F.R.C.P.(C)
Allan S. Kaplan, M.D., F.R.C.P.(C)

♦ ♦ ♦ ♦ ♦ ♦ ♦ ♦ ♦

This chapter describes an approach for the chronic anorexia nervosa patient that is modeled on programs for the chronic schizophrenic population. The goal is not cure but rather enhanced social integration and quality of life. Paradoxically, this de-emphasis on the eating symptoms appears to have been helpful for many of the patients, highlighting the dimension of control commonly described as a feature of patients with anorexia nervosa. This work demonstrates the usefulness of the group modality per se as a containing and supporting force.—The Editors

L ittle is known about the optimal treatment and management of patients chronically ill with anorexia nervosa (AN). However, this group represents a significant proportion—approximately one-third—of those with the illness (Theander 1985). Long-term follow-up studies in Sweden (Theander 1985), Great Britain (Morgan and Russell 1975), and the United States (Halmi et al. 1975) document the alarming morbidity and mortality for patients chronically ill with AN. The Swedish study found the total mortality from AN or suicide was 18% in a series drawn from a systematic search of somatic and psychiatric clinics within a defined region in Sweden over 33 years. Of additional significance are the lost years of productivity and development for those who did recover.

Our clinical setting in a metropolitan teaching hospital has provided care for a large number of such high-risk patients. Many of these patients have been treated intensively and repeatedly over a number of years. For some patients, treatment aimed at weight gain is experienced as imposed and punitive. The eating disorder, AN, has become an identity that is tenaciously valued in opposition to the wishes of caregivers, family, and friends. Hence a core of patients with relatively intractable AN has emerged. Characteristically, these patients are socially isolated, with few or no peer relationships.

In recognition of the limitations of traditional treatments, an alternative psychotherapeutic management has been developed. This utilizes as its rationale the model used for the continuing care of patients with schizophrenia (Wasylenki et al. 1981). The model is centered around the establishment of a supportive psychotherapy group of unlimited duration for patients suffering the same illness. The group focus is on the problems of daily living and quality of life issues, as opposed to symptomatic issues such as weight gain and improved eating. The working hypothesis for the group is that for chronically ill underweight patients with AN, a group format focused on quality of life issues other than those involving weight could lead to improved psychosocial functioning. Furthermore, improved physiologic status (i.e., weight gain) might be facilitated by avoiding entering into a power struggle over the responsibility for eating and physical well-being.

Literature Review

There are no reports on the long-term management of patients chronically ill with AN. There is abundant literature on inpatient management with weight restoration as the treatment goal (Agras and Werne 1977; Bruch 1974; Harper 1983), but the special needs of the patient who is repeatedly admitted with little amelioration of symptoms over years has not been addressed.

Group treatment of AN has also received little attention. There have been few units where groups of AN patients are treated together. The effects of starvation, expressed through the physical and psychological manifestations of the illness, are generally considered a contraindication for intense psychological treatment (Kaplan and Woodside 1987). The psychological manifestations of the illness are also cited as contraindications for the group treatment of AN patients (Hall 1985). Poor self-esteem and hypersensitivity to the feelings of others, particularly to criticism, may result in mobilization of pathological anxiety in a group setting. Competition with other patients for low weight or for the strongest anorexic identity may also become more pronounced in a group setting.

In contrast, Lieb and Thompson (1984) have reported on the positive effects of the introduction of a group format on an inpatient setting. The group decreased the patients' isolation, helped them develop a more cohesive sense of identity, and provided an opportunity for accomplishment through cooperation with others in a group. The researchers concluded that in their sample of four patients over nine sessions, the group decreased denial and facilitated the direct expression of feelings. Polivy and Garfinkel (1984) similarly found group psychotherapy a helpful adjunctive treatment to inpatient individual therapy. Their impression was that group therapy benefited the older patients with AN of the bulimic subtype with longer histories. Inbody and Ellis (1985) have described the specific psychological difficulties of patients with eating disorders as they emerged in an outpatient group of seven young people with AN or bulimia nervosa (BN). These difficulties included dealing with body distortion, fear of weight gain, perfectionism, isolation, magical thinking, and cognitive distortions. They believe group therapy provides a unique benefit for these patients as measured by weight gain, improved Beck Depression Inventory scores (Beck et al. 1961), and subjective report.

The Continuing Care Group

Theoretical Considerations

The effects of chronic illness on psychosocial functioning are of increasing concern to mental health professionals (Bachrach 1981). The continuing care model, usually in the form of ongoing support in a clinic setting, has been successfully applied to the schizophrenic population (Wasylenki and Goering 1984). It was this success with a population of chronically ill psychiatric patients that led us to pilot a similar model of treatment with patients chronically ill with AN. Control issues, particularly around weight changes, would be circumvented in a milieu that accepts low weight as the norm. Attention to nonweight related issues such as social isolation, self-esteem, fears of maturity, loss of aging parents, and efforts at personal productivity would be the focus of treatment. The objective was to provide treatment in those areas that were ego-dystonic for the patients, rather than engage in a highly resistive battle over weight gain. By their chronicity, these patients had demonstrated their capacity to defeat standard approaches to treatment. It was hoped that this treatment would lead to an improvement in their psychosocial functioning and, paradoxically, possible weight gain.

Referral Process

Patients were referred to the Continuing Care group for AN by psychiatric consultants attached to a large tertiary care hospital with specialized services for the treatment of AN. Patients were to be treated concurrently by a physician. In fact, these patients had a multitude of health care professionals involved in their care, including individual psychotherapists, nurses, nutritionists, and vocational and residential case workers. All patients were female with a DSM-III-R diagnosis (American Psychiatric Association 1987) of AN with or without bulimia. On entry into the group, all patients were visibly emaciated, with a mean duration of illness of at least 5 years. Intensive inpatient and outpatient treatments had not altered the course of illness.

The formal referral process requested a psychiatric consultant affiliated with the hospital to forward a psychiatric history to the group leader. Very often, in practice, the patient herself initiated the referral after speaking with her therapist, or more often, after speaking with current or former members of the group. Patients associated with the hospital maintain a vigilant network, keeping track of each other's physical status and circumstances, and more importantly, the resources they share. At the time of referral, most patients were well known to the group leader, who had worked in both the inpatient setting and the day hospital, or to colleagues with whom the group leader kept in close contact.

Before being included in the group, each patient was assessed, given an orientation, and prepared for group through an interview with the group leader. A capacity to relate to other anorexic women was assessed by considering issues such as denial, competitiveness, and willingness to self-disclose. Denial of the illness was assessed by discussing previous experiences in treatment and the extent to which the patient's illness was known to those around her. The patient was told that the group was for women chronically ill with AN who want support in living with the illness. Previous inpatient treatment had usually offered enough exposure to other AN patients to give the patient knowledge about her tendency to compete with others with the eating disorder. Patients readily admitted that they were very concerned about the risk of a recurrence of such competition for a low weight. Whenever this tendency was acknowledged, a verbal contract was made between group leader and patient to watch for competitiveness developing and in that event to terminate participation in the group. Furthermore, the patient's reaction to being described as chronically ill was viewed as a measure of current denial of the illness.

Men were excluded from the group to facilitate the discussion of sexual concerns should they arise. At the time of referral, patients were chronically stable at a low weight. Women who were premorbidly very heavy and had restricted food intake to a lower yet more "normal" body weight were refused based on the difficulties they experience in being in a group with underweight women. Women who were currently abusing alcohol and/or medications were also deferred until abstinent.

This process of anticipating the difficulties in bringing AN patients together in a group reassured them that the illness was well understood by the group leader. It implied that they could be more "real" in the group and not have to distort or deny their situation. Finally, new members were asked to describe their own concerns about being in the group. This was often the key to the difficulties that might be reenacted in the group. For example, one patient said she dreaded the tendency for patients to go into great detail over their attempts to lose weight by purging and exercise. Later, in group, she displayed this very behavior. Another patient said her greatest concern was that she would start to improve, gain weight, and with that would flee the group. Once such difficulties were expressed, the group leader and the patient agreed to discuss them with the group as they arose in order to prevent the acting out of these anxieties in the group. Systematic pregroup preparation has been effective in decreasing patient anxiety, forging a therapeutic alliance, increasing patient self-disclosure, and developing hopefulness regarding treatment (Bader et al. 1981; Yalom 1985). The assessment procedures described above apply this general process to the chronic anorexic population.

A formal history of the eating disorder was intentionally de-emphasized during assessment, as it had already been developed in great detail during previous hospitalizations. Because the focus of the group was to be on supportive interpersonal functions, preference was given to elaboration of psychosocial issues. Details concerning weight and emphasis on the "illness" were not as pertinent for the group. A self-report history of the illness along with other measures assessing social support will be described in greater detail later in this chapter.

Group Composition

The first 18 women treated in the continuing care group all met DSM-III-R diagnostic criteria for AN, with four also meeting criteria for BN. Two also presented with obsessive-compulsive disorders antedating the eating disorder. Three women had concomitant medical illnesses: diabetes, Turner's syndrome, and hemangioma of the small intestine. Three other women had seizure disorders or osteoporosis as a consequence of their eating disorders.

Baseline demographic information supports the description of these women as chronically ill (Table 13–1). On average, the women were approximately 30 years of age with a mean duration of illness of nearly 13

Table 13–1.   Demographic features of the group for anorexia nervosa

Characteristic	Mean ($n = 18$)	$\pm$ SD
Age	29.17	5.14
Height (in)	64.44	2.75
Weight as percent of MPMW	74.40	8.08
Highest weight as percent of MPMW	103.49	20.69
Lowest weight as percent of MPMW	59.62	10.18
Marital status		
Single	72.2%	
Married	22.2%	
Divorced	5.6%	
Employment status		
Employed	38.9%	
Unemployed	38.9%	
Disabled	22.2%	

Note. MPMW = Matched Population Mean Weight.
Source. Metropolitan Life Insurance Company 1954.

years. The mean presenting weight was 74% of average. Severity of illness was documented by the Eating Attitudes Test (EAT-26; Garner and Garfinkel 1979) showing the continuing care sample to have a higher score than an average anorexic sample (Table 13–2). Persistent attempts at weight control in the form of food restriction (100%), laxative abuse (83%), vomiting (88%), and exercise as a means of weight control (88%) was described in the Diagnostic Survey for Eating Disorders (DSED; Johnson 1985). Other demographic features demonstrated that the sample was representative of other AN populations in that they were well-educated, one-third had been married, one-third lived in the parental home, one-third lived alone, and one-sixth lived in psychiatric group homes. Vocational status reflected impairment in the area of productivity: one-third were fully employed, one-quarter were on long-term disability from work, and the remainder were involved in volunteer work, studying, or sporadic part-time employment.

    Psychosocial functioning was measured by two scales. The Miller So-

Table 13–2.   Patient scores on the EAT-26

Score	Mean $(n = 17)$	$+$ SD
Total	36.41	15.93
Dieting	20.00	11.30
Bulimia	7.71	4.34
Oral Control	8.41	5.09

Note. EAT = Eating Attitudes Test.
Source. Garner and Garfinkel 1979.

cial Intimacy Scale (Miller and Lefcourt 1982) required the patient to describe her most intimate relationship with a nonfamily member in terms of depth of the relationship and frequency of contact within the relationship. Compared to a female student sample (Table 13–3), the continuing care group sample described a paucity in intimate relationships, and one-fifth said they had no intimate relationships.

The Social Adjustment Scale (SAS-SR) (Weissman et al. 1978) is a 42-item self-report scale that measures performance over the past 2 weeks in six major areas: work (as a worker, homemaker, or student), social and leisure activities, relationship with extended family, role as a spouse, role as a parent, and membership in a family unit. The questions in each area assess the patient's performance at expected tasks, the amount of friction

Table 13–3.   A comparison of Miller Social Intimacy Scale scores

Sample	n	Mean	$\pm$ SD
Current AN	13	112.2	38.4
Married clinic[*]	15	133.8[a]	20.8
Unmarried student[*]	130	139.3[b]	26.8
Married student[*]	17	156.2[b]	7.3

*Miller and Lefcourt 1982.
[a]SD from current AN sample $P < .07$.
[b]SD from current AN sample $P < .01$.

with others, and finer aspects of interpersonal relations, inner feelings, and satisfaction. The SAS has been widely used with both psychiatric and non-psychiatric female populations. Based on this scale, the continuing care sample described themselves as having social adjustment problems comparable to a sample of acutely depressed female patients and a sample of female alcoholic patients (Table 13–4). In contrast, the social adjustment of a female population with schizophrenia was much less impaired. Similar findings regarding persistent social maladjustment in eating disorder populations have been reported (Herzog et al. 1987; Johnson and Berndt 1983; Norman and Herzog 1984; Norman et al. 1986).

Patient compliance with the self-report questionnaires became a confounding issue in the documentation of this treatment. The majority of these women have been subjects in a multitude of studies over the past 15 years and were unwilling to repeat the experience. It is also our impression that because the group leader was not a physician, the patients saw the group less as a medical treatment warranting scientific investigation and more as a group for themselves. In fact, the group experience seemed to be split off from prior or current medical/psychiatric treatment. Issues concerning shame, denial, and exploitation could have been playing a part in the reticence patients felt when asked to document their lives on paper.

Group Structure

The Continuing Care Group met weekly for 1 hour at the Eating Disorder

Table 13–4.   A comparison of Social Adjustment Scale (SAS) scores

Sample	n	Mean	± SD
Current AN sample	16	2.54	.73
Bulimic women[*]	80	2.23[a]	.44
Acutely depressed women[**]	155	2.53	.46
Alcoholic women[**]	19	2.36	.50
Schizophrenic women[**]	35	1.95[b]	.66
Community sample of normal women[**]	277	1.61[b]	.34

[*]Norman and Herzog 1984.
[**]Weissman et al. 1978.
[a]SD from current AN sample $P < .05$.
[b]SD from current AN sample $P < .01$.

Day Hospital. The initial group met early in the morning; however, when the need arose, a second evening group was established to accommodate working patients. Business around meeting times, holidays, or a change in membership took place at the beginning of each session. Concerns about absent members was addressed foremost, with members letting each other know about any out-of-group contacts since the preceding session. Medical problems, most often secondary to AN, were the most common reason for absenteeism. Very often the group leader was contacted before the group by the patient. This information was then passed onto the group. Following this business of the group, each member took a turn discussing her week with the leader actively prompting discussion and feedback from everyone.

The members were actively involved in decisions affecting the group. Examples included deciding whether or not to meet when the therapist was on holidays, willingness to take in new members following the termination of a senior member, scheduling issues such as the time, length, and day of the group, allowing visitors at group meetings, and processing of information from the self-report questionnaires.

Group Process

Group cohesion was quickly established as an result of the densely homogeneous nature of the group. However, those features that contributed to feelings of universality such as emaciation, chronicity, dependency, and social isolation were also the very features that propelled a number of members to view their symptoms as increasingly ego-dystonic as they confronted their symptoms by seeing them in others. Differentiation within the group quickly took two directions: either one competed to become thinner and more ill than the others, or one competed to succeed within the group by taking steps toward health through weight gain or through increased participation in noneating behaviors such as work.

The safety of the group through its tolerance of the symptoms and unconditional acceptance inevitably came to represent the illness and something that would need to be forsaken for health. Only in the context of the unconditional nature of the group could the control issues around the illness center on the patient and her illness as opposed to the patient and health care providers. Losing the group was to lose the illness, and this presented a risk to the patient should she choose to remain identified with the illness. This risk was viewed as the primary contraindication for the group and was a concern to some of the physicians who continued to see the patients individually at the same time as these patients were in group.

One patient was able to comment on this risk, and not only left the group but the entire hospital system, including her psychiatrist, as a way of throwing aside the illness. In follow-up several years later, she was at normal weight and living and working independently.

Although patients came into the group knowing it was for the chronically ill, they persisted in hoping that one day they would recover. They were very curious about the self-report questionnaires. Compliance in filling these questionnaires out increased dramatically when the results were incorporated into the group so that members could look at themselves as compared to subjects who were not anorexic. A genetic study, attempting to demonstrate a biologic causality for the illness, drew outrage from the group who insisted their illness was of their own choosing—and their own undoing. The group norm was to view the symptoms as something they were trying to overcome; however, the group shied away from trapping itself into behavioral goals that would inevitably lead to disappointment or another forum for control struggles.

Of most value to the members was the process of sharing themselves with others in a supportive, nonjudgmental environment. Existential themes were repeatedly expressed. Death was always close—their own deaths as well as those of their aging parents, dying grandparents, or friends with eating disorders. This fear was defended against by the sense that they were uniquely invulnerable—or uniquely protected by parents or health care providers. The fear and profound sadness of real or anticipated losses repeatedly emerged, particularly when group members became ill. Tremendous relief was expressed by the voluntary admission of members to hospital. During a 5-year period, there were no involuntary admissions of the members.

Letting go of those who can protect leaves one free and responsible for one's choices and life situations. Typically, group members expressed great doubt about their own personal effectiveness and their ability to function in a less structured adult world. Making decisions involved the possibility of offending or displeasing others. Very often, it was the desire to please others, as opposed to responding to internal desires, that paralyzed these patients. Validating their wishes in whatever way possible in the group was an empowering process. Respecting their wishes, yet asking them to look at the consequences and then make choices, was a way that most control issues were circumvented.

The social aspect of the group addressed the most distressing aspect of the illness—isolation. For many of the members, the group was their only social contact outside of medical appointments. In the case of one member, the group was her only social contact apart from her divorced parents. Her situation was particularly striking in that before entering the group she had spent almost the entire previous 2 years in hospital, usually under a certificate of involuntary admission. When her case was presented at psychiatric rounds and she was reported to be lost to follow-up, staff were amazed to hear that she had actually been attending the group regularly and maintaining a level of stability both in terms of mental status and physical health unparalleled in the past 5 years. However, she refused to have anything to do with psychiatrists and would speak only with the peer group. We propose that giving these women an opportunity to relate in a way meaningful to each other is the most therapeutic factor of the group. We discuss this later in the chapter.

Finally, a comment about the nature of conducting such a group: the issues that faced the patients were also those of the leader. Would the patients return from week to week, or would they die? Would this group be special enough to sustain their hope and the leader's hope for them? Would the caregiver be powerful enough to keep them alive? Would the leader let the group take responsibility for themselves, or impose a kind of dependency that recapitulated that of the families of origin? Was the leader herself replenished from week to week sufficiently to feed their craving for social contact? These concerns were discussed in regular supervision with an outside expert—an important arrangement for such work.

Outcome Measures

As outlined in Table 13–5, a number of members made gains while in the Continuing Care Group. These gains may have occurred regardless of the group. However, these were women who had been the recipients of sophisticated specialized care for over a decade and for whom there was little expectation of change except increased dependence and chronicity. More than half had improved social lives, and 40% had improved social functioning. One-third increased their weight by 10%. One-third were rehospitalized during the group. However, the nature of these hospitalizations was somewhat changed as they were not precipitous or against the

Table 13–5. Outcome measures ($n = 18$)

10/18	(55.5%)	Increased social contact
7/18	(41.1%)	Improved vocational functioning
6/18	(33.3%)	Increased weight by 10.5% (95.9–106 lbs)
6/18	(33.3%)	Rehospitalized
1/18	(5.5%)	Dropout
5/18	(27.7%)	Successful termination

patients' will. Often they entered the hospital with clearer goals for themselves, and an orientation to use the hospitalization as a means to getting on with their lives as opposed to staving off death. Successful termination was defined as someone who anticipated leaving, felt she had made gains, and worked through the process of saying goodbye to group members.

Discussion

The group served several important functions for the patients. The most important was the feeling of acceptance and intimacy they felt could only come from being with those who were like themselves. For women whose sense of self-esteem, capacity to trust, and sense of personal effectiveness is severely damaged, the opportunity to be helpful to others is often the only way they have of connecting at an interpersonal level. Properties described in the self-help literature clarify this process (Gartner and Reissman 1977). This perspective suggests that those who help are helped the most. Altruism functions to overcome egocentricity, and the ideological perspective of self-help keeps norms, attitudes, and sanctioned responses in the direction of health. Rubel (1984) has reviewed the history of self-help approaches in the treatment of eating disorders and has emphasized the importance of providing a safe place for the exchange of support, information, and a bridge for social contact.

There is no doubt this forum for support is fraught with danger, particularly for the person with AN who can only relate in a competitive manner through her weight. However, as an adjunctive treatment, the Continuing Care Group psychotherapy experience can possibly sustain the hope and quality of life needed to turn the anorexic process around. This raises questions about specific treatment approaches for this group of patients and the need to be innovative and possibly to look beyond the medical model for approaches to their long-term care.

References

Agras S, Werne J: Behavior modification in anorexia nervosa, in Anorexia Nervosa. Edited by Vigersky RA. New York, Raven, 1977

American Psychiatric Association: Diagnostic and Statistical Manual of Mental Disorders, 3rd Edition, Revised. Washington, DC, American Psychiatric Association, 1987

Bachrach LL: Continuity of care for chronic mental patients: a conceptual analysis. Am J Psychiatry 138:1449–1456, 1981

Bader B, Bader L, Budman S, et al: Pre-group preparation model for long-term group psychotherapy in a private practice setting. Group 5(3):43–50, 1981

Beck AT, Ward CH, Mendelson M, et al: An inventory for measuring depression. Arch Gen Psychiatry 4:561–571, 1961

Bruch H: Perils of behavior modification in treatment of anorexia nervosa. JAMA 230:1419–1422, 1974

Garner D, Garfinkel PE: The Eating Attitudes Test: an index of the symptoms of anorexia nervosa. Psychol Med 9:273–279, 1979

Gartner A, Reissman F: Self-Help in the Human Services. San Francisco, CA, Jossey-Bass, 1977

Hall A: Group psychotherapy for anorexia nervosa, in The Handbook of Psychotherapy for Anorexia Nervosa and Bulimia. Edited by Garner DM, Garfinkel PE. New York, Guilford, 1985

Halmi KA, Brodland G, Rigas C: A follow-up study of 79 patients with anorexia nervosa: an evaluation of prognostic factors and diagnostic criteria. Life History Research in Psychopathology 4:290–291, 1975

Harper G: Anorexia nervosa, in Inpatient Psychiatry. Edited by Sederer LI. Baltimore, MD, Williams & Wilkins, 1983

Herzog D, Keller MB, Lavori PW, et al: Social impairment in bulimia. International Journal of Eating Disorders 6(6):741–747, 1987

Inbody DR, Ellis JJ: Group therapy with anorexic and bulimic patients: implications for therapeutic intervention. Am J Psychother 39:411–420, 1985

Johnson C: Initial consultation for patients with bulimia and anorexia nervosa, in The Handbook of Psychotherapy for Anorexia Nervosa and Bulimia. Edited by Garner DM, Garfinkel PE. New York, Guilford, 1985

Johnson C, Berndt DJ: Preliminary investigation of bulimia and life adjustment. Am J Psychiatry 140:774–777, 1983

Kaplan AS, Woodside DB: Biological aspects of anorexia nervosa and bulimia nervosa. J Consult Clin Psychol 55:645–653, 1987

Lieb RC, Thompson TL: Group psychotherapy for four anorexia nervosa inpatients. J Group Psychother 34(4):639–642, 1984

Metropolitan Life Insurance Company: Metropolitan Life Tables. New York, Metropolitan Life Insurance Company, 1959

Miller R, Lefcourt H: The assessment of social intimacy. J Pers Assess 46:514–518, 1982

Morgan HG, Russell GFM: Value of family background and clinical features as predictors of long-term outcome in anorexia nervosa: four-year follow-up study of 41 patients. Psychol Med 5:355–371, 1975

Norman DK, Herzog DB: Persistent social maladjustment in bulimia: a one year follow-up. Am J Psychiatry 141:3, 1984

Norman DK, Herzog DB, Chauncey S: A one-year outcome study of bulimia: psychological and eating symptom changes in a treatment and non-treatment group. International Journal of Eating Disorders 5(1):47–57, 1986

Polivy J, Garfinkel PE: Group treatments for specific medical problems: anorexia nervosa, in Helping Patients and Their Families Cope with Medical Problems. London, Jossey-Bass, 1984

Rubel JA: The function of self-help groups in recovery from anorexia nervosa and bulimia. Psychiatr Clin North Am 7(2):381–394, 1984

Theander S: Outcome and prognosis in anorexia nervosa and bulimia: some results of previous investigations, compared with those of a Swedish long-term study. J Psychiatr Res 19:493–508, 1985

Wasylenki D, Goering P: A framework for continuity of care. Perspectives in Psychiatry 3(6):1–5, 1984

Wasylenki D, Plummer E, Littmann S: An aftercare program for problem patients. Hosp Community Psychiatry 32:493–496, 1981

Weissman MM, Prusoff BA, Thompson WD, et al: Social adjustment by self-report in a community sample and in psychiatric outpatients. J Nerv Ment Dis 66:317–326, 1978

Yalom ID: The Theory and Practice of Group Psychotherapy. New York, Basic Books, 1985

Appendix

The Road to Recovery

◆ ◆ ◆ ◆ ◆ ◆ ◆ ◆ ◆

Among the many sources utilized in the preparation of this manuscript, we would like to give special acknowledgment to three:

Garner DM, Rockert W, Olmsted MP, et al: Psychoeducational principles in the treatment of bulimia and anorexia nervosa, in Handbook of Psychotherapy for Anorexia Nervosa and Bulimia. Edited by Garner DM, Garfinkel PE. New York, Guilford, 1985, pp 513–572
National Eating Disorder Information Centre: Eating Disorders: An Overview. Toronto, Ontario, NEDIC, September 1988
National Eating Disorder Information Centre: Understanding and Overcoming an Eating Disorder. Toronto, Ontario, NEDIC, September 1988

The Road to Recovery

A Manual for Participants in the Psychoeducation Group for Bulimia Nervosa

Authors
(in alphabetical order):

Ron Davis, Ph.D., C.Psych.
Sarah Dearing, B.A.A.
Joan Faulkner, M.S.W.
Karin Jasper, Ph.D., M.Ed.
Marion P. Olmsted, Ph.D., C.Psych.
Carla Rice, B.A.
Wendi Rockert, B.A.

Address for correspondence:

Ron Davis, Ph.D., C.Psych.
Director, Eating Disorder Outpatient Clinic
The Toronto Hospital
College Wing, 1-328
200 Elizabeth Street
Toronto, Ontario M5G 2C4 Canada

Table of Contents

Introduction

Welcome to the Psychoeducation Group for bulimia nervosa—and congratulations for taking the first step along the road to recovery by joining the group! You probably have a number of questions about the group and we will try to address some of the more common ones here that participants from previous groups have asked. If you have other questions, please ask your group leader at the next meeting.

What can I expect from the Psychoeducation Group?

The group is a series of meetings designed to help you learn about the nature of your eating disorder and about specific methods for overcoming it. By attending the meetings and reading this manual, you will acquire information about a number of issues relevant to the process of recovery from an eating disorder. Some of the more important issues covered in the group and in this manual include:

♦ The multidetermined nature of eating disorders;
♦ Factors that can predispose, precipitate, and perpetuate an eating disorder;
♦ Physical and psychological problems associated with an eating disorder;
♦ Dangers and relative ineffectiveness of purging;
♦ The regulation of body weight and the consequences of dieting;
♦ The association between dieting and bingeing;
♦ The nondieting approach to eating;
♦ Effective coping with eating difficulties and other problems in living;
♦ Challenging troublesome attitudes and feelings;
♦ Feeling better about your body; and
♦ Maintaining healthy attitudes and eating behaviors after the group.

How can I derive the most benefit from the group?

In order for you to derive the full benefit of the group, it is important for you to attend each and every meeting because new information is presented at each meeting which you would otherwise miss out on. In our experience, this can cause confusion for the participant who misses a meeting because the next one builds upon information learned in the previous one. In the event that your absence from a meeting is unavoidable, please inform your group leaders in advance, even if this means making a quick phone call. Unexplained absences from the group are often a sign that the participant is having difficulties which need to be addressed, not avoided. In addition to regular attendance, it is important for you to read the corresponding chapters in this manual that are assigned at each meeting; however, the manual is not a substitute for group attendance. The group leaders will lead the presentations and, while questions and comments of the participants are certainly encouraged, you should not feel obliged to reveal personal information about yourself. While self-disclosure is an important aspect of many group therapy experiences, it is not an expectation of this Psychoeducation Group. Nevertheless, it is vitally important that group leaders be aware of the frequency and severity of eating symptoms during your participation. Therefore, we expect you to complete the Weekly Symptom Summaries and turn one in to your group leaders at each meeting. The Weekly Symptom Summary is not a "progress report;" you are asked to be honest and accurate in recording your eating symptoms rather than to underreport them in the belief that "progress" is expected of you.

Will the Psychoeducation Group help me?

The Psychoeducation Group has been in operation since 1986 and more than 100 participants have been in the groups thus far. Through direct feedback and suggestions from past participants, the group has been adapted to meet the needs and interests of new participants in ways that make the experience as helpful as possible. For any one participant, we cannot predict ahead of time how beneficial the group will be, but we can give you some suggestions that might increase your potential to benefit from the group.

1. Attend all the meetings, read this manual, and try to relate what you learn to your own situation. Self-knowledge is a key aspect of change!
2. Consider the period of time that you are involved in the group as a personal experiment—a period of time in which you should allow yourself to keep an open mind about what you learn and about what you can do to facilitate your own recovery.
3. Be a risk-taker. Confront your beliefs and your fears in a calculated way and at a pace that is comfortable for you. Try the suggestions the group leaders make and observe what happens in an objective manner. Then decide if the outcome justifies your considerable investment in the recovery process. We believe it will!
4. Take credit for any changes you make in your eating behavior and in the way you view yourself as a person. After all, changes come about through your own persistent efforts in examining your beliefs about food, weight, shape, and the underlying issues that may perpetuate your eating disorder.

Should I be seeing other health professionals while I am participating in the Psychoeducation Group?

It is important for you to be under the ongoing care of a physician who knows that you have an eating disorder. The reason is simple. As you will learn, significant physical problems can result from the eating disorder, and it is vital that your medical needs be attended to by a physician. In addition to your physician, if you are currently receiving treatment for your eating disorder from other health professionals (e.g., psychologist, psychiatrist, dietitian, social worker, counselor, nurse), please inform your group leaders. If you would like to begin treatment with another health professional in addition to your physician, we recommend that you hold off until you have completed the Psychoeducation Group and then decide what to do on the basis of what your needs might be at that time.

1

Overview of the Eating Disorders

◆ ◆ ◆ ◆ ◆ ◆ ◆ ◆ ◆

ana's day begins with a trip to the washroom for her morning weigh-in, a ritual which she has completed for almost a decade. As on most mornings, the scale sets the tone of her mood for the day, and it won't be a happy one because she weighs more than she did yesterday. Lana resolves to be good today by getting through on as few calories as possible. Her weigh-in tonight before bedtime will tell her just how "good," "in control," or "successful" she has been. Dressing is a dreadful time. Standing in front of the mirror, she examines her image and, feeling very fat, scans her wardrobe to find that safe outfit that won't betray to the world how fat she feels today. Breakfast is out of the question this morning.

At lunchtime Lana feels tired, jittery, but in control because she had a small salad and resisted the temptation to share in the pizza her co-workers were having for lunch. The afternoon drags on as she becomes preoccupied with thoughts about her weight and the pizza she turned down. She begins to feel ill-at-ease and withdraws from the world around her into a world of confusing thoughts and feelings about herself and about that pizza. On the drive home she detours into a fast-food restaurant with almost no forethought as she has done on countless evenings. At home she gulps the pizza in a frenzied manner with no regard for its taste beyond the first slice. The painful feelings in her stomach are almost as intense as the anxiety and guilt that she now feels. After a trip to the washroom, her day ends with the resolution that this is absolutely the last time she will binge, the same resolution she has made a thousand times before.

Lana is a unique individual with her own set of strengths, life experiences, and goals for the future. Yet, like so many other women, Lana suffers from an eating disorder that significantly affects how she thinks, feels, and behaves. The disorder is called *bulimia nervosa*, a problem that is affecting more and more people. It is estimated that 2–3% of adolescent and young adult women suffer from this problem (Garfinkel and Goldbloom 1988). A related eating disorder called *anorexia*

283

nervosa is present in about 1% of the young female population. Anorexia and bulimia affect people across all race and social class lines and, while the most common age of onset is between 14 and 25, eating disorders do occur in a wide age range. Approximately 90% of those suffering from eating disorders are women so, for simplicity, feminine pronouns are used throughout this manual.

In this chapter, you will learn about many of the attitudes and behaviors that characterize the two eating disorders, anorexia nervosa and bulimia nervosa. You will also learn how the eating disorders can affect your physical and emotional well-being.

We began this chapter with a story about a woman whose day is marked by a struggle with food, weight, and shape. You may identify with part of her struggle, or you may find that it describes many of the days you have been having lately. Of course, like Lana, you are a unique person whose story cannot be duplicated with exactness. By virtue of having an eating problem, you do however have certain issues in common with others who also have an eating disorder. These are the issues that we have attempted to outline in this manual. As you read the manual, put a star beside a point that you find confusing or one that requires more elaboration than is given here. Bring it up at the next meeting where your group leaders will try to discuss the issue in a way that is more meaningful for you.

The Features of the Eating Disorders

The core features of anorexia nervosa and bulimia nervosa are summarized in the table below where it can be seen that both disorders share two common elements: extreme concerns for weight and shape, and attendant practices of weight control. The additional symptom of binge eating is present in bulimia nervosa, and maintenance of a low body weight is present in anorexia nervosa. For people who maintain a low body weight and binge eat, their problem is referred to as anorexia nervosa of the bulimic subtype. Let's review each of these four core features in turn.

Core Features of Anorexia Nervosa and Bulimia Nervosa			
Feature	Anorexia nervosa (restricting subtype)	Anorexia nervosa (bulimic subtype)	Bulimia nervosa
Extreme concerns for weight and shape	present	present	present
Practices of weight control	present	present	present
Maintenance of a low body weight	present	present	absent
Episodes of binge eating	absent	present	present

Source. Adapted from Fairburn & Garner (1986).

1. Extreme Concerns for Weight and Shape

Concerns for weight and shape are by no means unique to someone who has an eating disorder but appear widespread among North American women who live in a society that places a premium on their slenderness. Yet for the individual with an eating disorder, weight and shape are of such fundamental importance in determining her self-worth as to render most, if not all, other pursuits secondary to achieving thinness. Much of her thoughts are filled with concerns related to the proportion and size of her body, with the overriding conviction that thinness is happiness and fatness deplorable. Here we will have a look at some of the common thoughts and feelings surrounding issues of food, weight, and shape.

The need to assert control over food intake and body weight. Those with eating disorders commonly feel a strong need to control their food intake and weight. They believe eating means failing in their rigorous attempt to assert will-power over their body and its appetites. They often set up a series of elaborate rules surrounding their eating habits and believe that if they break one of these self-imposed rules, chaos will follow. Control and self-discipline become forces that perpetuate the eating disorder and are often the only means by which those with eating disorders can make themselves "feel good."

As an individual with anorexia or bulimia, you may feel as though you are unable to stop starving, exercising, or purging, and that you may never begin to eat normally again. You may even feel that giving into your hunger means that you have "lost control," that you have "failed," and you end up feeling badly about yourself for breaking your strict dietary rules. Such "losing control" may lead you to punish your body in one way or another—through a new round of dieting, purging, or exercising—in order to repair the "damage" you've done.

♦ ♦ ♦ ♦ ♦ ♦ ♦

It is vitally important for you to understand you don't have the control you are struggling so hard to maintain. If you are letting your eating disorder tell you when, where, and what to eat (if it allows you to eat at all), then the eating disorder has you in its control. It is essential for you to realize you have lost confidence in your body's ability to regulate food intake and weight. By attempting to gain control over food and weight, you have lost touch with your body's ability to regulate itself.

♦ ♦ ♦ ♦ ♦ ♦ ♦

Fears of eating and weight gain. Eating can be extremely frightening for anyone with an eating disorder, particularly since most are terrorized by the possibility of gaining weight. You may attempt to manage this fear in a variety of ways: refusing to eat entirely; eating only diet foods; or purging the food, through laxatives or vomiting, that you would not otherwise allow yourself to eat. It is crucial to understand that you *can* learn to eat again. Through normal eating, your fears surrounding food and weight will gradually decrease. In Chapter 4 of this appendix, you will learn how to normalize your eating through the *nondieting approach*.

Anger toward the body. Those with eating disorders often feel angry with their bodies because they feel constantly betrayed by them. Despite self-starvation, purging, and exercising, the body is determined to defend its weight. You will learn about this "set point" concept in Chapter 3 of this appendix.

You may feel it is necessary to your well-being that you become or remain thin. If you believe that your body is not conforming to this wish, then you may feel angry and frustrated with it. Others may assure you that you look fine or even too thin. They don't seem to understand that you still feel fat and uncomfortable with yourself.

♦ ♦ ♦ ♦ ♦ ♦ ♦ ♦

You should try thinking about why you feel uncomfortable with your body size. Body dissatisfaction is often a clue that there are deeper feelings of personal distress.

♦ ♦ ♦ ♦ ♦ ♦ ♦ ♦

A sense of personal ineffectiveness. Someone with an eating disorder may feel so insecure about her own strengths and accomplishments that she finds weight control to be the one area in which she knows clearly whether she is performing well or not. Without such a secure measure of success, she may feel lost and inadequate. We all need barometers or guideposts to tell us how we are doing in life. However, for someone with an eating disorder, the weighing scales, fit of her clothes, or tape measure often provide a more powerful message about personal effectiveness than a school grade or a performance appraisal at work.

Eating disorders generally develop during periods of change when individuals feel unable to meet the demands, challenges and stresses of a new situation. As a way of coping with these changes, someone at risk of developing an eating disorder will focus her attention on food, weight, and shape issues. So much time and energy is invested in controlling food and weight that other challenges cannot be adequately addressed and dealt with.

You may have decided that changing your body will help you make important decisions and help you to cope with the demands of your world. You may have thought that changing your shape would allow you to assume a new "healthy" identity. With this you hoped would come the confidence necessary to live with other changes in your life. There may have been brief periods of time when you have been less preoccupied with eating, as a result of traveling, involvement in a project that was particularly important, or by starting a new relationship. These, however, are not permanent solutions, and you may have found your attention swinging back, perhaps to feelings of low self-worth, and certainly to your problems around food and weight.

♦ ♦ ♦ ♦ ♦ ♦ ♦ ♦

It is important to realize there are a number of emotional concerns that the eating disorder cannot resolve. Some of the problems may have even been created by the chaos of the eating disorder. That is why it is so critical for you to work on normalizing your eating behavior before these emotional concerns, if they exist, can be meaningfully addressed.

♦ ♦ ♦ ♦ ♦ ♦ ♦ ♦

A drive for perfection. Those with eating disorders may believe that achieving anything less than personal excellence means complete failure. Many have trouble accepting a performance that is less than perfect because they feel it reflects upon their worth as a person. They tend to judge themselves by what they do and how others respond to their achievements, not by who they are. If you feel this way, then you may perceive your weight and appearance in these all-or-none terms as well. You may feel as though you can't settle for anything less than the "perfect" shape because you believe weight is under your personal control.

◆ ◆ ◆ ◆ ◆ ◆ ◆ ◆

It may surprise you to know weight is not a factor you are free to determine. Because of this, efforts to feel good about yourself that are based solely on success at weight control will ultimately not work. Instead, you can learn to base self-esteem more broadly, anchoring it in self-awareness and acceptance.

◆ ◆ ◆ ◆ ◆ ◆ ◆ ◆

Confusion and guilt. Many individuals with an eating disorder tend to be confused about who they are and what they want. Their desire to be thin represents a need to "create" a successful, beautiful, and intelligent person. Even if others perceive these qualities in them, they may still feel as though they are impostors.

You may feel guilty and confused about leading what you perceive to be a double life. To the world you may attempt to appear poised, confident, and in control of your body, but on the inside, you may feel insecure and confused because of chaotic eating habits. You may temporarily feel euphoric when you are "successful" at restricting your intake and losing weight. However, breaking any of your rules around food and weight may devastate you and cause you to diet more strenuously to make up for these "mistakes."

Those with eating disorders often feel guilty and ashamed if they eat in front of others, or if they eat anything other than the "good" (e.g., diet) foods. The eating disorder is seen as a shameful secret that cannot be shared.

◆ ◆ ◆ ◆ ◆ ◆ ◆ ◆

It is essential to understand that weight control will not help you to sort out inner confusion or permanently raise self-worth. Dieting will only serve to perpetuate the eating disorder and distract you from addressing the underlying emotional issues.

◆ ◆ ◆ ◆ ◆ ◆ ◆ ◆

We have outlined above some of the common attitudes and feelings that individuals with eating disorders have about weight and shape issues. These concerns typically reflect the presence of broader issues that the person may be struggling with in her life. We have only touched upon some of the possible underlying issues that compel individuals with eating disorders to manipulate their weight and shape in the belief that thinness will bring about lasting happiness. It is the strength of this conviction that provides the fuel, or becomes the driving force, for the second hallmark feature of anorexia nervosa and bulimia nervosa: extreme practices of weight control.

2. Practices of Weight Control

Recent surveys confirm what we already know: body dissatisfaction and weight control are extremely common, particularly among women in contemporary society. Although most women would like to weigh less, very few go to such extremes to control weight as fasting, compulsive exercising, self-induced vomiting, and the misuse of laxatives and diuretics. Such practices of weight control are the rule rather than the exception among those with an eating disorder.

Caloric restriction. Dieting is the most common method of weight control among individuals with eating disorders. It takes on many forms, from following a diet plan in a book, attending commercial weight reducing clinics, to the most extreme form of outright fasting. Meals are skipped, portions are reduced, and certain food categories are banned, particularly those with a connotation for being "fattening."

There is nothing mysterious about diets. They all lead to the restriction of calories below that which your body demands for healthy functioning. When the restriction is severe enough, the body turns to its built-in energy stores and utilizes the adipose (fat) tissue to make up for the energy deficit. Consequently, one begins to lose weight.

◆ ◆ ◆ ◆ ◆ ◆ ◆ ◆

The body is equipped to handle short-term caloric reductions without much problem. Sustained caloric restriction is, however, met with many internal changes in the body. One consequence is binge eating. Bingeing is a natural consequence of caloric deprivation, and the bingeing symptom will persist as long as you continue to diet.

◆ ◆ ◆ ◆ ◆ ◆ ◆ ◆

Self-induced vomiting. Self-induced vomiting is a method by which many with an eating disorder attempt to avoid the unwanted calories ingested during a binge episode. Vomiting typically begins as a way of regaining control after overeating but results in an even greater breakdown in control since the vomiting "legitimizes" bingeing. The bingeing-vomiting cycle usually escalates and the individual may get to the point where she feels she must vomit any food which she fears will lead to weight gain. Vomiting leads to electrolyte disturbances that can pose significant health risks. Moreover, vomiting often fails to remove all calories from the stomach, so frequent bingeing and vomiting may not actually produce weight loss (Garner et al. 1985).

Laxatives and diuretics. These are dangerous and ineffective substances for avoiding calories. Laxatives primarily affect the emptying of the large intestine, which occurs *after* calories have already been absorbed in the small bowel. Diuretics merely rid the body of water and can cause an individual to become seriously dehydrated. These substances can also produce electrolyte disturbances leading to potentially serious medical complications (to be discussed later in this chapter).

Exercise. Without a doubt, exercise provides benefits to both the body and the mind; however, it has contributed to the increased pressure on women and men to achieve unattainable bodies. In 1983, the Canada Fitness Survey reported that two-thirds of active women ranked weight control as an important motivator for exercising (Canada Fitness Survey 1983). Many of those with an eating disorder often use exercise to burn off calories, a form of purging. Others will not allow themselves to eat unless they fill their quota of exercise for the day. One of the dangers of excessive exercise in combination with restrictive dieting is the intense strain placed on the heart. It is also important to note that exercise never fully compensates for the decline in metabolic rate that results from excessive dieting.

3. Maintenance of a Low Body Weight

Anorexia nervosa involves self-imposed starvation to the point where the individual maintains a weight that is well below a level necessary for healthy functioning. Many attain this low weight by reducing from a higher level during their teens or young adult years. Others start dieting at an earlier age and therefore fail to gain as they become taller and older. It is absolutely necessary for those with anorexia nervosa to restore their body weight to a biologically optimal level in order to overcome the many effects of starvation. This weight is referred to as the set point, or natural weight and we will discuss this in Chapter 3 of this appendix.

Many individuals who have developed bulimia nervosa are also below their set point, or natural weight, even though they may appear to be of normal weight, unlike the emaciated appearance of people who are anorexic. Yet, they too will not experience relief from acute caloric deprivation and the urge to binge until they achieve a healthier weight. Others with bulimia nervosa are close to their natural weight, but fail to recognize this because of their chaotic relationship with food. Although the periods of restricted intake between binge episodes cause them to experience the effects of semistarvation, their binge eating allows their bodies to maintain a weight that is often near or even above their natural weight range.

◆ ◆ ◆ ◆ ◆ ◆ ◆ ◆

In overcoming anorexia nervosa or bulimia nervosa, it is essential not to focus on weight gain. The focus should be on normal eating and getting well. It is important to realize that eating is not an indulgence to feel guilty about or afraid of; it is a basic requirement of life.

◆ ◆ ◆ ◆ ◆ ◆ ◆ ◆

4. Episodes of Binge Eating

This eating symptom is a feature of bulimia nervosa, although about one out of every two individuals with anorexia nervosa also regularly experience this symptom. An episode of binge eating is one in which the individual consumes an excessive amount of food in an uncontrolled manner, after which she feels self-disgust, guilt, or anxiety about possible weight gain. The speed of eating and type and quantity of food eaten are all experienced as beyond one's control. Binges typically involve calorie dense carbohydrates that are usually avoided except when binge eating. The eating is almost always done in secrecy and often ends only at the point of running out of food, being interrupted by others, or becoming painfully full with swelling of the abdomen. The eating may be preceded by strong food cravings, particularly for high-calorie food mainly in the form of carbohydrates (e.g., sweets, bread, ice cream, pastry, potato chips). The eating may also be preceded by feelings such as anxiety, depression, frustration, or boredom. These moods may be the result of an unpleasant experience such as an argument with someone, doing poorly on some task, or finding it difficult to fill unstructured time. During the binge, one is distracted from these unpleasant thoughts or feelings, but they invariably return when the binge has ended.

Most people with the binge eating symptom are perplexed and guilt-ridden about their chaotic eating behavior. Many regard themselves as "emotional eaters" and view their binges as temporary lapses in rigid self-control over food intake which occur when they are upset. Indeed, people frequently experience a worsening of mood just prior to binge eating. On the basis of this association between mood and binge eating, many people come to construe their binge eating as a method of coping with distressing thoughts and feelings. In most cases, this is a misconception of the mechanisms that really underlie binge eating. Negative moods trigger a binge *only* if the person is a chronic dieter. In a nondieter, even the most stressful situation or intense feeling will not lead to an episode of binge eating. It is also important to note that the feelings which often precede binge eating may be a direct consequence of a deprived nutritional state in the form of low levels of blood glucose.

Binge eating is a natural response to chronic dieting and sustained efforts to maintain a lower body weight. Without exception, individuals with this eating symptom are avid dieters who attempt to restrict both the quantity and type of food they consume in their pursuit of thinness or avoidance of fatness. Consequently, entire meals are often skipped. When meals are eaten, the amount and type of food is calorie sparing. The individual typically begins the day with a strong resolve to be a "good dieter" in terms of how much she will consume, but as the day progresses, mounting hunger and food cravings lead to increased preoccupation with food. Eventually this gives way to uncontrolled eating in the form of a binge if circumstances permit. This vicious cycle of undereating and overeating becomes self-perpetuating because the individual will once again resolve to be a good dieter tomorrow only to find herself binge eating at some point.

Nutritional deprivation can be habit forming. This means those with eating disorders develop relationships with food and eating habits that are difficult to escape. Thus, it is the process (dieting), not the substance (food) that is addictive. You "lose control" because you are deprived and not because you are addicted to a particular food. Your body actually needs the foods you think you are losing control over.

◆ ◆ ◆ ◆ ◆ ◆ ◆ ◆

It is essential for you to understand that once you normalize eating, you won't become compulsive with carbohydrates, desserts, and your "bad" foods because you won't be depriving yourself of them.

◆ ◆ ◆ ◆ ◆ ◆ ◆ ◆

From our review of the above four features of the eating disorders, it is clear that anorexia nervosa and bulimia nervosa are very similar. Specifically, extreme concerns about weight and shape, and practices of weight control are central to both disorders. In anorexia nervosa, the obsessive drive for thinness leads the individual to maintain a very low body weight, often to the point of emaciation. In bulimia nervosa, body weight is not dangerously low, but it is not necessarily at a healthy, natural weight either. The central features of bulimia nervosa are recurrent episodes of binge eating and the sufferer's attempt to counteract the fattening binge through self-induced vomiting, use of laxatives or diuretics, strict dieting or fasting, or vigorous exercise. About one in three individuals with bulimia nervosa has a prior history of anorexia nervosa. Among those with anorexia nervosa, about half engage in restricting only, while the other half regularly engage in the bulimic symptom as a consequence of their severe dietary restriction.

Relationship of Eating Disorders to Depression

A depressed mood, often involving self-deprecating thoughts and actions, appears to be common among sufferers of an eating disorder. Depression negatively affects areas of personality and interpersonal functioning, influencing the way we feel, the way we think, and the way we act. Some of the common signs of depression are

♦ Overwhelming feelings of sadness or being blue, down in the dumps;
♦ Loss of interest in most things previously considered pleasurable;
♦ Feelings of guilt, helplessness, and hopelessness about the future;
♦ Social withdrawal;
♦ Thoughts of self-harm;
♦ Diminished level of energy;
♦ Inability to concentrate; and
♦ Sleep difficulties.

For some individuals with an eating disorder, depression may have preceded the onset of their disorder. For others, depression occurs and persists following weight loss or chaotic eating patterns. Depression is a common by-product of semi-starvation that often improves when weight is restored and the eating is normalized.

Physical Complications

Estimates of the death rate for eating disorders range from 5% to 20% (Garfinkel and Goldbloom 1988). The most serious medical situation is the emaciated anorexic individual who induces vomiting, abuses laxatives, and engages in a vigorous exercise program. This combination of weight control methods increases the person's risk for heart problems through muscle wasting or perhaps an electrolyte disturbance. Many sufferers experience any number of distressing physical problems that are actually by-products of their eating disturbance. The discussion of the medical factors connected with eating disorders will be separated into two sections: complications of starvation, and complications of bingeing and purging (Kaplan 1988).

Starvation Related Complications

Most starved individuals have a lowered heart rate and low blood pressure. This may lead to dizziness upon getting up from a lying to a standing position and can result in blackouts. Starvation can also result in a reduction of the efficiency of the bowel, significant delays in stomach emptying, bloating, constipation, satiety problems, and abdominal pain. For the individual with anorexia or bulimia, this physical discomfort can help to make her feel more "fat" and guilty over eating, thus prohibiting her from normalizing her eating or triggering a purge.

Irregular menstruation, or loss of periods, is most common in underweight individuals but can also occur in women who are starved but still maintain a "normal" weight. Reduced body temperature is also a result of starvation, causing an intolerance to cold temperatures. This is a common complaint among starved and underweight individuals.

Complications Related to Bingeing and Purging

The stress of binge eating, self-induced vomiting, the use of large amounts of laxatives and/or diuretics, and excessive exercise place an individual in medical danger. Strenuous overexercising is a potentially dangerous activity in which anorexic or bulimic patients often engage.

Electrolyte imbalances.   Among other common physical effects of purging are the loss of protein and essential substances such as potassium, sodium, and chloride. Nerves and muscles (including the heart) need these elements, called electrolytes, in balance in order to function properly. Hypokalemia (low levels of potassium) can occur very quickly and is characterized by fatigue, muscle weakness, muscle spasms, irritability, and depression. Severe hypokalemia can cause irregular heartbeats and convulsions and may result in death due to heart or kidney failure.

Gastrointestinal problems.   Individuals with bulimia frequently have gastrointestinal complaints: bloating; fullness; and abdominal distress of varying degrees of severity, including constipation. Repeated vomiting may cause painful inflammation of the throat or esophagus and may also result in tears in the lining of the esophagus. The abuse of laxatives causes stomach discomfort, cramping, and often constipation and leaves the person weaker because her body has not had the opportunity to absorb fat, protein, and calcium through the walls of the intestine.

Nutritional deficiencies.   Nutritional deficiencies may occur as purging prevents appropriate absorption of protein, carbohydrates, and fats as well as fluids.

Swelling.   The use of laxatives has a minimal effect on caloric absorption and thus, on weight loss. Any weight loss that occurs following the use of laxatives or diuretics (water pills) is the result of fluid loss. Once dehydration occurs, however, there is often rebound fluid retention for 48 to 72 hours. This leads to swelling, which often makes the individual feel bloated and fat, which in turn helps to perpetuate the cycle of restricting food, bingeing, and purging.

Dental problems.   The loss of enamel and dentin on teeth is a common result of frequent vomiting, as are numerous cavities. Brushing teeth after vomiting does little to prevent this from happening, as it only serves to rub the acid into the teeth.

Chapter Summary

In this chapter, you have learned about the core features of the eating disorders and many of the emotional and physical problems that can accompany them. If any of the issues raised in this chapter are confusing to you, bring them up at the next meeting where your group leaders will try to discuss the issue in a way that is more meaningful for you. We will have more to say about the physical and emotional effects of dieting and starvation in Chapter 3 of this appendix.

2

The Multidetermined Nature of the Eating Disorders

◆ ◆ ◆ ◆ ◆ ◆ ◆ ◆ ◆

I t is difficult to outline what causes anorexia nervosa and bulimia nervosa as both eating disorders are *multidetermined*, meaning there is a combination of societal, individual, and family factors that play a role in the development and perpetuation of an eating disorder. Rather than interpreting these as distinct causal factors, it is best to see them as factors that make a person vulnerable to the development of an eating disorder.

Eating disorders are not solely disorders of eating. Rather, they develop as a result of multidetermined and self-perpetuating problems in the perception and expression of how an individual sees herself in the world (Bruch 1978). Some individuals are unable to effectively deal with the stresses and challenges that accompany life and, given certain precipitants or stresses, the vulnerable individual may turn to dieting as a "solution" to the problems and challenges she faces. The effects of semistarvation resulting from this dieting only magnify the underlying problems and entrench her in an eating disorder (see figure).

In summary, a person is *predisposed*, or made vulnerable, to the development of an eating disorder as a result of a combination of factors (societal, individual, and family). The eating disorder is *precipitated* by a stressful event or time of life, and then *perpetuated* by many of the original causal factors, as well as the effects of the eating disorder itself. The following sections will explore many of the predisposing factors.

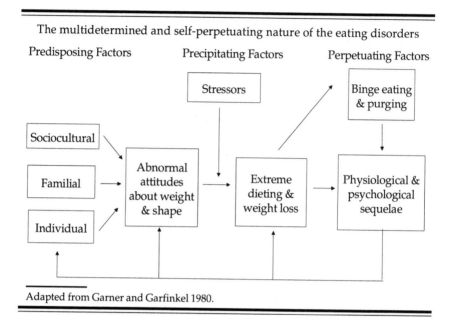

The multidetermined and self-perpetuating nature of the eating disorders

Adapted from Garner and Garfinkel 1980.

Sociocultural Factors

Society's Pressures to be Thin

A 1984 *Glamour* survey asked readers to answer the question, "What would make you happiest?" A full 42% of the respondents put weight loss at the top of their lists. Success at work ranked second (22%), a date with "a man you admire" ranked third (21%), and hearing from an old friend ranked fourth (15%) ("Feeling Fat in a Thin Society" 1984). Obviously, weight had a significant effect on the self-esteem and happiness of these women.

And why not? The media "promises" that women with low weights and svelte shapes will be happier, more sophisticated, better at their careers, more socially successful, and generally will lead a better life. Yet it is absurd to think success should be directly linked to weight. How do abilities improve with weight loss? They don't. But women sometimes define themselves by the acceptability of their bodies—abilities, intelligence, and personality having less to do with their perceived value as a person. Society clearly communicates that one of the most important roles for women is to look attractive. The media perpetuates and reinforces this and implies that the totality of women is expressed through their bodies; one glance at someone encompasses their whole being.

A woman's attractiveness is also tied to her ability to maintain a youthful appearance—in particular, maintaining a body shape resembling that of a prepubescent female. It is essential for women to adopt other yardsticks for measuring self-worth and for improving their feelings in this area. Youthful appearance will fade over the years, and bodies inevitably lose their youthful shape. However, skills and knowledge will always be valued and can always be improved upon.

Changing Roles for Women

Women today are bombarded with the message that they must become "super-women." Aside from possessing the all-important perfect body, they must also have perfect careers and perfect marriages and must be perfect mothers. Current role models are portrayed in unrealistic television or advertising images: thin, wealthy, sexy, beautiful, successful women. Women feel they must have it all and live up to the "modern women" seen in the media. At the same time, women continue to be socialized to be caregivers and nurturers, roles that strongly conflict with the new role of being initiators who assert their own needs.

Feelings of ineffectiveness can become a pervasive problem for women who face role conflicts. Whereas men tend to attribute problems to external factors instead of themselves and take personal credit for success, women tend to blame themselves if something goes wrong and credit external factors for success (e.g., "I was lucky"). They want their bodies to match the unrealistic ideals they are bombarded with through the media, and they believe it is due to some fault of their own that they don't "measure up." This thinking is undoubtedly harmful to their self-esteem.

With all of the stress involved in trying to "have it all," some women may feel their lives are out of control. Body weight is sometimes viewed as the one area of their lives over which they can assert personal control. Or perhaps they believe that by obtaining the perfect body, the perfect career and marriage will follow. For others, dieting and eating disorders offer an escape from daily pressures through an all-consuming obsession with food. Manipulation of weight and shape becomes a full-time occupation that diminishes one's capacity to effectively meet the challenges of life.

It has only been in this century that societies in the West have become so preoccupied with thinness. Before that time there were realistic models in local communities to emulate, not just image after image of thin fashion models. The relentless pursuit of thinness in the 20th century can be compared to the use of corsets in the Victorian era. At that time, women caused themselves severe harm by wearing corsets so tight that they broke their ribs. The processes are the same; there is an attempt to mold shape, be it through corseting or dieting, in search of an unrealistic ideal of beauty.

What is "over" weight today was considered beautiful and healthy in the 17th or 18th century, and even nowadays, for most of the world, body fat is widely accepted. Some theorists say that whereas body fat was once a sign of affluence, indicating the individual had ample food to eat, today in Western societies, because access to food is taken for granted, thinness has become the status symbol.

A study of women who were *Playboy* centerfolds and Miss America Pageant contestants has shown their average body weights and shapes progressively diminished between 1959 and 1979: bust and hip measurements have become smaller, and waist measurements have become bigger. Over these same 20 years, however, there was an increase in the average weight for women in the general population, particularly those in young adulthood. The "ideal" body shape, as determined by *Playboy* and the Miss America Pageant, is getting thinner while actual women are getting larger. This creates a vast disparity between the ideal and the real for most women (Garner et al. 1980).

Women diet in an effort to resolve this disparity. A 1978 Nielsen survey reported that 56% of females age 24–54 periodically dieted, 76% of them for reasons of appearance rather than health (Nielsen 1979). The Canadian Weight Gallup Poll conducted in 1984 showed only 17% of women in Canada "eat what they want" (Gallup Canada 1984). More than 80% of women dislike their bodies ("Feeling Fat in a Thin Society" 1984). Dieting and weight control have thus become a concern for females from nine-year-olds (King et al. 1986) to the very old (Health and Welfare Canada 1988). And why not? Women are constantly told to diet and to feel guilty for eating. A survey of women's magazines from 1969 to 1978 found the number of diet articles had nearly doubled from the previous decade (Garner et al. 1980). This is further exacerbated by the fact that the vast majority of women exercise, not usually for physical fitness, but for weight control (Canada Fitness Survey 1983). Health is really not the primary goal of diet and exercise in our culture; beauty is. Health concerns are only used to give legitimacy to these practices.

The Glorification of Eating Disorders

Anorexia nervosa is not glamorous but has nevertheless become associated with intelligence, upper social class, achievement, and perfection. The self-control, perfectionism, obsessiveness, and need for achievement that are characteristic of individuals with eating disorders are highly valued traits in our society. One myth that has developed over the years is that eating disorders only affect "rich little girls." In reality, both anorexia and bulimia affect individuals from all socioeconomic and racial groups. They also affect individuals of all ages and both men and women. Through glamorization, anorexia and bulimia are made to appear less serious and widespread than they actually are.

People often joke about wanting to "get a mild case of anorexia." It is not a joking matter. Someone suffering from anorexia nervosa or bulimia nervosa is obsessed with food and eating, with little or no time left over to be good at what she does at work or school. She begins dieting to be "more popular" or attractive, but due to the nature of eating disorders—the attitudes and beliefs about food and eating, and the intense fear of weight gain, coupled with the psychological and physical effects of starvation—she only becomes further socially isolated and less content with herself.

♦ ♦ ♦ ♦ ♦ ♦ ♦ ♦

The pursuit of thinness never leads to lasting happiness. In fact, the natural human goals to pursue happiness and greater personal contentment become less achievable as one becomes more entrenched in the eating disorder.

♦ ♦ ♦ ♦ ♦ ♦ ♦ ♦

Your goal for happiness must be recognized and encouraged, not your eating disorder. You need to learn strategies to pursue happiness in life, and realize the pursuit of thinness denies you the very things you hope to achieve.

♦ ♦ ♦ ♦ ♦ ♦ ♦ ♦

Prejudice Against Obesity

Prejudicial practices against the obese are among the few remaining socially sanctioned prejudices. If we ever hope to understand eating disorders, we will have to understand the stigma society places on obesity. Similarly, the elimination of eating disorders requires that we eliminate this prejudice. There are four widely shared, inaccurate stereotypes about obesity that perpetuate prejudice against heavy people.

"The obese eat more than the nonobese." In 19 out of the 20 studies conducted before 1979, obese people were shown to eat the same or less than people who were nonobese, thereby disproving the view that obese people are heavy because they eat more (Wooley and Wooley 1979).

"The obese have more psychological problems than the nonobese." Several studies have shown that obese people have no more and no fewer emotional problems than nonobese people. Personality and level of adjustment also appear to be similar for both groups *despite* the fact that the obese must deal with tremendous social pressure against them.

"Moderate obesity is associated with increased mortality and morbidity." Some studies have extrapolated the health risks associated with extreme obesity to those who are moderately obese as well. But the Framingham study (Sorlie et al. 1980) showed the highest mortality or death rate for women was for those who were underweight. The lowest mortality rates were for women who were 10% and 20% over average weight. Although increased blood pressure and death due to heart disease may be associated with being "over" weight, there is speculation that it is the effects of dieting, losing weight, and then regaining the weight that accounts for the increase in blood pressure, and consequent heart disease.

"Long-term treatment through dieting is successful." Several long-term follow-up studies have shown that the success rate of diets over time is dismal at best. It has been estimated that only 5% of obese individuals maintain a weight loss of at least 20 pounds for 2 years or more (Garner et al. 1985). If diets work, why is there a new best-selling diet book on the market each month? Why do weight-loss centers have repeat customers? Most people believe it is merely a matter of poor self-control. This belief ignores the facts about dieting and only perpetuates women's feelings of low self-worth around weight "control" issues.

Individual Factors

Who Develops an Eating Disorder?

It is virtually impossible to outline "the profile" of an individual at risk to develop anorexia nervosa or bulimia nervosa. The ways in which starvation and eating disorders actually affect personality make it difficult at times to separate those aspects of personality that are a result of the eating disorder from those that are part of the true personality, from before the onset of the eating disorder. However, there are individual traits that may serve to predispose an individual to develop an emotional problem or to have difficulties coping with stress.

Problems With Autonomous Functioning

A possible predisposition to anorexia nervosa and bulimia nervosa is the difficulty some individuals have with autonomy—in other words, in experiencing a sense of personal identity. This leaves the individual unable to function separately from the family or other external "guideposts." Bruch (1973) has related a vulnerability to eating disorders to difficulties with autonomy and mastery over one's body that she describes as "personal ineffectiveness." This feeling of ineffectiveness may result in difficulties when the individual is placed in situations where there are new expectations (e.g., a change in school, job, neighborhood, intimate relationship). For the individual vulnerable to eating disorders, these situations set the stage for her body to become a symbol and source of autonomy, control, and identity. She may then misinterpret thinness as a sign of specialness, and weight loss and deprivation from food as indications of self-control (Garner and Davis 1986).

Self-Esteem Deficits

People develop beliefs or images about who they are that constitute their "self-concept." The degree to which individuals approve of their self-concept is known as "self-esteem." The less similar their self-concept is to what they would consider to be ideal, the lower their sense of self-esteem (Tschirhart and Donovan 1984).

Levels of self-esteem vary widely through both sexes; however, it is more often women who have lower self-esteem. Self-esteem among women is often not generated internally, but linked to external factors such as appearance, performing for others, and responding to the needs of others for approval. An individual may feel so insecure about her relationships and performances that she concentrates on weight as the one area in which she is assured of "success" and acceptability. Women with a particularly low sense of self-esteem during a crucial period of their lives may turn to appearance oriented criteria to raise this faulty sense of self-worth. The tragedy is that dieting efforts will neither help sort out problems nor permanently raise self-worth.

Individuals with eating disorders use weight and shape as essential means of assessing their worth. Once in the cycle of an eating disorder, some individuals have reported that it is too "scary" to give up. The anorexia or bulimia or the thinness has become their identity, or it alone is what makes them feel "special."

As a result of poor self-awareness, many individuals with eating disorders tend to be confused about who they are, where they belong, and what they want. They may allow and encourage parents or intimate friends to make decisions for them because of internal confusion and fear that their choices will not meet with parental or peer approval. Quite often what the anorexic or bulimic individual projects to the world does not reflect her inner reality of fear, insecurity, and confusion.

Drives for Perfectionism and Self-Control

Perfectionism is common among those with eating disorders. Many sufferers attempt to alleviate their underlying feelings of ineffectiveness by pressuring themselves to strive for perfection. They often believe that anything less than perfection is not good enough; if they can't do something exactly right the first time, in many cases, they are afraid to attempt it at all. These attitudes are carried over into feelings about food, weight, and shape: many individuals believe they must maintain the perfect or "ideal" body at any cost.

A woman may believe that changing her body will help her make important decisions and establish interpersonal effectiveness, and help her to cope. She may also believe that changing her shape will enable her to transform herself and assume the confidence necessary to deal with other challenges in her life. Her desire to be thin is, in many cases, the need to create a new identity: a successful, beautiful, and intelligent one.

Surprisingly enough, perfectionism actually reinforces feelings of ineffectiveness, setting an individual up for repeated failure. Each time she sets an unrealistically high expectation in her drive for perfection, the woman reinforces her feelings of inadequacy because the goals she has set are usually impossible to attain. Perfectionism stresses being free of fault instead of being a capable individual. In emphasizing flawlessness, perfectionism simply doesn't allow for being human. And, given that body weight is not something we can easily or permanently alter, women who try to achieve the "perfect" body inevitably fail because they can't master their biology.

It is common for those with anorexia and bulimia to believe it is necessary to maintain rigid control over their bodies and their lives. This may result from feelings of powerlessness and of being controlled by outside forces. Messages received from family members or through cultural institutions such as the media often influence whether or not an individual feels powerful, effective, or capable. If underlying feelings of powerlessness develop and are not resolved, they will surface at times when the individual feels situations are beyond her control and may cause her to use weight manipulation as a coping mechanism, as a way to feel in control. As one woman put it: "You view every single day as a battle against food; each morning is the beginning of a new struggle against your weight, and the end of each day is a short-lived success or a repeated failure in the fight for control."

One of the most frustrating and damaging aspects of this behavior is that individuals with eating disorders don't have the control they are struggling so hard to attain. Cycles of starvation and deprivation control the individual and dictate when, where, and how she will eat. It is crucial for you to understand that you can learn to eat again and that *normal eating* is the key to getting back the control in your life.

Fear of Maturation

Eating disorders often develop in adolescence during a period of numerous changes: sexual, physical, and emotional. There are changes arising from the transition from childhood to adolescence, and once again accompanying the move from adolescence to adulthood. Some individuals are simply unable to deal with these changes. Both these periods are generally accompanied by some weight gain, which could act as a precipitating factor. It has been noted that early puberty and a tendency toward being "over" weight at a young age may be a predisposition to developing an eating disorder (Garfinkel et al. 1987).

The fear of maturation and the increased independence this requires may result in an individual seeking out a way to deal with her fears or avoid them. Individuals who develop an eating disorder in adolescence often seem "stuck in childhood" and may not have had the type of encouragement to help them develop the thinking of an adult. Instead, they often think like a child in extremes (good vs. bad, all vs. none). They view themselves as either obese or thin and can't see the middle ground of a healthy weight. This dichotomous way of thinking serves to perpetuate the eating disorder.

Family Factors

Some people tend to lay the blame for the development of eating disorders on poor family communication and relationships. In fact, whether eating disorders are caused by poor family relationships or actually cause some of the problems in the family can be difficult to say. Seeing one's child starve herself would result in complex feelings and behavior in most families; anger, anxiety, and guilt are common emotions (Garfinkel and Garner 1982). In addition, it is not unusual to see struggles for control between parent and child if the child has been starving herself.

It is far too simplistic and unfair to say an individual develops an eating disorder because of her family situation. The importance of looking at anorexia nervosa and bulimia nervosa as multidetermined disorders must be emphasized. There is a combination of forces in play that may lead to the development of an eating disorder. Although familial characteristics may predispose someone to an eating disorder, it is their interaction with an individual's constitutional makeup and the cultural factors that determine whether this predisposition will result in an eating disorder.

Families tend to reflect larger social conflicts, attitudes, and ideology. Women may learn the social conflicts about roles and functioning through the family. Thus, low self-esteem and a sense of personal ineffectiveness can be engendered in the family. Attitudes about weight can also be passed on among the family members. There is some concern that the incidence of eating disorders will increase among the next generation of young women as the parents of today are the most weight obsessed ever.

Certain family characteristics have been identified that may predispose an individual to developing an eating disorder. These include:

♦ Lack of conflict resolution;
♦ Parental overprotectiveness;
♦ Rigidity, unbendable rules, no compromise is possible;
♦ Blurring of generation boundaries (e.g., daughter taking on many of the roles usually associated with mother);
♦ High parental expectations;
♦ A family history of depression or alcoholism; and
♦ A history of sexual or physical abuse.

Again, it is important to note that family problems on their own do not produce anorexia nervosa or bulimia nervosa. They may, however, represent one among many vulnerability factors.

Chapter Summary

Eating disorders are not solely disorders of eating. Rather, the eating disorder may be the manifestation of underlying difficulties with autonomy and identity. Some individuals are unable to effectively deal with the stresses and challenges that accompany life and, given certain stresses, the vulnerable individual may turn to dieting as a perceived solution to the problems and challenges she faces. As will be shown in the next chapter in this appendix, however, the physical and psychological effects of dieting only magnify the predispositions and problems and entrench an individual in an eating disorder.

3

The Regulation of
Body Weight and the
Consequences of Dieting

♦ ♦ ♦ ♦ ♦ ♦ ♦ ♦ ♦

There are certain physical responses to dieting that serve to precipitate and perpetuate eating disorders. The human body is not concerned with the "ideal" that society dictates. In fact, in most cases the body may actually fight it, making it difficult for individuals to reach and/or maintain their perceived "ideal" weight through dieting (Bennett and Gurin 1982). The truth of the matter is that the vast majority of dieters fail to maintain significant weight loss in the long run. Given this fact, we need to understand why dieting is so ineffective in producing permanent changes in weight. Unfortunately, most women see the struggle and the failure at dieting as evidence for their lack of willpower, or in some cases as a sign of general worthlessness. This may drive them to drastic measures in their attempts to lose weight. Among individuals with some of the other predispositions to an eating disorder, dieting is typically the first step along the road to developing an eating disorder.

Effects of Starvation

Whether it is a result of restricting intake or bingeing and purging, anorexic patients, bulimic patients, and restrictive dieters are nutritionally deprived. Even though individuals with bulimia nervosa may be at a statistically "normal" weight, they are suffering to a certain degree from the effects of deprivation. This deprivation comes about in two ways; from the long-term restriction of calories and the subsequent loss of weight, and in the short run, from skipping meals or not eating enough during the day. This observation is alarming to most people with bulimia nervosa who believe the exact opposite: that they are consuming far too many calories and should be able to eat much less. Every aspect of our functioning requires nutrients as well as calories. When not getting enough, the body reacts in a variety of ways both to try to conserve energy and to prompt the person to eat. As we will see in the following sections, many of the symptoms observed in women with eating disorders are actually the result of not getting enough calories.

In a classic study conducted at the University of Minnesota in the 1940s, completely healthy male volunteers were exposed to a 6-month "starvation" diet in which they ate approximately one-half of their usual intake (Keys et al. 1950). This restriction resulted in weight loss of, on the average, 25% of body weight, which is equivalent to that in anorexia nervosa and often even in bulimia nervosa. Although there were many individual differences in the way these men responded, it was concluded that when food is restricted and weight loss occurs, individuals will experience significant physical and psychological changes *that eventually reverse during nourishment and weight restoration.*

Changes in Eating Attitudes and Behavior

Like many individuals with an eating disorder, the men in the Minnesota study became preoccupied with thoughts about food and eating as a result of starvation. Not only did they spend a great deal of time planning how they would eat their ration of food, but they became completely absorbed in eating once mealtime came around. The men had difficulties focusing on day-to-day activities because intrusive thoughts of food and eating interfered with their concentration. Much of their experience became centered around food; they dreamt and talked about food, many began reading cookbooks and collecting recipes, and some even changed careers and entered food-related occupations. The consumption of tea and coffee and gum chewing became so excessive that these substances had to be limited by the researchers conducting the study.

Bulimia

All of the men experienced an increase in hunger during weight loss. Although for some this did not affect adherence to the diet, for others the urge to eat became overwhelming and some men experienced episodes of binge eating. During the nourishment phase, many of the volunteers lost control of their eating and ate more or less continuously once they started to increase their calories. The investigators wrote:

> Subject no. 20 stuffs himself until he is bursting at the seams, to the point of being nearly sick and still feels hungry; no. 120 reported that he had to discipline himself to keep from eating so much as to become ill; no. 1 ate until he was uncomfortably full; and subject no. 30 had so little control over the mechanics of "piling it in" that he simply had to stay away from food because he could not find a point of satiation even when he was "full to the gills." . . . Subject no. 26 would just as soon have eaten six meals instead of three. (Keys et al. 1950, p. 847)

Even after 3 months of refeeding the men often complained that they felt hungrier after eating a large meal. Although most of the men had normalized their eating patterns after about 5 months, some continued to have difficulties stopping eating, and for a subset this persisted after more than 8 months of nourishment.

Remember that these men were placed on a semistarvation diet as part of an experiment; they did not lose weight because they wanted to be thin. Binge eating in these men cannot be explained by a desire to punish themselves, or by a theory of addiction to food. Sometimes, psychological themes become superimposed on binge eating or can trigger specific episodes, but this only happens in the context of significant dietary restraint. The important point here is that there are marked differences between people in their response to starvation. For reasons that are still unknown, some individuals develop bulimia that may continue for many months after dietary restriction is relaxed.

Psychological Responses to Starvation

♦ Preoccupation with food
♦ Impaired concentration and memory
♦ Loss of interest and motivation to engage in activities previously enjoyed
♦ Depression, mood swings
♦ Irritability, anxiety, apathy
♦ Sleep disturbance

Over the course of the starvation period, some of the men experienced depression, outbursts of anger, irritability, anxiety, and apathy. They became progressively more withdrawn and isolated and less interested in spending social time with others. Even interest in sex declined. Not only were there changes in personality and temperament but also difficulties with concentration, alertness, and judgment. What is so surprising about this is that these were otherwise healthy men who did not show signs of emotional disturbance prior to weight loss. In fact, on a variety of screening tests, these volunteers were more psychologically robust than the average person prior to the starvation phase of the study. Once again, although some of the volunteers seemed to adjust fairly well, others developed psychological disturbances in response to losing weight. After normal eating was restored, it took some time before the emotional changes returned to normal levels, suggesting that weight loss and prolonged food deprivation, rather than short-term caloric restriction, are linked to these disturbances.

Physical Responses to Starvation

♦ Disruption of menstrual function in women
♦ Gastrointestinal discomfort and constipation
♦ Lowered metabolic rate, feeling cold
♦ Cardiac changes
♦ Thinning of scalp hair, growth of lanugo (downy hair)
♦ Dehydration
♦ Muscular weakness

Not surprisingly, the body's response to severe caloric restriction is a general slowing down of bodily functions. Of particular importance to our understanding of the effects of food deprivation is the decrease in basal metabolic rate, which is the rate at which the body burns calories while at rest. At the end of the starvation phase, the men's metabolic rate had dropped by about 40% from normal. This means that it becomes harder to lose weight while eating the same amount of food because the calories are being burned more slowly. The body adapts to having too few calories by trying to conserve energy; it uses incoming nutrients to maintain the basic physical processes that are necessary for survival. Metabolism sped up once the volunteers were refed, with the greatest recovery in metabolic rate seen in those who were eating the largest amount of food. It seems that once metabolism has been suppressed, it needs a "fuel injection" in order to get the wheels turning more quickly.

Importance of the Starvation Study for Understanding Bulimia

Many of the behaviors noted in the Minnesota starvation study are common features of eating disorders, directly related to starvation and not to emotional instability. You may have experienced many of these symptoms yourself and not been aware that your psychological experiences and physical concerns were, in large part, the effects of nutritional deprivation. Because many of the symptoms that have been thought to cause these disorders may actually result from undernutrition, it is vital that weight be stabilized or restored and nutrition improved as the essential first part of recovery. It is only after the effects of starvation have been removed that possible issues independent of the eating disorder can be accurately dealt with. Normalizing eating not only stabilizes emotional state, but relief from the preoccupation with food frees up one's capacity to focus on these other underlying issues.

One could argue that all of the starvation effects described here are understandable in light of the amount of weight lost by these men. You may be looking at your own weight history and find that you have never lost that amount of weight. As you will learn later in this chapter, the same metabolic changes and tendencies to overeat occur in women who diet, regardless of their actual weight or weight loss.

During refeeding, a temporary "rebound" effect was observed in the men's body weights and percentage body fat. On the average, after 8 months, they gained back to their original weight plus about 10%; over the next 6 months, their weight gradually declined. As they restored their eating, a large percentage of the weight gained was in total body fat. Many individuals with bulimia nervosa and anorexia nervosa "feel fat" during the recovery process; it is important to remember that for these men the increase in fat during refeeding was only temporary. They returned to their original levels of total body fat and body weight by the end of the 1-year follow-up period.

The starvation study shows that the body does not simply reprogram itself to maintain a lower weight obtained by dieting. Similarly, just as the body "fights" weight loss by slowing metabolic rate, it is equally rigorous in defending gains above a certain level. In studies where normal weight individuals were overfed by as much as several thousand calories a day, they did not gain as much as would be expected given the amount of food they had eaten. In one study, male prison volunteers were fed double their usual intake over a 6-month period with the goal of gaining 20–25% of their weight (Sims et al. 1968). Although the first few pounds were gained fairly easily, the total amount of weight gained was about 75% less than that expected considering the number of calories they were eating. For the majority of men it proved to be a tremendous undertaking to reach the goal weights of the study, because their metabolism sped up to burn off most of the excess calories they were consuming.

When overfeeding is discontinued, weight, for the most part, returns to the original level. The body reacts to excess calories by burning up extra energy through a process called "diet induced thermogenesis." Although there is some debate about the importance of this in people, it certainly plays a major role in energy regulation in animals.

For people who are not dieting, it is very difficult to push weight significantly up; it takes thousands of extra calories to produce weight gain. Think about people you may know who are not always restricting their intake. Think about how much their weight seems to fluctuate. Weight remains quite stable over long periods of time in individuals who do not closely monitor their food intake against energy output. A little arithmetic shows that if you consistently ate 100 calories more than usual each day, you might expect to gain about 10 pounds over a year. That is equivalent to only an ounce of cheese, one piece of bread with butter, or a large apple eaten as a snack! The fact is that although most people's calorie intake does vary from day to day, their weight stays pretty much the same, give or take a few pounds.

Set Point Theory

Just as individuals have a predetermined height, there is a "set point" weight that the body tries to defend, one which it appears cannot be permanently changed through restrictive dieting (Bennett and Gurin 1982). This set point will fluctuate by 5 to 10 pounds in most people and should be viewed as a range, rather than a specific weight. The notion of set point makes sense from an evolutionary perspective since animals most certainly would have died when food was scarce if there was not an internal mechanism for regulating weight. This theory helps explain why dieters fail to keep weight off in the long run and why some people eat more than most without gaining weight.

Many individuals with bulimia nervosa are below their set point for body weight and will not experience relief from deprivation and the urge to binge until they achieve a healthier weight. Other individuals with bulimia nervosa are close to their natural weight but fail to recognize this because their eating patterns are so chaotic. Although the periods of restricted intake between binge episodes cause them to be affected by the effects of semistarvation, their binge eating allows their bodies to maintain a weight that is, in some cases, near their natural weight range.

It is common for those with eating disorders to find that, although they resolve to restrict their intake during the day, they end up consuming many more calories later during a binge (because of extreme biological pressure to eat). For some people, the cycle of dieting and bingeing may actually cause them to gain weight beyond what they would weigh if they were eating normally and allowing their body to do what it is already equipped to do—regulate weight.

Factors influencing set point. Just as different people have different heights, we also have different natural weights. Some people naturally have a lower set point than others. There is much debate about where this mechanism exists and exactly how it is defended. We do know that any one individual's set point depends on hereditary factors (Price 1987; Stunkard et al. 1986).

During development, at certain times such as adolescence or pregnancy, set point appears more flexible, and there are a number of factors that influence the "setting." Stress level, age, cigarette smoking, and exercise appear to have some impact on regulated weight. However, the effect of any of these factors is quite small, and one must seriously question whether a few pounds is worth, for example, the life-threatening dangers of cigarette smoking.

Set point and weight loss. The set point concept challenges many culturally shared stereotypes about obesity. We have no difficulty accepting that height is unchangeable. It would be ridiculous to expect short people to grow or tall people to shrink because a certain height may be considered more attractive! Being heavy is like being short. In an ideal world, many women would certainly prefer to be 5' 6" rather than 5' 0" or 6' 0". If there was a surefire way to attain that height, we would likely see clinics specializing in height change. And if there were no complications or side effects to the methods, and if the results were permanent or at least easy to maintain, the attendance at these clinics by people unhappy with their height would make sense. Unfortunately, "treatment" programs for obesity fail to achieve long-lasting weight reduction, and the consequences for even trying can be devastating to emotional and physical well-being.

One of the few long-term studies of the effectiveness of "therapeutic fasting" found that almost all of the 121 individuals were able to lose weight initially (Johnson and Drenick 1977). Although most maintained the loss for 1 year, 50% of the group regained all of the weight lost within 2 years. Nine years later, only 6% weighed less than they did originally, and more than 25% weighed more than they did before the fast. These results, along with those from many similar studies, argue against the popular notion that all one needs is willpower to successfully lose weight. Your own diet histories are the most powerful testimony to the extreme difficulty in keeping off unwanted weight. You have probably tried every method available for losing weight: commercial programs, grapefruit diets, fasts, and so on. Each new diet promises to be the one that will finally work.

Even if you have been able to maintain a weight loss, your attendance here in the Psychoeducation Group illustrates the drastic methods you need to use to keep it off and how much suffering this causes. It is not simply a matter of motivation because you would likely top the scale for wanting to lose weight; rather, it is evidence of the body's attempt to maintain a set level.

Dieting and the Energy Output Side

We now know a lot about the effects of dieting that may help to explain some of the profound frustration of trying to lose weight. At the beginning of embarking on a diet, it may be relatively simple to lose a few pounds as a result of water loss. But as you may have found, the dieter, regardless of her weight, often reaches a "plateau" where further weight loss is difficult, even when eating very little.

The body adapts to caloric deficits by slowing the metabolic rate to conserve energy. Dieting can result in reducing metabolic rate by an incredible 15–30% (Garner et al. 1985; Thompson and Blanton 1984). This means that you can continue eating the same low number of calories on your diet and not lose any further weight. One study showed that when caloric intake was reduced from 2,000 to 1,500 calories a day, the amount of weight lost was cut in half each month (Apfelbaum et al. 1971).

The longer one diets, the more the body will fight against further weight loss.

Women who have lost a substantial amount of weight but can't seem to lose more have been found to have very low metabolic rates, lower body fat, and have lengthy dieting histories compared to women who are able to reduce further in weight (Miller and Parsonage 1975).

It is not only the length of dieting that affects metabolic rate but also the cycling between dieting and nondieting. With each new diet, weight is lost more slowly and is later regained more readily than on the previous diet (Bennett and Gurin 1982). With repeated attempts to restrict intake, it takes longer for metabolic rate to recover and metabolism drops more readily when there is a return to dieting.

Weight is gained more easily after dieting. When starved rats are refed, they gain as much as 18 times more weight than nonstarved animals fed the same amount (Boyle et al. 1978)! Women hospitalized with anorexia nervosa gain weight at a rate much higher than would be predicted by the number of calories consumed during renourishment.

Your current eating patterns virtually guarantee that you won't lose a significant amount of weight. Many women with bulimia nervosa achieve a weight from this process that is higher than their weight before the dieting started in the first place. When you can convince your body that it won't be restricted of energy, your metabolism will catch up to your intake and your body will reassume the self-regulating process of controlling your weight.

These facts are important in understanding the effect of your eating cycles. Like many individuals with eating disorders, you may either start your day eating as little as you can and end up bingeing later, or go in cycles of days of dieting followed by days of bingeing. Weight loss will become more difficult each time you embark on a new diet or start a new day of restriction, and the calories eaten during the inevitable binge are less likely to be burned as fuel and more readily stored as fat.

Dieting and the Energy Input Side

Just as we saw with the volunteers in the Minnesota starvation study, many of the differences between individuals in the way they respond to food have less to do with their actual weight and more to do with whether or not they are dieters. In one study, college women were classified as dieters or nondieters. Under the guise of a "taste experiment," they drank either one milkshake, two milkshakes, or no milkshakes and were then asked to "taste and rate" several flavors of ice cream. The real purpose of the experiment was to see what effect these "preloads" had on later ice cream consumption. The results were surprising—the dieters ate more following a preload than they did after no milkshakes. On the other hand, nondieters ate the most when they were not given a preload, less after one milkshake, and still less after two milkshakes. Nondieters seemed to regulate their intake well in this situation, whereas dieters "counterregulated" by eating more if they had already eaten and less if they had not (Herman and Mack 1975).

This seemingly paradoxical pattern may sound familiar to many of you. In fact, it has been proposed that mechanisms similar to those that produce this "counterregulatory" eating in normal dieters also play a role in bulimia nervosa (Polivy and Herman 1985). One theory to explain why the dieter eats more following a preload is because she has already exceeded the number of calories prescribed by her diet; since she has already "blown it," she feels that she may as well continue eating.

Many individuals with bulimia nervosa have rigid all-or-none rules about "good" and "bad" foods. Eating even a small amount of a "bad" food can often trigger a binge. Usually the foods eaten during binge episodes are the very foods that are avoided when dieting. You may be thinking that there is something inherent in higher calorie food that leads to overeating; that higher calorie foods are somehow more "addictive." Further research has shown that it is the dieter's belief that the preload is high in calories that "disinhibits" eating, regardless of the actual caloric content of the food eaten.

Depression, anxiety, and the intake of alcohol have all been found to increase eating in dieters (Polivy and Herman 1983). The effect of all of these factors makes sense in light of the caloric deprivation experienced when dieting. It requires considerable mental effort to maintain self-control in the face of mounting biological pressure to eat. Any event that interferes with this effort, such as eating a "fattening" food or feeling stressed, may temporarily lead to the breakdown in one's resolve to diet.

Chapter Summary

Binge eating is a natural response to chronic dieting and sustained efforts to maintain a lower body weight. Without exception, individuals with this eating symptom are avid dieters who attempt to restrict both the quantity and type of food they eat in their pursuit of thinness or avoidance of fatness. Consequently, entire meals are often skipped. When meals are consumed, the amount and type of food eaten is calorie sparing. The individual typically begins the day with a strong resolve to be a "good dieter" in terms of how much she will consume, but as the day progresses, mounting hunger and food cravings lead to increased preoccupation with food. Eventually this gives way to uncontrolled eating in the form of a binge if circumstances permit. This vicious cycle of undereating and overeating becomes self-perpetuating because the individual will once again resolve to be a good dieter tomorrow only to find herself binge eating at some point.

For all individuals with eating disorders, this vicious cycle is perpetuated by an extreme dietary stance toward food. This stance is characterized by rigid rules which dictate what, when, and how much they allow themselves to eat in the service of promoting weight loss or preventing weight gain. These rules are usually characterized by a dichotomous, all-or-none style of thinking about food, and when they are perceived by the individual to have been broken, it frequently triggers an episode of binge eating. Consuming even a small quantity of "forbidden food" often leads to the thought "I have blown my diet; now I will satisfy my food cravings and continue to eat—tomorrow I will start my diet again." It is only once the individual begins to interrupt this pattern by eating normally that urges to binge subside and metabolism has the opportunity to recover from its suppressed level.

4

Developing a Healthy Relationship With Food: The Nondieting Approach

$$\blacklozenge \ \blacklozenge \ \blacklozenge \ \blacklozenge \ \blacklozenge \ \blacklozenge \ \blacklozenge \ \blacklozenge$$

In order to overcome your eating disorder, you must begin to normalize your food intake. Because intensive and prolonged dieting has likely caused you to suffer from the effects of deprivation, you must begin thinking about normalized eating as the only means of reversing many of the physical symptoms of the eating disorder, and as the most crucial step in overcoming it. When you begin practicing a program of nondieting, hunger and satiety sensations begin to normalize while the other effects of deprivation will gradually dissipate. In particular, the frequency of binge-eating episodes will gradually decrease.

Nondieting Means:

♦ Eating in response to hunger and learning to stop when you feel full, rather than eating according to personal dietary rules;

♦ Allowing yourself to eat normal portions of food from all the food groups;

♦ Eating protein, fat, and carbohydrate, including the calorie-dense foods that you undoubtedly avoid;

♦ Eating the equivalent of three nondieting meals a day; and

♦ Eating at least 1,500 calories a day.

The key to nondieting is persistence. Remember, your eating behavior is not something that suddenly developed. It has taken a long time for your current relationship with food to evolve, and you must expect it will take a reasonable amount of time to change. Your eating behavior may be so closely connected to your feelings of well-being and self-worth that you will not be able to challenge and change your eating habits overnight.

It is important not to become discouraged if you work on nondieting yet experience some setbacks. If you have bulimia nervosa, you may feel an urge to binge for a period of time even after normalization, but the desire dissipates with time and continued normalization of food intake.

If you are unable to eat 1,500 calories a day, begin normalizing by gradually increasing your intake. Perhaps in this way you can reduce the fear surrounding normalized eating.

◆ ◆ ◆ ◆ ◆ ◆ ◆ ◆

It is impossible to fully recover from anorexia or bulimia while dieting. Dieting leads to deprivation which, in turn, creates fears of eating and causes bingeing and purging behaviors. To overcome the physical effects of an eating disorder, it is absolutely essential to begin practicing a program of nondieting.

◆ ◆ ◆ ◆ ◆ ◆ ◆ ◆

What is a Nondieter?

A nondieter is one who eats pretty much what she wants when she wants without the fear of uncontrolled weight gain. In other words, a nondieter eats according to biological need rather than according to how much she prefers to weigh. Nondieters begin to eat when they are hungry and stop eating when they are full, the latter called satiety. For a long time, you have probably not paid attention to your hunger signals and may in fact be confused about what hunger really is for you. By the same token, you may not know when you have achieved physical fullness or satiety because of years of eating calorie sparing amounts of food. Adopting a nondieting stance toward food ensures that you will eventually come to detect when you are hungry and when you are full, and eat according to these physical cues. Achieving this state may take a little time so it is vitally important that you begin to eat in a "mechanical" fashion.

What is Mechanical Eating?

Those recovering from eating disorders learn they must follow a program of mechanical eating until they can respond to hunger and satiety cues. Mechanical eating means establishing and sticking to a pattern of nondieting that includes eating breakfast no later than an hour after you awaken, having lunch 3–4 hours after your first meal, and dinner in the early evening. Meals must be treated as medicine and given the highest priority in your day. You should eat according to your predetermined schedule of intakes and *not* according to appetite or personal dietary rules. It is very important not to skip meals. Simply put, skipping meals during the day sets you up for a nighttime binge.

◆ ◆ ◆ ◆ ◆ ◆ ◆ ◆

Your goal is to eat three nondieting meals each day: one in the morning, one around noon, and one in the early evening, as well as occasional snacks in between.

◆ ◆ ◆ ◆ ◆ ◆ ◆ ◆

What is a Nondieting Meal?

A nondieting meal is one in which an independent observer would probably conclude that you were not eating calorie sparing foods and not on a diet. If you have trouble with this concept, think about what another female, who you know is not actively dieting, eats in a typical meal. This will invariably include a wide variety of foods from the different food groups in an amount that is enough to sustain her for part of the day. You may find it helpful to draw up a meal plan in the morning or a day in advance in which you outline when and what you would like to eat during each of the three nondieting meals. This plan will help protect you from *undereating* in situations where

♦ You become confused about how hungry you might be and therefore question your need to eat;
♦ The choice of available food is too great to make on-the-spot decisions about what you want; and
♦ The available food is too limited, in which case you can shop ahead of time or plan to go somewhere where the supply is sufficient.

This plan will also help protect you from *overeating* in situations where you have consumed a healthy, nondieting meal and yet still feel you want more. In this situation, you can fall back on your meal plan to control how much you eat during any given meal because you may not yet be able to rely on your satiety cues. These cues will come in time through your sustained efforts at nondieting. To help you better understand some of the amounts and varieties of food composing a nondieting meal, a few examples are given at the end of this chapter.

When you begin to normalize your eating, your stomach may distend or swell after you eat and take a while to empty because your body isn't accustomed to digesting normal amounts of food. Your stomach will return to its normal size as the food is digested. You can minimize distention by avoiding foods that are particularly difficult to digest. You may want to avoid raw foods for the first few weeks of nondieting (e.g., cook vegetables instead of eating them raw).

You may also experience abnormal bowel movements because your bowels aren't used to normal amounts of waste or because you may have been abusing laxatives. However, the problem will correct itself as your system becomes accustomed to a regular pattern of eating. If you are having problems with constipation during the period of normalization, make sure that you drink plenty of fluids and eat high-fiber foods. If you are constipated for several days, consult your doctor. Avoid laxatives, however!

Control of Bingeing During the Washout Phase

Those working to overcome their eating disorder have often experienced problems with overeating when beginning to normalize their eating behavior. This is due in part to the fact that they haven't yet learned to respond to fullness cues. We refer to this period of the recovery process as the washout phase: Nondieting while possibly experiencing gastrointestinal problems (e.g., prolonged bloating after a meal, impaired satiety sensations, and perhaps having urges to binge). It is important to avoid overeating as it may lead to bingeing and the urge to purge. If you are anorexic, it may lead you to develop bulimic symptoms.

Bingeing Can be Avoided by:
♦ Following the program of mechanical eating. You won't be allowing the feel-

ings of hunger to mount through the day because you will be eating at regular intervals; and

◆ Leaving the eating area when you have finished your nondieting meal.

You may still feel an urge to binge or purge even after the first few weeks of normalized eating. Although the impulse will lessen as you and your body become more accustomed to nondieting, there are specific things you can do to cope with the urge. One useful technique is to rehearse a series of coping phrases to repeat when you feel the urge to binge.

◆ "This urge is strong now, but I know it will reduce to a tolerable level in a little while so I must just ride it out."

◆ "One reason I want to keep eating beyond the meal I just consumed is because my stomach is not yet signaling to me that I am full. In an hour or so I will feel satisfied so there is no need for me to binge now."

◆ "I know that part of my problem is that I get confused between real emotions and my urges to binge eat. The urge I feel right now is not a physical one because I have nourished myself today with regular nondieting meals."

The most effective prevention technique is to continue eating your nondieting meals even though you may feel a strong urge to restrict your food intake. If you are experiencing difficulty eating a normal meal, you might repeat one or more of the following phrases to yourself.

◆ "This food will not lead to uncontrolled weight gain."

◆ "Eating nondieting meals is a necessary part of getting better."

◆ "I know that my hunger and satiety cues are confusing to me, so I must eat mechanically rather than how I feel I should eat."

◆ "Eating this nondieting meal will prevent me from binge eating tonight."

◆ "I must take food as though it were medicine."

More Coping Strategies for the Washout Phase

Many who recover from an eating disorder have developed ways of coping with eating during their nondieting efforts. The list below contains some of the more common and helpful suggestions they have come up with.

Start breaking your dietary rules slowly. If you have a rule that says you can't eat breakfast, try beginning to eat a little bit: a piece of fruit, an egg, some bread—anything. Then leave the eating area at the point when you are starting to feel uncomfortable. This will protect you from giving in to the urge to binge and will help you to break some of the rules you have constructed around eating.

Eat more of the foods you already allow yourself and gradually begin to introduce the foods you haven't allowed yourself in the past. Even if you can only initially accept small portions of nondieting foods—bread, pasta, chocolate, peanut butter, meat—allowing yourself to eat them at all is the first step. If you binge on certain foods, it is important to introduce those foods into your diet in normal amounts and to practice not bingeing on them. This will serve to inoculate you against future binge eating of such foods.

Begin trying to eat regular, standard portions. This is all part of trying to break those dieting rules that control your eating behavior. If you have difficulty in knowing what a standard portion of food is, copy the amounts eaten by a nondieting person or use restaurant portions as a guide.

Start thinking about throwing out your diet foods. This might include eating regular salad dressing instead of diet dressing, drinking soda or fruit juice in place of diet drinks, and using sugar instead of artificial sweetener.

Initially it may be easier for you to eat five or six smaller meals a day instead of three larger ones. Because it may be difficult for you to digest normal portions, eating smaller amounts more often may make it easier to increase your intake comfortably. If you are afraid that a nondieting meal will set off a binge episode, try eating until you've reached a comfortable limit, then stop. Leave the table and repeat the process again a few hours later. This procedure may help you to avoid bingeing. You will discover that the amounts you can comfortably eat will increase. Before you know it, you will be able to cope with a regular meal and not fear bingeing.

Eat in nonthreatening environments. If you don't feel comfortable eating with others, then schedule your meals alone. It may take a while for you to feel comfortable about eating in public. However, it is important not to use this as an excuse for not eating. Sometimes it is good for individuals with eating disorders to try eating in restaurants or other public places. The meals are composed of nondieting amounts of food, and a public place may provide a greater inhibition from bingeing. Try to relax when you eat. Listen to music, read a book, and try to sit down. Make the atmosphere as comfortable as possible.

Find ways to distract yourself after you have finished a meal. You   don't want to sit and think about the fact that you have food in your stomach. Take a walk, call a friend. Some people find it helpful to keep a list of these distractions to refer to.

Give yourself other pleasures. This is particularly important if you feel the urge to binge or are upset about your weight. Make a list of the ways you can reward yourself. Start thinking about the things you can afford (in terms of time or money) and implement them when you are feeling low. Taking a long hot bubble bath, seeing a movie, visiting a museum or art gallery, writing letters, or reading a book are all ways of giving yourself some pleasure.

Learn to exercise for pleasure, not to burn calories. The key is not to approach exercise as a way of punishing your body or of losing weight. Walking, swimming, and movement classes are all good forms of physical activity that will promote feeling positively about your body. Exercise does help to lower your set point, but only marginally (by 5% in some studies). A healthy balance seems to involve a program of moderate, enjoyable physical activity coupled with normalized eating.

Stop weighing yourself. The scale will only upset you and sabotage your attempts at normalization. Instead of focusing on your weight, concentrate on eating normally and giving up your obsession with food. Remember, eating normally will not necessarily make you obese. There are many weights between excessive thinness and obesity, one of which you will naturally settle at. Keep in mind that your natural weight range is not one number. When you reach your natural weight, it will fluctuate about 5–7 pounds up or down from time to time.

Get rid of your unrealistically "thin" clothing. Clothes can sometimes act as a scale does in helping you to monitor your weight. If your more tight-fitting clothes become too small, try to see it as an indication that you are getting well.

Keep a private journal. Record what you eat, when you eat, if you binge, purge, and exercise, and how you feel. You may be able to detect patterns. Record the information right after you finish eating. This will help you to judge whether or not you are eating properly, what you should increase, and when you should be eating more. Recording your feelings may also help you discover what emotions tend to trigger a binge, and when you are most vulnerable to restricting intake.

Stop purging. Purging through vomiting, laxative abuse, or vigorous exercise is very hazardous to your health. Moreover, they legitimize the binge by reducing the anxiety or guilt associated with the inevitable weight gain. When you eliminate purging altogether, you tremendously reduce your chances of bingeing (assuming, of course, that you are eating regular nondieting meals).

Treat each meal as an independent event. Your goal is to complete each meal, and your decision to eat must not be influenced by what you have already eaten or what you plan to eat later on in the day.

Treat food as though it were medicine. Think of your nondieting meals as medicine and give them the highest priority just as you would if you were prescribed a medication for a physical problem. Remember, the best "medicine" for an eating disorder is nondieting.

Sample Nondieting Meals

PLEASE NOTE: THIS IS NOT TO BE USED AS A DIET—IT IS A GUIDE. BE FLEXIBLE. THE IDEA IS TO ENSURE YOU FOLLOW CANADA'S FOOD GUIDE. THE FOLLOWING MEAL PLAN IS DESIGNED ONLY TO GET YOU STARTED ON YOUR WAY. THE TOTAL DAILY INTAKE IS IN THE 1,500–2,000 CALORIE RANGE.

BREAKFAST

1 protein:	2 oz. cheese *or* 2 eggs *or* 2 tbsp. peanut butter
1–2 carbohydrates:	1–2 pieces of bread with butter *or* 1 bagel with butter *or* 1 cup of cereal with milk *or* muffin

1 fruit or juice

LUNCH

1 protein:	2–3 oz. of cheese *or*

	3–4 oz. of salmon, tuna, chicken, or egg, mixed with mayonnaise or mustard, *or* sliced meats
1–2 carbohydrates:	1–2 slices of bread *or* 1 cup of beans, cereal, pasta, *or* 1 cup rice *or* 1 potato
2 or more vegetables:	1 tossed salad with dressing *or* stir-fried, cooked, or baked vegetable with sauce

1 fruit or juice

Meal Suggestions for Lunch:

A) Sandwich with bread, mayonnaise, cheese (or meat or mixture of meat and cheese) *with*
   vegetables on sandwich, or in side salad with dressing *with*
   fruit or juice
   optional: yogurt/milk/soup
B) Quiche with vegetables, cheese, or meat (or mixture or meat and cheese) *with*
   side salad with nondiet dressing *with*
   fruit or juice
C) Soup *with*
   large salad with cheese or meat (or combination) *with*
   roll or bun *with*
   fruit or juice
   Optional: Milk or yogurt (especially if there is no cheese or meat on the salad)

DINNER

1 protein:	3–4 oz. serving of meat or fish—hamburger, salmon, tuna, chicken, meatballs, meat sauce, etc. (if you wish to decrease the meat, you must increase the amount of carbohydrates), *or* 2–3 oz. serving of cheese *or* 2 eggs *or* beans or tofu (usually found in Chinese, Mexican, or Middle Eastern cooking)
1–2 carbohydrates:	1–2 pieces of bread *or* 1/2 to 1 cup of pasta (if you decrease meat or other protein you must increase carbohydrate) *or* 1/2 to 1 cup of rice (amount depends, once again, on protein intake) *or* potato with butter *or* bun
2 or more vegetables:	side salad *or* 3/4 cup of 2 different vegetables, 1/2 cup of three different choices, *or* 1-1/2 cups of mixed vegetables

Meal Suggestions for Dinner:

A) 1–2 vegetables or 3/4 cup each (or above options) *with*
   1/2 cup of rice, corn, or pasta, or potato with butter *with*
   4 oz. of meat, chicken, or fish prepared with butter and sauces (or decrease
   amount of meat and increase potato, rice, or pasta)
B) Hamburger on bun *with*
   side of vegetables or vegetables on hamburger (with french fries occasionally)
C) 1 cup of spaghetti and meat sauce or lasagna *with*
   salad and dressing or other side of vegetables
D) Sandwich (as described above) *with*
   soup and/or salad
E) Chinese, Mexican, or Middle Eastern food (same portion as a nondieting person)

SNACKS

1–2 snacks a day—These are necessary because nondieting people sometimes become hungry between meals. These are not to be eaten instead of a meal.

> nuts or granola
> cheese and crackers
> fruit yogurt
> peanuts
> fruit

DESSERTS

3–4 times a week—After a meal, or as a snack, not in place of a meal.

> a few cookies
> a piece of cake or pie
> 2 scoops of ice cream
> 1 chocolate bar

Chapter Summary

Complete recovery from your eating disorder will come about only when you achieve freedom from dieting. Consequently, you must work hard at becoming a nondieter so that you eventually eat pretty much what you want when you want without irrational fears of uncontrolled weight gain. This involves eating in a mechanical fashion in the form of three or four nondieting meals per day. A nondieting meal involves a wide variety of food in amounts that are not calorie sparing. Your goal is to consume not less than 1,500 calories per day spread over regular nondieting meals that you may have to plan in advance to protect yourself from undereating and overeating. With sustained efforts at nondieting, the frequency and intensity of your urges to binge eat will decrease in a short period of time. Along with this you will experience relief from troublesome gastrointestinal problems and the return of normal hunger and satiety sensations. Remember, persistence in your nondieting efforts will pay off for you in the long run; in the short run, it will require considerable effort on your part and it may not be fun, but it will be worth it! The goal is to achieve physical and emotional well-being.

5

Effective Coping: Attitudes About Weight, Shape, and Dieting as Impediments to Recovery

♦ ♦ ♦ ♦ ♦ ♦ ♦ ♦

From previous chapters in this appendix, you have learned that normalized eating is the only way to overcome the physical and psychological effects of deprivation that result from strict dieting. Eating normally is a necessary but insufficient first step on the road to overcoming an eating disorder. You may believe "intellectually" that many of these principles make sense. As you reflect back upon your own dieting history, you may recognize the link between being deprived of food and bingeing. You may have set a personal goal of being able to eat normally and get through the day without bingeing and without being so preoccupied with food. But you may at the same time have difficulties letting go of the fantasy of what life would be like if you were thinner. You may wonder how you can replace the good feelings you have about yourself when you exert control over your eating.

You may be afraid of relinquishing "control" and giving up dieting. For many individuals with anorexia nervosa or bulimia nervosa, weight loss is a sign of being in control, a barometer to measure how well one is doing. Personal control and feelings of effectiveness are certainly desirable goals that are universal. We all struggle with finding ways of feeling in control of our lives and being in control of what happens to us.

But although the goal of feeling in control is normal and admirable, attempting to achieve these feelings through dieting is ultimately self-defeating. Since dieting inevitably leads to bingeing, any good feelings that result are always short-lived and can never really be counted on. There is always at the back of your mind the fear and risk of losing control. Real lasting control comes from making choices. When you choose to do one thing rather than another based on your own personal values, goals, likes, and dislikes, you are in the driver's seat. Making decisions and choosing options is often difficult and sometimes frightening. It takes a lot of practice to feel comfortable and confident in your choices. In this section, you will learn about some strategies to develop more enduring feelings of control, and to interrupt the loss of control that occurs during a binge.

More Strategies for Interrupting Bingeing or Purging

Bingeing or purging can become an almost habitual response to emotional upset or eating "forbidden" foods. You may have had a bad day at work or an argument with a friend and automatically find yourself in the midst of a binge. It is critical to break this cycle and to begin to examine what you are upset about. Practice using these strategies as soon as you feel the urge to binge or soon as possible after you have started eating. Remember, *these strategies will only be helpful if you have started to normalize your eating* and are experiencing some relief from the physical and psychological effects of food deprivation.

Distraction

The impulse to binge may be interrupted by distracting yourself from eating. In order for distraction to be effective, it must involve an activity which is powerful enough to override your anxiety for the moment. Listening to loud music, making a phone call to a friend, engaging in vigorous activity, or going for a walk are some ways of diverting your attention away from an urge to binge or purge.

Delay

Similarly, by delaying bingeing or purging, many people find that the strong urge to engage in these behaviors subsides in a short period of time. One way to delay is to construct a short list of activities that you must perform before bingeing or purging. These activities should be as enjoyable as possible. An example would be to listen to a favorite song and spend 10 minutes on a hobby or watching television. It may be helpful to write the list of prebinge activities on a cue card that can be referred to during a high-risk moment. Another method of delaying involves setting a specified amount of time that you must wait before engaging in the behavior that you are trying to avoid. Once you have practiced these strategies, you can try filling the delay interval with some of the steps to problem solving described later on in this chapter. When you are working out delay strategies for yourself, remember not to make the task too difficult. You may want to start with a short delay interval and gradually increase it over the following weeks.

Practicing Coping Phrases

It is often helpful to repeat coping phrases to yourself both at the early stages of gaining control over eating and at later stages to overcome temporary lapses in control. Depending on the situation, this involves rehearsing phrases such as the ones suggested here:

♦ "This one chocolate bar will not make me fat."
♦ "Vomiting now only increases its likelihood later."
♦ "Eating three meals a day is a necessary part of getting better."
♦ "Bingeing will not make my problems go away."
♦ "I will feel worse about myself if I binge."

If you have tried these strategies and still have an overwhelming urge to binge or purge, it is crucial to get back on track by eating normally during the next scheduled meal. Remind yourself that *you are still further ahead than before*—you were able to exert some control by simply putting off bingeing or purging for a period of time.

Binge Eating as a "Coping Mechanism"

Since binge episodes often occur in the context of emotional upset, many individuals view their bingeing as a "coping mechanism." You may not have learned how to deal with stress in healthier ways. You may even have experienced a sense of relief from stress during or after a binge. Even after eating is normalized, many find that they occasionally binge when feeling distressed. This does not mean that you are back to square one; rather, it is evidence that the process of recovery is not uphill all the way. It may have taken many years for you to develop your eating disorder, and it may take a long time to overcome it. It will be easier to deal with "slips" if you are prepared for them and if you learn some strategies to make them less likely to occur.

The first step is to understand the meaning that bingeing in response to stress may have for you. Some common themes described by individuals with eating disorders are discussed here.

"I sometimes binge to avoid dealing with things."

For some people who are flooded by overwhelming feelings, a binge may serve as a powerful distraction from the confusion or distress they are experiencing. However, the binge only serves to interrupt the confusion; it is a short-term "bandage," not a long-term solution to the problems they face. Inevitably, the problems that trigger the binge return and this leads to a self-perpetuating cycle of bingeing to get rid of negative feelings. One disadvantage of avoidance is that it doesn't give you the opportunity to develop skills to deal with problems more effectively. The other disadvantage is that it is like pushing a snowball down an icy mountain. When problems are not examined, they continue to grow until they seem completely unmanageable. As long as you avoid dealing with the real issues that bother you, you will not be able to look at things from a different perspective.

Often underlying the idea that avoiding uncomfortable feelings will make them go away is the belief that you should not have those feelings in the first place. You may believe that it is acceptable for other people to have negative emotions, like anger or jealousy, but that you are not allowed to have them. Or you may believe that you should be able to cope well under almost all circumstances, only to chastise yourself for imperfect coping. Many individuals with eating disorders have perfectionistic ideas about what effective coping is. Think about people you know and how they seem to deal with problems. Do they always have problems under control? How often do they get angry?

"I binge when I feel overwhelmed."

Bingeing in response to feeling overwhelmed is paradoxical because the guilt and self-condemning thoughts which follow a binge only add to distress. The binge heightens the feelings of personal ineffectiveness and loss of control that you may have experienced before the binge. Many individuals with eating disorders describe being flooded with feelings and have great difficulty identifying either what the feelings are or the reasons they have those feelings.

It is important to remember that feelings are always linked to the way we view situations in our lives. For example, you would probably have little reaction if someone pointed a pencil at your head. On the other hand, you would likely be terrified if that person pointed a gun at your head. The difference between the two situations is that a gun has a certain meaning to you—it represents significant danger.

In the same way, you will probably be very upset by criticism if you believe that you should always be perfect and never make mistakes. If you believe that it is acceptable to make mistakes, you will react to criticism as though it is a pencil, not a gun. Negative feelings, which are often potent triggers for binges, are signals to you about the way you think about yourself.

Challenging Attitudes

Although stress is often a reaction to the demands of everyday living, some of the "stress" that may precede a binge is the direct result of unrealistic thinking about oneself and other people. As you become aware of how this works, you can learn ways of challenging your attitudes to reduce the anxiety that is produced by unrealistic thinking. For example, people who accept a less-than-perfect performance as part of being human are not overly distressed when they make a mistake. It is only when you expect yourself to behave perfectly at all times that normal transgressions are experienced as failures. You not only believe that you have failed, but conclude that you as a person are a failure.

Those with eating disorders often share particular attitudes, beliefs, and opinions that affect the way they perceive themselves in relation to the world around them. One's belief system influences the kinds of relationships formed with others. It also determines how we cope with conflicts and problems in life. Such belief systems form the underlying causes and perpetuate the eating disorder. These thinking patterns, combined with especially difficult conflicts that individuals face at particularly vulnerable times of their lives, give rise to the attempted solution: *the false solution of weight control.*

Many of the thinking patterns common to those with eating disorders are described below. It is important to note some of these patterns stem from before the onset of the eating disorder, whereas some arise with the eating problem and serve to perpetuate it.

All-Or-None Reasoning

It is common for individuals with eating disorders to engage in dichotomous reasoning, or thinking in extremes. You may believe that if you can't be ultrathin, then you are going to be overweight. This way of thinking permeates all aspects of some individuals' lives. There is simply no intermediate ground for those who think in extremes; you may feel that you must either exist in a state of absolute control or utter chaos will follow.

You may believe that if you begin to eat normally you will lose all control and end up extremely overweight. When you think this way, you are thinking in extremes; ultrathinness and obesity are simply not the only alternatives. You now know that your body functions best at its natural weight range, which is somewhere in between ultrathin and obese.

One technique that may help you to avoid all-or-none reasoning is to begin recognizing all of the possible solutions to a problem. Even if you can't immediately implement any of the alternatives you come up with, at least you can begin recognizing that there are options. One good place to start is with your eating disorder; begin normalizing and prove to yourself that obesity is not the only alternative to thinness. We will outline some guidelines for looking at options later on in this chapter.

Personalization

Because their sense of self-worth is often dependent on what others think, many individuals with eating disorders have the tendency to personalize opinions and events that others would interpret impersonally. In believing themselves to be the focus of outside events, they reinforce their feeling of failure and their belief that others disapprove of them.

One technique that may help you is "decentering." It involves applying the same standards to others as you apply to yourself and seeing if you come to similar conclusions. For example, this is a common belief during the process of recovery:

"I can't go out because I've gained 5 pounds and everyone will notice how fat I am." One of the stumbling blocks to maintaining normal eating is real or imagined weight gain. Some people may gain weight when they stop dieting and others may simply "feel fat" after eating normal amounts. The idea that others are scrutinizing your behavior is a common one among individuals with eating disorders and often extends beyond food and weight. In order to view situations from a more objective standpoint, it is often helpful to ask yourself some questions. Do you really notice when someone has lost or gained a few pounds? Since you may be particularly sensitized to the issue of weight, it may be true that you pay some attention to other people's shape. Even if you do notice such fluctuations in others, is it a catastrophic event for them? How much time do you spend thinking about it? What do you really infer about the person? It would be nice if we were the object of other people's preoccupations, but most people are pretty busy with their own concerns in life.

Overgeneralization

Many women with eating disorders believe that if something turns out badly once, then it will always happen that way. Many tend to assert absolute control over their familiar environment and avoid exploring the unknown because they are afraid of a "negative" outcome. Individuals recovering from eating disorders have learned that if an undesirable experience results from a particular situation, the outcome doesn't always repeat itself.

If you began normalizing in the past, you might have rapidly gained a small amount of weight, and become so frightened by the possibility of obesity that you immediately stopped your efforts at normalization. You now know that your body was working to counter the effects of deprivation and was storing up calories because your metabolic rate was low. Just because you gained a small amount of weight did not mean that you were going to become obese, even though you thought it did. You overgeneralized.

Magical Thinking

It is common for those with eating disorders to establish causal relationships between what others would perceive to be unrelated events. Many believe that thinness equals happiness and success, that high-calorie foods are bad for the body, that individuals can only eat as much as they burn off in exercise or they will get fat, that perfection is necessary for self-fulfillment, and that self-discipline is a great achievement.

You may now hold some of these beliefs, but when they are examined more closely, do they make sense?

♦ If you have experienced ultrathinness, have you really become happy and successful? Or has it caused you to become more careful about your weight and even more fearful of obesity?

♦ You now know that high-calorie foods provide essential fuel for your body, so how can they be "bad"?

♦ Have you ever asked yourself why complete self-discipline is a great achievement? Does it really make you happy?

In tying happiness, success, self-fulfillment, and self-worth to thinness, self-discipline, and food restriction, you have virtually ensured the survival of your eating disorder. However, once you can begin to recognize that losing weight is not a necessary condition of self-esteem and self-fulfillment, then you can begin thinking about getting well and getting on with life!

Catastrophizing

Many women with eating disorders gauge how they feel about themselves by others' reactions. Although you may subscribe to the idea that it is not possible to be liked by everyone, you may privately believe that it would be awful if you did not gain another's acceptance. When your self-esteem is so intimately connected to external guideposts such as approval from others, your feelings about yourself are not under your own control.

It is easy to understand how this connection can develop. Women are reinforced for doing things that please other people, and this reinforcement feels good. The problem occurs when we don't feel good about ourselves unless our behavior pleases others: we end up sacrificing our own needs in order to get that prized reinforcement.

◆ ◆ ◆ ◆ ◆ ◆ ◆ ◆

When was the last time you did something that you really didn't want to do in order to make someone else happy? What do you think would have happened if you had said no? Would it really be as catastrophic as you imagined? Even if you did not like the consequences, was there anything you could have done to cope with the situation? When you demand of yourself that something must or must not happen, the inevitable result is upset.

◆ ◆ ◆ ◆ ◆ ◆ ◆ ◆

Problem Solving

Problematic situations are a normal part of everyone's life. When we disagree with parents, when we are choosing between two jobs, or when we don't like a friend's behavior, we may be faced with a problem. Scenarios like these only pose problems if there is no good response immediately available to us. The tendency to think in all-or-none terms may prevent you from seeing the range of solutions to a problem situation.

Because problems are inevitable, emotional distress and self-defeating behavior can often result from an ineffective approach to handling problems. You may recognize that you are more likely to binge or restrict when you are upset about a problem in your life. Or an equally common feeling is when you may feel frustrated or angry and not realize that this is because you are experiencing some kind of conflict. Particularly when it comes to our relationships with others, we may find ourselves in the midst of a problem before we understand what the problem is.

It is important to remember that not every problem can be solved and that not every solution is satisfactory. However, developing effective skills in problem solving can increase one's feelings of control and one's ability to cope with problem situations that inevitably arise.

◆ ◆ ◆ ◆ ◆ ◆ ◆ ◆

One of the most important points to learn about coping more effectively is to stop and think before doing, rather than acting impulsively on the first idea that you think of or resigning yourself to the problem and doing nothing. The strategies of delay and distraction teach you to do this—to stop and think before acting.

◆ ◆ ◆ ◆ ◆ ◆ ◆ ◆

The very first step in effective coping is to develop and explore attitudes toward life's problems. Be willing to take some risks and think about your situation from new perspectives rather than being locked into only one way of seeing your world. After we outline some of the other steps to problem solving, you may want to experiment with a specific problem you have been having lately.

Step 1. Identify and Define the Problem

You come home after a long day at work. You feel tired and drained and at the same time quite anxious. Your first urge is to go into the kitchen and eat. This is a signal to you that something may be bothering you and that you need to stop and translate your vague sense of distress into more specific and concrete details that are manageable.

Go over in your head some of the events that occurred that day. Just by reviewing the details of the day, you may begin to identify the problem that is bothering you. Let's say that you had an argument with a co-worker. What thoughts and feelings did you have about the argument? Consider not only the actual events that occurred but also your internal reactions to the situation. Think about all of the aspects of the situation that are relevant. For example, you may have had previous disagreements with this person. You may have had difficulty getting your work done because of your disagreement. You may have not let the other person know how you saw the situation and feel that you let your co-worker "walk all over you."

As you go over the specific relevant details, you may be able to define the problem and formulate some goals. In this example, your goals may be the following:

♦ To have a better relationship with your co-worker; and
♦ To act more assertively with people at work.

It is vital that you establish realistic goals for yourself. If you set your goals impossibly high, you will never be satisfied with the results.

Examine the conflicts in the situation. One conflict may be the desire to assert your feelings and opinions versus feeling uncomfortable asserting yourself.

Step 2. Identify Alternative Ways of Coping With the Problem

You may have already thought of possible solutions just by identifying the problem and formulating goals. You may feel "stuck," or you may only think of one or two extreme alternatives (e.g., you find yourself thinking in all-or-none terms). Good solutions to a problem are more apt to be found if you follow three principles:

♦ Defer judgment. Think of all possible alternatives before you rule any out. Consider even the most unlikely solutions as an exercise in learning the in-betweens.
♦ More is better. The more potential solutions that you consider, the more likely you will be to find one that is suitable. "Brainstorm" as much as you can.
♦ Start with the general and move to the specific. Identify a general strategy (e.g., talk to your co-worker) before you think of a specific plan to actually carry out a solution (e.g., exactly what you will say).

Step 3. Make a Decision

Once you have thought of all possible solutions, you need to determine the probable consequences of each. Keeping in mind that you may tend to see things in predictable ways, it is important to check that you are not overgeneralizing, magnifying the consequences, or personalizing.

If you find that it is hard to think clearly, you may want to take a few pieces of paper and write down each possible solution on a separate page. Consider what the pros and cons of each solution may be. In our example, some possible solutions and their consequences may be:

♦ Avoid contact with your co-worker. You may realize that this solution has some major drawbacks. At most workplaces, it would be almost impossible to avoid contact, particularly if you work on projects together. Previous experience may have also shown you that avoidance only creates more tension.

♦ Tell your boss that you are having problems with your co-worker. Consider whether this will help you to reach your goals of having a good working relationship and behaving more assertively.

♦ Talk to your co-worker. Think about the implications of this, and be realistic about what you can comfortably manage.

Making a decision is often an intuitive process; one of the possible solutions may emerge as the best alternative. Once you have chosen a general strategy for dealing with the problem, begin to plan out how you will carry it through. For example, if you choose to talk to your co-worker, you must work out how you will talk to him or her, what you will say, how to assert your opinions without sounding hostile, and so on. Be willing to take some risks and to do things that may be difficult.

Step 4. Carry Out the Solution and Evaluate Its Effectiveness

Once you have decided on a course of action and have carried it out, spend some time the next day reviewing the outcome. Did it meet your goals? Did what you expect to happen really happen? This final stage is important because it gives you the opportunity to check out whether your assumptions about the world are actually true. It also increases your repertoire of possible ways to handle difficult situations in the future.

Chapter Summary

Coping effectively is rarely as systematic as following a sequence of steps. Training yourself to approach problems with an eye to looking for alternatives and thinking realistically about the consequences is a more useful way to handle problem situations that inevitably come up. Think of these steps as a mental road map rather than a checklist. The next time you feel overwhelmed, accept that having problems is part of being human, stop and think about why you are distressed, and consider the realistic consequences of possible solutions to your problems. Try the solution and evaluate how well it has worked for you.

6

Developing a
Healthy Relationship
With Your Body

◆ ◆ ◆ ◆ ◆ ◆ ◆ ◆ ◆

F eeling more accepting of your body is one of the essential elements of recovering from bulimia. Working toward acceptance can be facilitated by looking at the sources of your current body image and "feeling fat."

What is Body Image?

Body image is the *representation* you make of your body to yourself and the *feelings and judgments* that you have about this representation. The representation includes how you perceive the actual size and shape of your body. If you over- or underestimate the size or shape of your body, this is called *body image distortion*. For example, you may believe that your body is larger than it actually is.

The feelings and judgments a person has about her representation of her body may include

♦ Approving or disapproving of her body;
♦ Judging her body to be bad (in a moral sense);
♦ Believing that other people judge her body negatively; and
♦ Being confused about sensations and feelings within her body.

When a person doesn't like her body or feels badly about it, this is called *body image disparagement* or *dissatisfaction*.

In our society, it is difficult for women to feel good about their bodies because so few women have bodies that naturally match the size and shape currently considered ideal. This very abnormal "ideal" body size and shape has encouraged the development of widespread body image dissatisfaction among women.

Displacement

For some women, body image dissatisfaction is only dissatisfaction about perceived body size or shape. For others, dissatisfaction with their bodies can be part of a more pervasive dissatisfaction with self. If a person is simply dissatisfied with her body, then changing it (e.g., changing its shape slightly through exercise) will make her feel satisfied. If she is also dissatisfied with herself, then changing her body will not make her feel satisfied—she will probably want to make more and more changes, always falling short of being really satisfied. To see how this can happen, it is important to understand the idea of displacement.

One example of displacement can be seen in the way little children use special blankets or teddy bears. Children under six often have one blanket or teddy bear that is very special to them, that they will not part with, even for washing, and which is most strongly held on to when they are unhappy or separated from their parents. One explanation for this phenomenon is that each child has displaced some of the feelings she has for her parent(s) onto the object (blanket or teddy). This is very useful because it allows the child to cope with upsetting feelings in the absence of the comforting parent. It allows the child to be separate from the parent and to keep the feelings of security associated with the parent close at hand by snuggling with the blanket or teddy. We might say that the child has taken the positive feelings of comfort and protection that originally arose in relation to the parent and displaced them onto the blanket or teddy. This is a very natural and adaptive way for the child to cope when separated from the parent.

Turning back to body image, you might be able to see how displacement can work within you. You can take feelings that first arise in relation to one aspect of yourself and displace them onto another aspect of yourself. Suppose that, as a result of a poor relationship, you feel unwanted. This is a difficult feeling to tolerate and also difficult to find a way to resolve. The feeling of being unwanted may be displaced onto your body so that you feel it is your body that is not desirable, instead of your whole self. The displacement allows you to solve a problem. Identifying your body as the problem may initially help you in several ways:

♦ It may diminish the power of the very negative feeling by localizing it;
♦ It may allow you to avoid an overwhelmingly painful idea by changing its nature; and
♦ It may allow you to believe that you now know how to deal with the feeling.

Although it may be very difficult to find a way to deal with the feeling that you are unwanted, it seems easy to deal with having a body that is unsatisfactory: you simply have to lose weight and exercise to re-shape your body until it is satisfactory. You may reason that as soon as your body is more ideal, people will love you and you will feel good about yourself because you are now lovable. It is here that the displacement fails.

How Displacement Fails

Displacement is not a foolproof tool to cope with distressing thoughts and feelings. Even for children who use teddy bears and blankets, there are situations in which their upsetting feelings really do require the presence of their parents for resolution (e.g., getting lost, a traumatic experience). There is a similar but more serious problem in the case of a person who has tried to change her body in order to feel more lovable. The effort to make her body more acceptable is endless.

◆ ◆ ◆ ◆ ◆ ◆ ◆ ◆

Because it really isn't your body that you originally feared was unwanted, fixing it won't make you feel that you are lovable, at least not for long. You will most likely feel that there is always something more about your body that needs fixing or improvement.

◆ ◆ ◆ ◆ ◆ ◆ ◆ ◆

Feeling Fat

Consider the possibility that when you "feel fat," you are actively displacing some feelings about yourself onto your body. Suppose, for instance, that you feel inadequate, ineffective, or out of control in your life, but have little idea about how to develop or strengthen feelings of effectiveness or being in control. You may *displace* these "bad" or intolerable feelings about *yourself* onto your *body*, resulting in your "feeling fat." Since fatness is, in our culture, often associated with inadequacy and being out of control, it is a likely candidate for displacement. The result of the displacement is that you will believe that you know what to do to feel better, more effective, and in control. You will simply LOSE WEIGHT.

We know, of course, that this won't work. You will never lose enough weight for long enough because weight or fat is not the real problem. Instead of solving your problem, you are likely to get stuck in a cycle of

◆ Disliking your body;
◆ Losing weight;
◆ Feeling a little better for a little while;
◆ Then feeling badly either because you gain weight or because something happens to make you feel ineffective or out of control in some other area of your life; and
◆ Then trying to lose more weight to feel better again.

This cycle is reinforced by the strong social pressure on women to be thin and our society's prejudicial attitudes about fatness.

How to Escape the Cycle

The key to escaping this vicious cycle is to break the displacement. In order to do this, you have to get to know yourself and your body enough to make some educated guesses about where displacement may be operating.

Get to Know Yourself

When you "feel fat," what dissatisfactions about yourself might this represent?

At-Home Exercise

Make a list of things about yourself you are most dissatisfied with, excluding any references to your body. Look at the list and ask yourself the following questions: Are these items rational? Would another person point these things out as problems for me? Am I being perfectionistic with personal

expectations so high that no mortal could ever reach them? Scratch off any items you think should not be on the list now. For each of the most significant items remaining on your list, enter something you could do to make yourself feel better. You might use the steps to problem solving discussed in Chapter 5 of this appendix. It is important to deal directly with the things about yourself that you feel dissatisfied with, but at a pace and with expectations that are possible to meet.

Get to Know Your Body

Women are used to experiencing their bodies visually and from the outside looking back at themselves, rather than kinesthetically, tactilely, and from the inside looking out. In fact, the tendency is for a woman to see a visual image of her body and to immediately compare it part by part with the media model of the ideal body. Her body becomes an object to be looked at, dissected, and compared, instead of being the place from which she acts as a whole and integrated person. How can you get to know your body better and begin to experience it as a whole, from the inside instead of as an appearance to be manipulated into the "right" shape?

Try a kinesthetic experience of your body. * Find a room that is large enough for you to walk around in, and wear comfortable clothing. Walk around the room as you usually walk and notice how you hold your body, what parts of your body you are most conscious of, and how you feel. Is there anything about your body that you are trying to camouflage? After a few minutes, stop and think of a time when you were angry. Walk around the room as you would if you were angry. How does this change the way that you hold your body, how you walk, and so on? Next, think of a time when you were ashamed. Walk around the room as you would if you were ashamed. How does this change the way that you hold your body, how you walk, and so on? Next, think of a time when you were proud. Walk around the room as if you were proud. How does this affect your posture, how you walk, how you hold your body, and so on? Now go back to walking the way you usually walk. What is different, if anything?

The way you move and feel in your body is probably more strongly affected by how you feel about yourself than how much you weigh. You can affect the way you move, and thereby the way you feel, by choosing an "affirmation" to move by. Make up a sentence that describes how you would like to move through the world (e.g., "I move with grace, confidence, and pride") and say it to yourself as you walk in your daily routine.

Try a visual experience that encourages seeing your body as a whole. Look in a full-length mirror and notice the usual judgments you make about various parts of your body ("good" and "bad"). Let them pass through your mind like birds flying through the air, acknowledging each one for its opinion as it flies by. Do this until there are no more "opinions" to be given. Then just look at your body as a whole, just being there. See if you can catch it just being there with nothing good or bad to say about it.

---

* Adapted from Hutchinson MG: Transforming Body Image: Learning to Love the Body You Have. New York, Crossing Press, 1985, p. 113, "Moving Attitudes."

Break the Connection Between How "Fat" You Feel and How You Behave

If you did the kinesthetic exercise above, you may have noticed that how you feel about yourself and your body has a lot to do with how you behave. Here is another way to look at this connection.

At-Home Exercise*

Imagine yourself at a party. There are lots of people, some of whom you know and some of whom you do not know. There is a table in the room with lots of food on it. Now imagine that you are growing very large. Now, even larger. How do you behave at the party. How are you dressed? Whom do you talk to? How do you stand? Walk? Do you eat food from the table or not? What is your mood? Are you comfortable? How do others react to you?

Now imagine yourself shrinking smaller and smaller until you are the thinnest woman in the room. How do you behave at the party now? How are you dressed? Whom do you talk to? How do you stand? Walk? Do you eat or drink? What is your mood? Are you comfortable? How do others react to you?

What differences are there for you in these fat and thin fantasies? You can learn from this exercise how you permit yourself to behave, based on how fat or thin you feel, as opposed to how fat or thin you really are. Perhaps you can permit yourself to experiment with behaving however you would like to, regardless of your size (actual or perceived).

Chapter Summary

Body image is the representation you make of your body to yourself, and the feelings and judgments you have about this representation. Displacing bad feelings about yourself onto your body may seem like the easy solution to feeling better about yourself through manipulation of your weight and shape. However, in the long run this is neither adaptive nor realistic and will only serve to perpetuate the bad feelings about yourself and your eating disorder. Get to know yourself. Get to know your body. Break the connection between how fat you feel and how you think, feel, and behave.

---

* Adapted from Orbach S: Fat is a Feminist Issue II: The Anti-Diet Guide to Permanent Weight Loss. New York, Berkley Publishing Group, 1987, p. 145.

7

The Road to Recovery

♦ ♦ ♦ ♦ ♦ ♦ ♦ ♦ ♦

You have been presented with much information and many recommendations for overcoming your eating disorder. You have learned that one of the most important tasks is for you to engage in a nondieting eating pattern for an extended period of time. It may be useful for you to review the following points often to encourage yourself that you are on the right path.

The Meals-Binge Connection

Binge eating is strongly related to food deprivation at other times of the day. The regular intake of a normal amount of food is the medicine that will help to protect you from future binges.

If at First it Feels Like Work, You're Probably Doing it Right

Interrupting symptomatic behavior will probably require considerable effort on your part for some time to come. You may have to restructure your day so that you are sure to have time and a suitable location for normal meals. As well, you may have to plan activities to distract yourself following each meal and at other times when you may be at the greatest risk of bingeing or purging. You may have to eat when you do not feel like doing so and you may have to tolerate the physical discomforts associated with the changes in your eating patterns (e.g., bloating, stomach upset, constipation, water retention). It is essential for you to remind yourself that overcoming an eating disorder can be hard work—but you *can* do it. Also remember that much of what you have to do now is a stepping stone on the way to recovery. The physical discomforts, the urges to binge or purge, and the effort required to eat a normal meal will all decrease dramatically over time. You will not have to work this hard forever.

Avoid Frequent Mind Changes

Although it is a good idea to consider the changes you are making in your eating pattern as a personal experiment, it is important that you commit yourself to the experiment for a reasonable period of time. It is not helpful to give yourself the option of turning back at each meal or at other times of difficulty or distress. Try to make the decision to try normalized eating as an experiment once, and then stick with it—even if the experiment with normalized eating lasts for 6 months, this is a very small portion of your whole life span. After the experiment is over, you can make an informed decision about what you want to do: You can always begin to diet and/or engage in other symptoms such as purging at that time, if that's the choice you make. At least by that point it will be an informed, personal choice on the basis of what you have learned from your nondieting experiment.

Don't Rush Out of the Short Term

Right now you may be using several rigid strategies to control your behavior (e.g., mechanical eating according to a schedule, immediately going out when you have an urge to purge, etc.). You will not have to use these strategies for the rest of your life, but don't pressure yourself to discard them too early. Although some of the things you are doing may be inconvenient at times, they are certainly not harmful. You should continue to apply these "short-term" strategies for as long as you even think you might need them. If you like the structure or security that your coping strategies provide, you may wish to continue them for even longer.

Make Sure You Are Satisfied

From a biological point of view, it is essential that you eat an absolute minimum of 1,500 calories each day (and more is normal) and that you include protein, carbohydrate, and satiety nutrient (e.g., fat) in your meals. Be sure that you are eating enough, in a normalized way, so that you are not left hungry for long periods of time. From a psychological point of view, it is important that any food you crave be available to you in a normal quantity. If you like donuts, you should plan to go to a donut shop, perhaps with a friend, and have one donut in a normal, enjoyable manner. Although this may be a difficult task for you, it is essential that you tackle it in a planned way when you feel ready. Remember that the ultimate goal is to be able to eat all kinds of foods, including "binge" foods, in normal quantities and to avoid depriving yourself of normal amounts of anything.

If You Slip Up

Many individuals who are recovering from an eating disorder will gain a lot of control over their eating and other symptoms, but still have occasional periods of difficulty. This pattern may be especially frightening to you if you are symptom-free for a period of time and then have an episode of bingeing or purging. Prepare yourself ahead of time to deal with "slips" by remembering that they are expected, and by reviewing the following points.

Recovery takes time. Applying perfectionistic and all-or-none expectations to recovery will only lead you to interpret any transgressions as failure. The road to recovery is rarely smooth and straightforward; sometimes "slips" occur even after months of normal eating. If you have an unanticipated bingeing or purging episode, remind yourself that this does not represent a personal failure. Rather than viewing a temporary lapse as a disaster that cannot be undone, think about the episode as a "slip" in your recovery process. A novice bike rider learns a great deal from her falls; she learns to take the next turn more slowly and to break earlier at stops. Use this episode as a learning experience. Were you cutting back on food before the binge occurred? What circumstances in your environment may have made the binge more likely? If you are prepared for the possibility of "slips" and recognize that they are part of the process of getting better, you will be better equipped to deal with them.

A slip is a specific, unique event in the here and now. A binge or purge episode is a specific episode that occurs at a specific time and place. Because it is just that, it does not tell you anything about how things will be in the future. Be aware of any tendencies to overgeneralize—a binge on Tuesday does not have to mean a binge on Wednesday. Nor does it indicate that any meals should be skipped or that attempts should be made to compensate for the binge in any way.

Each day is a new day. Each meal is a new meal. If you do have a binge or if you "overeat" at a meal, it is vital to get right back on track by eating normally at the next scheduled meal. Remember that it is normal for nondieting women to occasionally overeat and that the body balances this out over time. You will not gain weight over the long run by "going overboard" at one meal.

Reinforce yourself for progress made. If you used to binge every day and now binge three times a week, you have come a long way. If you feel fat and go to that party anyway, you are working on your attitudes about weight and shape. It is important to acknowledge changes in both the way you act and the way you think, no matter how small they may seem. You should evaluate your progress over a reasonable period of time. If you have just binged, it is not fair to evaluate yourself on only the last 2 hours. Consider how you have done over the last week, the last month, the last 3 months. Remember that no one does things perfectly and that you deserve credit for what you have done.

Your body may lag behind your behavior. It may take months to fully overcome the effects of years of dieting. Even after weeks of eating normally you may not be able to rely on internal sensations of hunger and fullness to guide your eating. The longer you continue to adequately nourish your body, the more opportunity your body has to recover its own built-in regulating functions.

Start planning and monitoring your eating if you find yourself slipping back into old eating patterns. It is vital to continue scheduling meals and snacks until a nondieting approach is almost automatic for you. Some people feel confused when presented with choices about what to eat. If this is the case, try to plan ahead as much as possible; if you are unsure about how much to eat, try modeling your eating after a nondieting person you know.

Additional Work

It is important to remember that the psychoeducation group you attended was designed to show you how to help yourself to overcome your eating disorder. We do not expect you to be fully recovered right now, but we do hope that you have started the process of recovery. With this in mind, it would be useful for you to reread this manual from time to time as a booster for both your memory and your motivation.

References

Apfelbaum M, Bostsarron J, Lacatis D: Effects of caloric restriction and excessive caloric intake on energy expenditure. Am J Clin Nutr 24:1405–1409, 1971

Bennett W, Gurin J: The Dieter's Dilemma: Eating Less and Weighing More. New York, Basic Books, 1982

Boyle PC, Storlien H, Keesey RE: Increased efficiency of food utilization following weight loss. Physiol Behav 21:261, 1978

Bruch H: Eating Disorders. New York, Basic Books, 1973

Bruch H: The Golden Cage: The Enigma of Anorexia Nervosa. Cambridge, MA, Harvard University Press, 1978

Canada Fitness Survey: Fitness and Lifestyle in Canada. Ottawa, Ontario, Canada Fitness Survey, 1983

Fairburn CG, Garner DM: The diagnosis of bulimia nervosa. International Journal of Eating Disorders 5:403–419, 1986

Feeling fat in a thin society. Glamour Magazine, February 1984, pp 198–201, 251–252

Garfinkel PE, Garner DM: Anorexia Nervosa: A Multidimensional Perspective. New York, Brunner/Mazel, 1982

Garfinkel PE, Goldbloom DS: Anorexia nervosa and bulimia nervosa: introduction, in Current Update: Anorexia Nervosa and Bulimia Nervosa. Edited by Garfinkel PE. Kalamazoo, MI, Upjohn, 1988, pp 3–9

Garfinkel PE, Garner DM, Goldbloom DS: Eating disorders: implications for the 1980's. Can J Psychiatry 32:624–631, 1987

Garner DM, Davis R: The clinical assessment of anorexia nervosa and bulimia nervosa, in Innovations in Clinical Practice: A Source Book, Vol 5. Edited by Keller PA, Ritt LG. Sarasota, FL, Professional Resource Exchange, 1986, pp 5–28

Garner DM, Garfinkel PE: Socio-cultural factors in the development of anorexia nervosa. Psychol Med 10:647–656, 1980

Garner DM, Garfinkel PE, Schwartz D, et al: Cultural expectations of thinness in women. Psychol Rep 47:483–491, 1980

Garner DM, Rockert W, Olmsted MP, et al: Psychoeducational principles in the treatment of bulimia and anorexia nervosa, in Handbook of Psychotherapy for Anorexia Nervosa and Bulimia. Edited by Garner DM, Garfinkel PE. New York, Guilford, 1985, pp 513–572

Gallup Canada: A report on the behaviour and attitudes of Canadians with respect to weight consciousness and weight control. Toronto, Ontario, Canadian Gallup Poll Limited, 1984

Health and Welfare Canada: Canada's health promotion survey: Technical report. Edited by Rootman I, Warren R, Stephens T, Peters L. Ottawa, Ontario, Minister of Supply and Services Canada, 1988

Herman CP, Mack D: Restrained and unrestrained eating. J Pers 43:647–660, 1975

Hutchinson MG: Transforming Body Image: Learning to Love the Body You Have. New York, Crossing Press, 1985, p 113

Johnson D, Drenick EJ: Therapeutic fasting in morbid obesity: long-term follow-up. Arch Intern Med 137:1381–1382, 1977

Kaplan AS: Medical aspects of anorexia nervosa and bulimia nervosa, in Current Update: Anorexia Nervosa and Bulimia Nervosa. Edited by Garfinkel PE. Kalamazoo, MI, Upjohn, 1988, pp 19–26

Keys A, Brozek J, Henschel A, et al: The Biology of Human Starvation. Minneapolis, MN, University of Minnesota Press, 1950

King AJC, et al: Canada health attitudes and behaviors survey: 9-, 12- and 15-year-olds, 1984–85. Ottawa, Ontario, Health and Welfare Canada, Health Promotion Directorate, 1986

Miller DS, Parsonage S: Resistance to slimming. Lancet 1:773–775, 1975

Nielsen AC: Who's Dieting and Why? Chicago, IL, A.C. Nielsen Company, 1979

Orbach S: Fat is a Feminist Issue II: The Anti-Diet Guide to Permanent Weight Loss. New York, Berkley Publishing Group, 1987, p 145

Polivy J, Herman CP: Breaking the Diet Habit: The Natural Weight Alternative. New York, Basic Books, 1983

Polivy J, Herman CP: Dieting and bingeing: a causal analysis. Am Psychol 40:193–201, 1985

Price RA: Genetics and human obesity. Annals of Behavioral Medicine 9:9–14, 1987

Sims EAH, Goldman R, Gluck C, et al: Experimental obesity in man. Transcript of the Association of American Physicians 81:153, 1968

Sorlie P, Gordon T, Kannel WB: Body build and mortality: the Framingham study. JAMA 243:1828–1831, 1980

Stunkard AJ, Foch TT, Hrubec Z: A twin study of human obesity. JAMA 256:51–54, 1986

Thompson JK, Blanton PD: The effects of dieting and exercise on metabolic rate. Behavioral Medicine Abstracts 5:v–viii, 1984

Tschirhart SL, Donovan ME: Women and Self-Esteem. New York, Penguin Books, 1984

Wooley SC, Wooley OW: Obesity and women, I: a closer look at the facts. Women's Studies International Quarterly 2:67–79, 1979

WEEKLY SUMMARY

NAME: _____

WEEK BEGINNING MONDAY _____

MONTH   DAY   YEAR

	MON	TUES	WED	THURS	FRI	SAT	SUN
Number of BINGE EPISODES							
Number of VOMITING EPISODES							
Number of LAXATIVES							
EXERCISE (minutes)							
OTHER (specify)							
NONDIETING MEALS*							

* A nondieting meal is one in which an independent observer would probably conclude that you were not consuming calorie sparing foods and not on a diet. A nondieting meal is not followed by self-induced vomiting.

WEEKLY SUMMARY

NAME: _____

WEEK BEGINNING MONDAY _____ MONTH DAY YEAR

	MON	TUES	WED	THURS	FRI	SAT	SUN	
Number of BINGE EPISODES								
Number of VOMITING EPISODES								
Number of LAXATIVES								
EXERCISE (minutes)								
OTHER (specify)								
NONDIETING MEALS*								

* A nondieting meal is one in which an independent observer would probably conclude that you were not consuming calorie sparing foods and not on a diet. A nondieting meal is not followed by self-induced vomiting.

Index

♦ ♦ ♦ ♦ ♦ ♦ ♦ ♦

Page numbers that are followed by a "t" refer to tables; those in italics refer to figures.